Home Healthcare Services and Technology Implications

Haşim Çapar
Dicle University, Turkey

Mehmet Aziz Çakmak
Mardin Artuklu University, Turkey

IGI Global
Scientific Publishing
Publishing Tomorrow's Research Today

Vice President of Editorial	Melissa Wagner
Director of Acquisitions	Mikaela Felty
Director of Book Development	Jocelynn Hessler
Production Manager	Mike Brehm
Cover Design	Jose Rosado

Published in the United States of America by
IGI Global Scientific Publishing
701 East Chocolate Avenue
Hershey, PA, 17033, USA
Tel: 717-533-8845
Fax: 717-533-7115
Website: https://www.igi-global.com E-mail: cust@igi-global.com

Library of Congress Cataloging-in-Publication Data

Names: Çapar, Haşim, 1989- editor | Cakmak, Mehmet Aziz, 1993- editor
Title: Home healthcare services and technology implications / edited by Haşim Çapar, Mehmet Cakmak.
Description: Hershey, PA : IGI Global Scientific Publishing, 2026. | Includes bibliographical references and index. | Summary: "The edited book explores the relationship between the development of home healthcare services and technological innovation in the field, addressing technological change and transformation of the new world, changes in population structure and related health needs. In particular, it focuses on how artificial intelligence and new algorithms will shape the growing expectations of healthcare services due to major changes in lifestyles"-- Provided by publisher.
Identifiers: LCCN 2025023123 (print) | LCCN 2025023124 (ebook) | ISBN 9798337330990 hardcover | ISBN 9798337331003 paperback | ISBN 9798337331010 ebook
Subjects: LCSH: Home care services--Technological innovations
Classification: LCC RA645.3 .H649 2026 (print) | LCC RA645.3 (ebook)
LC record available at https://lccn.loc.gov/2025023123
LC ebook record available at https://lccn.loc.gov/2025023124

British Cataloguing in Publication Data
A Cataloguing in Publication record for this book is available from the British Library.

Table of Contents

Detailed Table of Contents

The Dartmouth Conference held in 1956 marks the official birth of the field of artificial intelligence (AI). This meeting brought together pioneering scientists such as John McCarthy, Marvin Minsky, Claude Shannon, and Nathaniel Rochester to explore the question "Can machines think?" from an interdisciplinary perspective. The term "artificial intelligence" was used for the first time at this conference, and the idea that machines could imitate human-like intelligence was proposed. Prior to this, significant theoretical foundations had been laid by figures like Alan Turing, particularly with the "Turing Test," along with developments in logic, computability, neural network models, and cybernetics. The use of AI in home healthcare began with these foundational conceptual studies in the 1950s and has since evolved into today's integrated solutions, combining clinical decision support systems, remote monitoring technologies, wearable devices, social robots, and smart home innovations.

The widespread adoption of cloud computing and a variety of affordable client devices such as smartphones, sensors, wearable technology, and the Internet of Things (IoT) has transformed the way we collect data. The constant connectivity of these devices enables remote and continuous data access, making data-driven healthcare not only highly feasible but also executable from a distance. Data gathered from these devices enhances remote diagnostics and can be leveraged to deliver healthcare value in homecare settings, particularly for families and senior citizens. Health consultations can now be conducted remotely, and through coordinated collaboration within the healthcare business ecosystem, integrated healthcare solutions will improve well-being, especially for families and seniors. This chapter explores advancements in digital health, digital solutions for family and senior care, healthcare value creation, the digital healthcare business ecosystem, and recent case studies on digital healthcare innovations.

Human-Machine Interaction (HMI) is the interaction of patients, families and healthcare staff with technologies such as sensors, software and robots in home healthcare. It offers elderly and chronic patients the opportunity to live independently at home. Due to the aging population and the increase in chronic diseases, the desire of individuals to live independently in their own homes has stimulated the development of these technologies. In this context, HMI should be designed in accordance with the physical and cognitive capacities of the users, as well as to improve health outcomes. HMI consists of physical devices, social relationships and data layer. User-centered design and accessibility are important. Home care is supported by monitoring systems, security solutions and emergency assistance technologies.

In this chapter, a comprehensive evaluation of remote healthcare is presented, beginning with the definition of the concept and a detailed explanation of the key terms associated with it. Subsequently, the historical background of remote healthcare is examined and then the major benefits and the potential risks of remote healthcare are discussed. Furthermore, the possible challenges that may arise during the integration of remote healthcare services into national healthcare systems are addressed, alongside proposed solutions to these challenges. Afterward, future trends in remote healthcare are analyzed, with a particular focus on emerging issues likely to become prominent in the near future. The chapter concludes with a general evaluation, summarizing the main interests and insights. It is intended that this chapter will serve as a valuable resource for policymakers involved in decision-making processes related to remote healthcare, researchers conducting academic studies in this field, and all stakeholders engaged in the provision, utilization, and financing of remote healthcare.

As smart home technology becomes more prevalent, optimizing user interface (UI) design is essential to enhance user experience and unlock the full potential of home automation. This paper explores key factors that influence user interaction and satisfaction by analyzing challenges and opportunities in smart home UI design. Drawing on principles from HCI, cognitive psychology, and design thinking, we propose a framework emphasizing usability, personalization, and flexibility. We review current literature, assess emerging technologies like voice assistants, gesture recognition, and AI algorithms for proactive UI optimization, and provide actionable insights to guide future smart home UI development.

The integration of digital technologies into healthcare has transformed home-based nutrition support. Tele-health, especially tele-nutrition, has become essential for delivering personalised dietary counselling and monitoring by overcoming geographical and logistical barriers. This chapter examines the development and implementation of tele-nutrition, particularly in home enteral nutrition (HEN) and chronic disease contexts. Drawing on current evidence, it discusses how mobile applications, wearable technologies, AI-based systems, and hybrid care models improve clinical outcomes, patient engagement, and continuity of care. The chapter also addresses barriers such as limited digital literacy, regulatory inconsistencies, and social inequalities, alongside ethical concerns like informed consent and algorithmic transparency. Policy implications are analysed in relation to reimbursement systems, licensure frameworks, and the legal responsibilities of clinicians. The chapter concludes with strategic recommendations for integrating tele-nutrition into public health infrastructures and outlines research priorities focused on long-term effectiveness, patient-reported outcomes, and inclusive design. By synthesizing multidisciplinary evidence, this chapter provides a comprehensive roadmap for the sustainable integration of tele-health in home-based nutrition support, reinforcing its relevance in achieving equitable, person-centred, and technology-enabled dietary care.

This chapter explores the increasing importance of home healthcare technologies in facilitating tourism participation among elderly and disabled populations. As the global aging demographic expands, the tourism sector must adapt to accommodate diverse accessibility needs. The chapter highlights how emerging technologies such as wearable healthcare devices, smart city infrastructure, and mobile navigation applications support greater autonomy and mobility for individuals with disabilities. Drawing on key statistical projections and academic literature, it addresses the concept of accessible tourism, the challenges disabled travelers face, and the role of inclusive technologies in overcoming physical and digital barriers. In doing so, this chapter emphasizes not only the social equity benefits but also the economic potential of integrating inclusive practices into tourism systems.

Nowadays countries are entering a period where their social profiles are increasingly dominated by the elderly population. Due to increasing demand and limited personnel resources, home healthcare services are becoming increasingly difficult to manage. Technological applications are used to prevent disruptions that mentioned here. This section evaluates the effects of technological applications on home healthcare services and management. In order to make this assessment, studies on home healthcare services and technologies which emerged with Health 4.0 were examined. All technologies that used in home healthcare services have effects in terms of saving costs and resources, as well as providing convenience to people who have difficulty accessing services, and increasing patients' quality of life. When these are considered in terms of healthcare management, they will provide savings in the health economics, efficient use of limited resources and the provision of accessible, patient-focused services with no boundaries.

Preface

The convergence of healthcare and technology has led to a paradigm shift in how medical services are delivered, particularly in the context of home-based care. As global populations age and chronic illnesses become more prevalent, there is a growing need for accessible, cost-effective, and personalized healthcare solutions. Home healthcare, once seen as a supplementary service, has evolved into a central component of modern healthcare systems. This transformation is made possible through the integration of digital health innovations, artificial intelligence, smart devices, telecommunication technologies, and user-centered interface design.

This edited volume, *Home Healthcare Services and Technology Implications*, brings together interdisciplinary perspectives on the technological, clinical, and managerial dimensions of home healthcare. The chapters offer both foundational context and forward-looking insights into how innovations are reshaping care delivery for patients, families, and healthcare professionals.

CHAPTER OVERVIEW

Chapter 1 introduces the conceptual and historical roots of artificial intelligence in healthcare, tracing its origin to the Dartmouth Conference in 1956. The chapter provides context for how early ideas in machine intelligence evolved into today's intelligent healthcare systems, laying the groundwork for AI-supported home healthcare.

Chapter 2 examines the digital transformation of home healthcare through a business ecosystem lens. By analyzing the role of cloud computing, smart devices, and continuous connectivity, the authors explore how coordinated digital health solutions create value, especially for families and the elderly.

Chapter 3 focuses on human–machine interaction in home settings. It discusses how sensors, software, and assistive robots enable individuals with chronic conditions or advanced age to live more independently. The chapter emphasizes the importance of designing systems that align with users' cognitive and physical capabilities.

Chapter 4 provides a comprehensive overview of remote healthcare. It covers definitions, historical development, benefits, risks, and integration challenges. The author also identifies key trends and future directions in remote healthcare delivery, making this chapter particularly useful for policymakers and healthcare administrators.

Chapter 5 explores emerging technologies in smart home interface design. The authors present a framework to improve usability and personalization by incorporating principles from human-computer interaction and cognitive psychology. Innovations such as voice assistants and AI-driven interfaces are examined for their role in improving user experience.

Chapter 6 delves into tele-nutrition and home-based nutrition support. The chapter discusses how mobile applications, wearable devices, and hybrid care models improve dietary management and clinical outcomes. It also highlights challenges related to equity, digital literacy, and ethical considerations.

Chapter 7 addresses the intersection of home healthcare and accessible tourism. As elderly and disabled populations seek more inclusive travel opportunities, the chapter explores how wearable health devices and smart infrastructure support greater mobility and participation in tourism.

Chapter 8 concludes the volume by examining the management implications of adopting technology in home healthcare. The author evaluates how Health 4.0 tools contribute to resource efficiency, cost savings, and improved service delivery. Strategic insights are offered for integrating these technologies within health systems.

Together, these chapters present a multi-faceted view of how home healthcare is being redefined by technology. The book aims to serve as a resource for healthcare practitioners, researchers, technologists, and policymakers who are shaping the future of care beyond traditional clinical settings.

Hasim Çapar
Dicle University, Turkey

Mehmet Aziz Çakmak
Mardin Artuklu University, Turkey

Chapter 1
1956 Artificial Intelligence Is Born

İlknur Arslan Aras
https://orcid.org/0000-0003-4030-0158
Yuksek Ihtisas University, Turkey

ABSTRACT

The Dartmouth Conference held in 1956 marks the official birth of the field of artificial intelligence (AI). This meeting brought together pioneering scientists such as John McCarthy, Marvin Minsky, Claude Shannon, and Nathaniel Rochester to explore the question "Can machines think?" from an interdisciplinary perspective. The term "artificial intelligence" was used for the first time at this conference, and the idea that machines could imitate human-like intelligence was proposed. Prior to this, significant theoretical foundations had been laid by figures like Alan Turing, particularly with the "Turing Test," along with developments in logic, computability, neural network models, and cybernetics. The use of AI in home healthcare began with these foundational conceptual studies in the 1950s and has since evolved into today's integrated solutions, combining clinical decision support systems, remote monitoring technologies, wearable devices, social robots, and smart home innovations.

1. INTRODUCTION

By the mid-twentieth century, the question "Can machines think?" had become a fundamental issue engaging both scientists and philosophers. Understanding history is not merely about exploring the past—it is also essential for anticipating future innovations and opportunities. The core dynamics that have driven technological progress for decades tend to persist in similar patterns, and development often unfolds along recognizable trends. In this context, gaining insight into the historical

DOI: 10.4018/979-8-3373-3099-0.ch001

evolution of artificial intelligence is particularly important for comprehending both the current role and future potential of AI in home healthcare services.

In 1950, the British mathematician Alan M. Turing directly tackled this question in his seminal article "Computing Machinery and Intelligence," proposing an experimental game—now known as the Turing Test—to determine whether a machine could be considered intelligent (Turing, 1950). Rather than asking "Can machines think?" Turing suggested assessing "whether the behavior of a machine is indistinguishable from that of a human being" through an "imitation game," thereby transforming the debate into a concrete test (Turing, 1950). During this period, Turing and other pioneering thinkers advanced the idea that the human mind could be understood through mathematical and information-processing models and that computers might perform complex cognitive tasks.

The 1950s witnessed the advent of digital computers and a rapid increase in computational power. Electronic machines developed during World War II demonstrated the potential to mechanically replicate human abilities in calculation and logical reasoning. These technical advances fueled optimism that "human intelligence could be modeled algorithmically." Concurrent research in cybernetics (Wiener, 1948) and automata theory investigated feedback control mechanisms and the theoretical foundations of computation, while McCulloch and Pitts (1943) argued that neurons in the human brain could be modeled as simple logical gates. Collectively, these efforts laid the conceptual groundwork for what would become artificial intelligence. However, at that time, the label "artificial intelligence" had not yet been coined; researchers referred instead to "thinking machines," "automatic machines," or "information-processing systems" (McCarthy, Minsky, Rochester, & Shannon, 1955).

In 1956, a workshop was convened at Dartmouth College in the United States, where these disparate ideas were brought together under a single roof, thus symbolizing the birth of a new research field. The Dartmouth Summer Research Project on Artificial Intelligence, as it became known, represented the first official use of the term "artificial intelligence" and was tasked with defining the discipline's boundaries. In this chapter, the conference's preparation, content, participants and initial outcomes are examined. Subsequently, the rapid developments and challenges of the late 1950s and 1960s are analyzed—particularly how criticism was provoked by the field's overoptimistic expectations and how funding was curtailed during the so-called AI winters". Finally, the lasting impact of the 1956 beginnings on the current state of AI and the development of AI in healthcare will be evaluated.

2. CONCEPTUAL FOUNDATIONS OF ARTIFICIAL INTELLIGENCE (PRE-1956 DEVELOPMENTS)

Figure 1. Publications by Wos categories

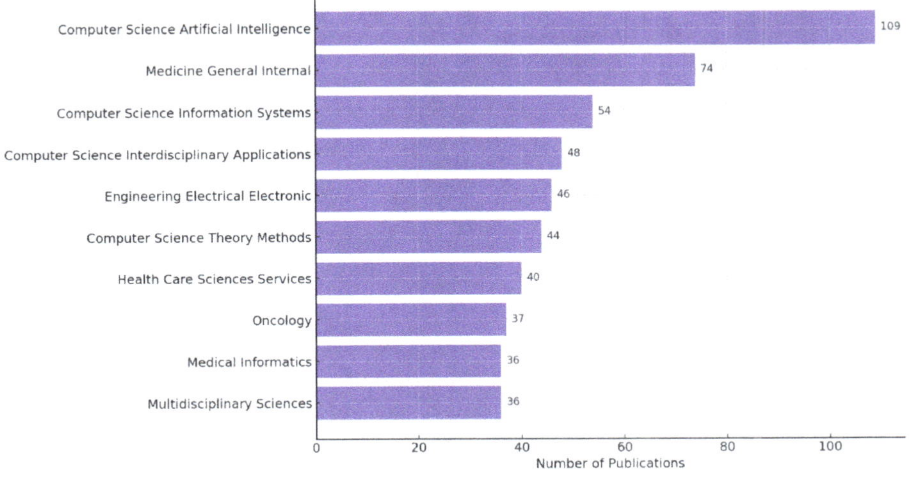

According to Figure 1, as of April 2025, a total of 1007 scientific publications were identified in the Web of Science database under the title search using the keywords "artificial intelligence" and "history." These studies span a wide range of disciplines, with the highest concentration found in the category of Computer Science Artificial Intelligence (109 publications, 10.82%). This is followed by medicine general internal (74 publications, 7.35%), computer science information systems (54 publications, 5.36%), computer science interdisciplinary applications (48 publications, 4.77%), and engineering electrical electronic (46 publications, 4.57%). Other notable categories include computer science theory methods (4.37%), health care sciences services (3.97%), oncology (3.67%), medical informatics (3.57%), and multidisciplinary sciences (3.57%). The distribution of these studies indicates that academic interest in the historical development of artificial intelligence is not confined to computer science and engineering domains alone. Instead, it extends meaningfully into fields such as medicine, healthcare services, oncology, cardiovascular systems, and interdisciplinary sciences. This reflects the increasing recognition that the history of artificial intelligence is relevant not only from a technical standpoint but also from clinical, systemic, and societal perspectives.

To understand the foundations of artificial intelligence, it is essential to review the scientific and philosophical developments that preceded 1956. The notion that human-made entities could exhibit intelligent behavior had long been discussed across a spectrum from philosophy to literature, but it did not fully transition into concrete scientific inquiry until the mid-twentieth century.

Figure 2. Timeline of AI history

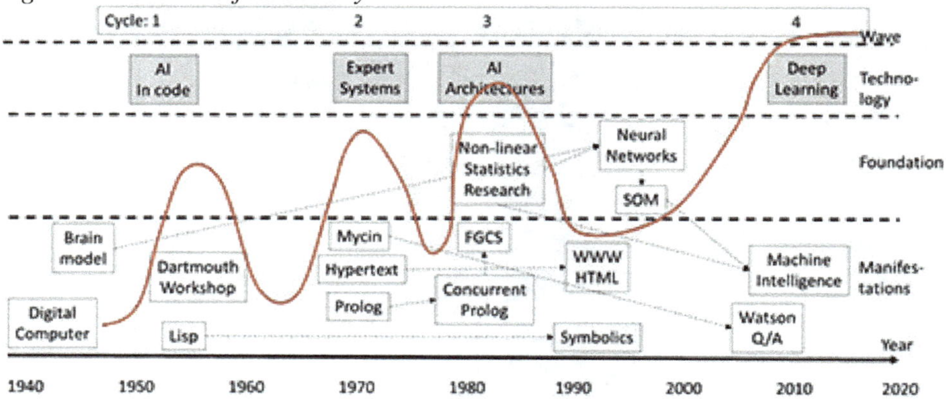

Figure 2 illustrates the cyclical nature of artificial intelligence development from the 1940s to the present, highlighting the fluctuations between periods of high expectations and subsequent disillusionment. The first wave, beginning with the invention of digital computers and the 1956 Dartmouth Workshop, focused on symbolic AI and coding intelligence, but soon entered a decline due to limited computational capabilities. The second cycle emerged in the 1970s with expert systems like Mycin and logic-based programming languages such as Prolog, yet the high cost and complexity of knowledge engineering led to another stagnation. The third wave in the 1980s centered around AI architectures and statistical research, but once again faced setbacks due to hardware constraints. Finally, the fourth and current wave, driven by deep learning, big data, and significant improvements in processing power, has resulted in practical applications like IBM's Watson, marking a period of tangible success. These four AI cycles, as shown in the figure, not only reflect technological progress but also demonstrate the influence of broader economic and societal trends. In the following section, each of these historical phases will be examined in greater detail to provide a comprehensive understanding of the evolution of artificial intelligence.

2.1. Logical and Mathematical Foundations

Philosophers and mathematicians in the seventeenth and eighteenth centuries were intrigued by the possibility of explaining human reasoning through symbolic manipulation. Gottfried Leibniz proposed a "universal calculus" whereby all thought could be reduced to mathematical operations, and George Boole's nineteenth-century development of Boolean algebra demonstrated that logical expressions could be represented algebraically. These historical ideas paved the way for binary logic and digital circuit design. In the early twentieth century, Alan Turing advanced the concept of computability by formally defining which problems a Turing machine could solve (Turing, 1936). Such works offered the first significant evidence that intelligent behavior might be modeled algorithmically.

2.2. Neural Network Models

Advances in neuroscience and information theory during the 1940s introduced the idea that intelligence could be understood on a neural basis. McCulloch and Pitts (1943) proposed a model showing that a single neuron could function like a simple logical gate and proved that sufficiently large networks of these units could compute any logical function. This result established a formal framework for modeling the biological brain. In parallel, Norbert Wiener's work on cybernetics explored feedback mechanisms in control systems, highlighting machines' capacity to adapt to their environment and self-regulate (Wiener, 1948). Together, these studies heralded the neural (connectionist) and cybernetic dimensions of artificial intelligence.

2.3. Computing and Algorithmic Developments

The post–World War II period saw the emergence of general-purpose electronic computers such as ENIAC and EDVAC, demonstrating that machines could perform not only numerical calculations but also logical decision-making and problem solving. In 1950, Claude Shannon discussed algorithms for enabling a computer to play chess, representing an early example of "intelligent" behavior through computation (Shannon, 1950). Concurrently, Arthur Samuel's checkers program, developed from 1952 onward, demonstrated that a program could improve its performance through experience—an insight that would later underpin the field of machine learning (Samuel, 1959).

2.4. Philosophical Approaches

Early work in artificial intelligence also grappled with philosophical questions. René Descartes, in the seventeenth century, argued that machines could never truly think because thought required a divine soul. Such objections persisted into the twentieth century. In 1950, Turing countered that no philosophical barrier prevented machines from thinking, although he acknowledged the difficulty of defining "machine" and "thinking" (Turing, 1950). His proposed "imitation game" reframed intelligence in behavioral terms: if a machine could convincingly imitate human responses to deceive an interrogator, it was reasonable to attribute thinking to the machine. By linking intelligence to observable behavior, Turing bridged philosophical debate with empirical experimentation.

In summary, by 1956, no formal discipline called "artificial intelligence" yet existed, but a substantial body of work in computing, algorithms, neural modeling, and philosophy had coalesced. It was now necessary to bring these strands together under a systematic framework to address the question, "Can machines truly exhibit intelligent behavior, and if so, how?" The Dartmouth Conference was designed precisely to meet this need, uniting experts from diverse fields to clarify and define the concept of artificial intelligence. From these early works in different disciplines, the theoretical and philosophical foundations of artificial intelligence were shaped; however, until the 1956 Dartmouth Conference, these studies were conducted separately. Dartmouth marked a turning point by bringing together this multidisciplinary knowledge to explore the conceptual and practical boundaries of artificial intelligence.

2.5. Turing's Influence and the Turing Test

Alan Turing, one of the most influential figures in AI, had already laid the groundwork before the Dartmouth Conference. His Turing Test, introduced in 1950, provided a benchmark for assessing machine intelligence. Turing argued that if a machine could convincingly imitate human responses in a text-based conversation, it should be considered intelligent (Turing, 1950).

The Turing Test, first proposed by Alan Turing in 1950, remains a fundamental milestone in discussions on artificial intelligence (AI). This test is designed to determine whether a machine can exhibit human-like intelligence by engaging in a conversation that will be indistinguishable as being with an actual human (Levesque, 2017). While the test has had a large influence on AI development, it has been faulted by numerous individuals and also has alternative ideas.

Moor (2001) explains that although humans indicate the Turing Test as being antiquated, AI continues to develop and the test is still reliable to assess the intelligence of a machine. Nevertheless, other scholars believe that successfully passing the Turing Test does not actually reflect intelligence at all. Rather, it reflects on a person's ability to imitate human replies (Shapiro, 1992). In this regard, Yampolskiy (2013) ranks the Turing Test as an AI-complete problem. That is, it is one of the hardest problems in AI creation.

There are also some researchers who suggest other tests of intelligence, instead of the usual Turing Test. For instance, the Winograd Schema Test is a better method since it demands reasoning, instead of pattern matching (Levesque, 2017). Marcus,

Rossi, and Veloso (2016) prefer creating several cognitive tests instead of depending on a single test.

Recent studies have tried to analyze how well the Turing Test fares with modern advanced AI models. For example, Mei et al. (2024) performed a study on comparing AI chatbots' behavior with humans and showed that modern AI systems can effortlessly trick human judges but do not really understand. French (2000) also suggests that while the Turing Test is important, no AI system has yet fully simulated human thought.

As AI becomes a part of everyday life, scientists argue if the Turing Test remains a good test of intelligence. While it has guided AI research in the past, ongoing debates suggest that we need more and improved ways to determine true machine intelligence. His ideas greatly impacted AI research and continue to be argued in the field today.

3. THE 1956 DARTMOUTH CONFERENCE: THE BIRTH OF ARTIFICIAL INTELLIGENCE

The Dartmouth Conference held in the summer of 1956 is widely regarded as the founding moment of artificial intelligence (AI) as a formal research field. Rather than a traditional academic conference, this event took the form of a several-week-long workshop titled the "Dartmouth Summer Research Project." The initiative was spearheaded by John McCarthy, a young faculty member in the mathematics department at Dartmouth College. In 1955, McCarthy proposed gathering a select group of leading scientists for a summer meeting to explore a new scientific frontier. It was McCarthy who coined the term "artificial intelligence," a phrase that would soon define an entire discipline. According to McCarthy and his colleagues, this terminology was deliberately chosen to avoid the ambiguous associations tied to existing terms like "cybernetics." Unlike these, "artificial intelligence" offered a neutral and inclusive conceptual frame (McCarthy et al., 1955).

3.1. Planning the Conference

On August 31, 1955, a formal project proposal titled *A Proposal for the Dartmouth Summer Research Project on Artificial Intelligence* was drafted and signed by John McCarthy, Marvin Minsky (then a young researcher at Harvard University), Nathaniel Rochester (a computer engineer at IBM), and Claude Shannon (a Bell Labs mathematician and the founder of information theory). The proposal suggested convening a 10-person research group for approximately two months at Dartmouth College in the summer of 1956. The document boldly stated the project's objective:

"The study is to proceed on the basis of the conjecture that every aspect of learning or any other feature of intelligence can in principle be so precisely described that a machine can be made to simulate it. An attempt will be made to find how to make machines use language, form abstractions and concepts, solve kinds of problems now reserved for humans, and improve themselves" (McCarthy et al., 1955).

This statement encapsulated the core assumption of early AI research: if intelligence could be described in formal, algorithmic terms, then it could be simulated by a machine. McCarthy and his collaborators argued that a carefully selected group of scientists working together intensively over a summer could make meaningful progress toward this goal.

3.2. Execution of the Conference

The proposal was submitted to the Rockefeller Foundation, which granted the necessary funding. The Dartmouth meeting commenced in June 1956. Among the invited participants were several young and brilliant researchers. McCarthy and Minsky remained on-site throughout the summer as primary organizers. Shannon and Rochester also joined, although for shorter periods. Allen Newell and Herbert Simon, based at Carnegie Tech in Pittsburgh and known for their work on human-like problem solving, arrived at the conference with a landmark contribution: *Logic Theorist*, the first program designed to replicate human reasoning (Newell & Simon, 1956).

Other participants included Raymond Solomonoff, who was interested in probabilistic inference and machine learning, and Oliver Selfridge, a researcher in pattern recognition. Although invited, Frank Rosenblatt—known for his work on neural networks—was unable to attend. Additional short-term contributors included cyberneticist W. Ross Ashby, neuroscientist Walter Pitts, and economist Herbert Simon.

Despite irregular attendance, the Dartmouth workshop sustained an environment of fruitful intellectual exchange from mid-June to mid-August. Participants engaged in daily discussions and explored how machines might learn, develop concepts, and solve problems. Notably, Newell and Simon demonstrated that their Logic Theorist program could prove 38 of the first 52 theorems from *Principia Mathematica*—a milestone showing that a symbolic AI system could rival human reasoning (Newell & Simon, 1956). Simon captured the excitement of this achievement when he exclaimed, "Over Christmas, Allen and I invented a thinking machine" (Crevier, 1993).

3.3. Atmosphere and Early Outcomes

The Dartmouth project fostered a genuinely interdisciplinary spirit. Participants from logic, linguistics, neuroscience, mathematics, and engineering collaborated to establish a shared terminology and methodology. McCarthy's discussions on a new programming language would later culminate in LISP, developed in 1958. Minsky contributed insights from neural learning mechanisms, including his SNARC simulator. Shannon expanded the debate beyond games like chess and checkers to broader strategies for programming general problem solvers. Rochester explored how IBM hardware could accelerate symbolic computation.

Although no single groundbreaking discovery emerged from the workshop, its greatest success was conceptual: artificial intelligence was now a distinct scientific field with a name, a goal, and a core community. By the end of 1956, many participants had returned to their institutions to form new AI research groups. McCarthy and Minsky later co-founded the AI Laboratory at MIT in 1959. Newell and Simon directed Carnegie Tech's computer science and brain research efforts toward AI. Indeed, nearly all who had attended or interacted with the Dartmouth meeting became key figures in the field's golden era of the 1960s.

Contributions of Key Participants

- **John McCarthy (1927–2011):** Originator of the term "artificial intelligence" and developer of LISP, McCarthy laid the foundation for the symbolic/logical approach in AI (McCarthy, 1959).
- **Marvin Minsky (1927–2016):** A pioneer in neural networks and later symbolic AI, Minsky's SNARC simulator and *Perceptrons* (1969) shaped both early optimism and later critiques of connectionism (Minsky & Papert, 1969).
- **Claude Shannon (1916–2001):** His ideas on game-playing algorithms and heuristic search strategies contributed a mathematical rigor to the problem-solving discussions (Shannon, 1950).
- **Nathaniel Rochester (1919–2001):** A key IBM engineer who attempted early simulations of McCulloch-Pitts neural networks and helped bridge theory and hardware (Rochester et al., 1956).
- **Allen Newell & Herbert Simon:** Creators of *Logic Theorist* and later *General Problem Solver*, they also developed the Physical Symbol System Hypothesis, a theoretical pillar of symbolic AI (Newell & Simon, 1997).
- **Ray Solomonoff (1926–2009):** Introduced ideas on probabilistic inference and later developed algorithmic information theory (Solomonoff, 1964).
- **Oliver Selfridge (1926–2008):** His "Pandemonium" model laid groundwork for multi-agent and perceptual AI systems (Selfridge, 1959).

- **Arthur Samuel (1901–1990):** Known for his checkers-playing program, Samuel's work inspired reinforcement learning approaches (Samuel, 1959).

Other influential figures such as Norbert Wiener and John von Neumann, though not directly involved, were well aware of the conference's developments. While von Neumann supported computational approaches, Wiener remained more skeptical about machines fully replicating human intelligence (Wiener, 1960).

3.4. Impacts and Outcomes of the Dartmouth Conference

Following the establishment of artificial intelligence (AI) as an independent field of inquiry, the Dartmouth Conference marked the beginning of a period characterized by dynamism and optimism in AI research. The immediate impacts and long-term consequences of the conference can be analyzed under several key headings:

3.4.1. Adoption of the Term "Artificial Intelligence"

Arguably the most immediate and visible outcome of the Dartmouth Conference was the widespread acceptance of the term "artificial intelligence" within scientific and public discourse. In the years following 1956, this term rapidly gained traction in academic publications, project proposals, and conference proceedings. For instance, a symposium held in New York in 1958 prominently featured "Artificial Intelligence" in its title and focused on AI methods. The adoption of this terminology gave the field a cohesive identity and enabled scholars from various disciplines to communicate in a shared language. Consequently, previously fragmented efforts labeled under cybernetics, automata theory, or computational neuroscience began to consolidate under a unified banner. The emergence of a shared literature, such as the influential early textbook *Computers and Thought* (Feigenbaum & Feldman, 1963), further amplified this terminological legacy by disseminating post-Dartmouth developments and accelerating interdisciplinary communication.

3.4.2. Establishment of AI Research Centers

Many researchers who participated in or were influenced by the Dartmouth Conference subsequently established AI-focused laboratories at their respective institutions. In 1959, McCarthy and Minsky founded the Artificial Intelligence Project at MIT; in 1963, McCarthy initiated the Stanford Artificial Intelligence Laboratory (SAIL); and in 1965, Donald Michie launched the Experimental Programming Unit at the University of Edinburgh, which later evolved into the Edinburgh AI Lab. These centers produced significant advances throughout the 1960s and institutionalized AI as a formal area of study. For example, MIT's AI Lab developed ELIZA (Weizenbaum, 1966), a milestone in natural language processing; SAIL pioneered the Shakey robot (1966–1972), the first autonomous robot capable of modeling its environment and planning actions; and researchers in Edinburgh focused on logical theories and pattern recognition systems. The interplay between institutional competition and collaboration helped propel the vision set forth at Dartmouth into diverse lines of development.

3.4.3. Funding and Project Support

A critical, albeit indirect, outcome of the Dartmouth Conference was the increase in financial support for AI research. Reports of the conference's success and subsequent findings attracted attention from both government agencies and the private sector. In the Cold War context, the U.S. Department of Defense's Advanced Research Projects Agency (ARPA, later DARPA) began funding AI projects in the early 1960s. In 1963, ARPA allocated substantial resources to AI initiatives at MIT and Carnegie Mellon University, enabling full-time research efforts. During this period, AI was widely regarded as a "technology of the future," and governments invested heavily in projects involving machine translation, intelligent assistants, and automated diagnostic systems. This level of support had been unprecedented prior to Dartmouth; the conference helped legitimize AI as a research objective worthy of strategic and financial backing.

3.4.4. Shaping of Theoretical Agendas

One of the Dartmouth Conference's most lasting impacts was its role in defining the research agenda of AI for at least a decade. The central themes discussed—natural language processing, game playing, automated theorem proving, learning algorithms, abstraction, and concept formation—became the dominant topics of AI research throughout the 1960s. Researchers divided these broad challenges into more tractable sub-problems, leading to the development of concrete projects. Automated theorem proving remained active after *Logic Theorist* and inspired new systems at SAIL and Stanford. Natural language understanding evolved from simple models like ELIZA to more advanced systems such as SHRDLU (Winograd, 1972), which could interpret and act on complex sentences within a limited world model. In game playing, chess programs received serious attention post-Dartmouth; Newell and Simon's team contributed significantly, and Richard Greenblatt at MIT developed MAC Hack (1967), a program capable of competing with chess masters. In machine learning, researchers pursued a range of techniques—Bayesian models and decision trees emerged in the late 1960s, inspired in part by the pioneering work of Arthur

Samuel. Despite methodological variety, all these efforts shared a common objective: to automate intellectual tasks modeled after human cognition, staying true to the vision articulated at Dartmouth.

3.4.5. Interdisciplinary Dialogue

The Dartmouth Conference exemplified the productive synergy that could emerge from interdisciplinary collaboration, bringing together scholars from computer science, mathematics, psychology, linguistics, and neuroscience. This collaborative ethos continued in its aftermath. At Carnegie Mellon, for example, psychologists and computer scientists worked together in Simon and Newell's lab; at MIT, Minsky engaged with neurologists, perceptual psychologists, and mathematicians on joint projects. This interdisciplinary approach also contributed to the emergence of cognitive science in the late 1960s—a field that fused AI research with studies of the human mind under a unified umbrella. Thus, AI came to be seen not merely as a branch of engineering but also as a theoretical tool for understanding human cognition. In many respects, the Dartmouth Conference can be credited with catalyzing this integration.

Taken together, the impacts of the Dartmouth Conference were overwhelmingly positive during the early phase of AI development. The period from 1956 to roughly 1970 can be considered the "first spring" of AI—a time when pioneers pursued bold new approaches with confidence, laying the groundwork for future breakthroughs. As the next phase of this history will show, however, this era of early optimism would eventually confront the practical limits and challenges of the real world.

4. EARLY APPLICATIONS OF ARTIFICIAL INTELLIGENCE (1956–1970)

Following the Dartmouth Conference in 1956, the field of artificial intelligence (AI) expanded rapidly, producing applications across a variety of subdomains. The period between 1956 and 1970 can be regarded as AI's "infancy" and "childhood." While this era saw remarkable successes, it was also marked by significant setbacks. This section reviews early AI applications by topic area:

4.1. Problem Solving and Logic

One of the first areas of focus inspired by Dartmouth was the ability of computers to perform abstract problem-solving. *Logic Theorist* (1956) by Newell and Simon and its successor, the *General Problem Solver* (1957–1959), demonstrated that computers could solve problems using symbolic logic and heuristic search techniques. GPS, designed to solve logical puzzles, introduced the concept of "state-space search" (Newell, Shaw, & Simon, 1959; Clark, 2003). These projects laid the groundwork for search algorithms (e.g., depth-first and breadth-first search) and heuristic methods in AI.

In the early 1960s at Stanford, John McCarthy worked to formalize problem-solving through mathematical logic involving states and state transitions. This effort led to systems like STRIPS (Stanford Research Institute Problem Solver) and *Planner*, developed in 1969 (Fikes & Nilsson, 1971). A major breakthrough came in 1965 with J. Alan Robinson's development of the resolution method, revolutionizing automated theorem proving and deductive inference. By the late 1960s, computers could prove mathematical theorems. Stanford's SAINT and SIN programs successfully solved integral calculus problems, and the TPP system at Argonne National Laboratory proved geometric theorems. These applications substantiated Dartmouth's core claim: computers could emulate human reasoning.

4.2. Games and Strategic Thinking

Games like chess became a popular benchmark for evaluating AI performance. Significant progress was made in this area beginning in the late 1950s. Claude Shannon's principles for chess move search (Shannon, 1950) were implemented in practical programs. In 1958, Alex Bernstein and colleagues developed the first full chess-playing program on the IBM 704. Though rudimentary, it generated legal moves and followed basic strategies. In 1962, MIT students under John McCarthy wrote a more advanced chess program.

The real breakthrough came in 1967 with Richard Greenblatt's *Mac Hack VI*, the first chess software to defeat a tournament-level human player. In addition to chess, AI researchers explored simpler games such as checkers (Samuel's program famously defeated a former U.S. champion in 1962), tic-tac-toe, and even rudimentary Go. Games provided an ideal testbed due to their well-defined rules and measurable outcomes. Game-playing programs facilitated the development of minimax search and alpha-beta pruning algorithms, which were later applied to broader decision-making problems (Newell & Simon, 1961).

4.3. Natural Language Processing

Understanding and generating human language was one of the most challenging goals in AI. In the 1950s, machine translation emerged as one of AI's first practical applications. Cold War tensions fueled interest in automatic translation between Russian and English. A 1954 demonstration by IBM and Georgetown University using a limited vocabulary generated great enthusiasm, with predictions that full automation was imminent.

Despite being discussed at Dartmouth, concrete advances in language processing were delayed. In the 1960s, researchers shifted toward rule-based systems. At Cambridge, Margaret Masterman's team experimented with semantic translation, while at MIT, Joseph Weizenbaum created *ELIZA* in 1966. This program used pattern-matching techniques to respond to typed user input, simulating a Rogerian therapist. Though simplistic, ELIZA was a landmark in natural language processing and revived interest in the Turing Test (Weizenbaum, 1966).

Another significant leap came in 1968 with *SHRDLU*, developed by Terry Winograd at Stanford (Winograd, 1972). This program could understand and execute English commands in a virtual "blocks world." For example, upon receiving the command "put the blue cube on the red cylinder," SHRDLU identified the objects and executed the action. It even asked clarifying questions in ambiguous situations. SHRDLU demonstrated that language understanding, visual perception, and planning could be integrated into a single system.

4.4. Vision and Perception

Giving machines the ability to see and hear like humans was an early goal of AI. In the early 1960s, simple programs were developed to interpret camera images. At MIT, Larry Roberts (1963) examined how to reconstruct 3D shapes from 2D images, identifying key problems in computer vision. In 1966, under Seymour Papert, MIT students attempted to write software to analyze and describe random images—a task that proved far more difficult than expected.

Nevertheless, some progress was made in constrained domains. Optical character recognition (OCR), such as reading handwritten ZIP codes, became practical by the late 1960s. Still, general-purpose visual perception remained one of AI's hardest challenges. Oliver Selfridge's *Pandemonium* model (1959) introduced multi-level feature detection but lacked broad application. In speech recognition, early efforts from the 1950s (e.g., Davis et al., 1952 at Bell Labs) gained momentum after Dartmouth. By the late 1960s, David Raj Reddy in Scotland and teams at IBM developed limited vocabulary speech recognition systems. Though success was modest, foundational algorithms such as k-nearest neighbors and basic neural networks emerged, laying the groundwork for future breakthroughs.

4.5. Robotics and Motion Planning

AI began extending beyond software to physical environments in the late 1960s. The Shakey project, launched at the Stanford Research Institute (SRI) in 1966, sought to integrate perception, reasoning, and action in a robotic platform. Shakey, a wheeled robot, mapped its environment with an onboard camera, planned its movements, and executed tasks like opening doors or pushing blocks (Nilsson, 1984). STRIPS, environment mapping, and object recognition all stemmed from this project.

At MIT, the *Hands-Up* project demonstrated a robotic arm stacking blocks (1969). These robotic systems combined perception (e.g., vision), reasoning (e.g., planning), and actuation (e.g., motor control), making them end-to-end implementations of AI. Through robotics, the abstract concept of "machine intelligence" began to take on a physical, real-world form.

4.6. Learning and Adaptation

Although symbolic AI dominated the 1960s, interest in machine learning persisted. Notable developments occurred despite limited focus. In 1967, Nilsson's group tested learning systems in game tree pruning problems. Donald Michie created the *MENACE* system for learning matchstick games using a physical box and beads—an early reinforcement learning prototype. Frank Rosenblatt's *Perceptron* algorithm (1957) stood out for its learnability. In 1960, he introduced the *Mark I Perceptron*, a system that could learn to recognize simple shapes (Rosenblatt, 1958).

However, in 1969, Minsky and Papert's book *Perceptrons* mathematically demonstrated limitations of single-layer neural networks, causing research in connectionism to stall. By 1970, learning remained an unresolved but increasingly crucial issue in AI, paving the way for machine learning to emerge as a central discipline in the 1980s and beyond.

4.7. General Assessment

By 1970, AI researchers had accomplished a range of "firsts" in simulating aspects of human intelligence: proving mathematical theorems, defeating humans in games, understanding natural language in restricted settings, perceiving simple objects, and planning physical actions through robots. These achievements inspired great optimism. Many believed that AI would reach human-level general intelligence by the 1980s (Simon, 1965; Minsky, 1967).

Yet early systems also revealed the limits of AI. Programs like SHRDLU functioned only in narrowly defined environments and could not process real-world language. Chess programs lacked generalization to other domains. These limitations planted the seeds of later criticisms and disappointments—issues that will be addressed in the next chapter.

5. CRITICISMS AND AI WINTERS

Although the field of artificial intelligence (AI) experienced rapid growth from 1956 to the late 1960s, it faced significant criticisms and stagnation by the early 1970s. This period, often referred to as the “AI winter,” denotes times when interest and funding in AI research significantly declined. This section examines the primary criticisms directed at AI and the resulting AI winters.

5.1. Unfulfilled Overoptimistic Predictions

During the initial years, AI pioneers made highly optimistic forecasts. For instance, Herbert Simon predicted in 1965 that “machines will be capable, within twenty years, of doing any work a man can do” (Simon, 1965). Similarly, Marvin Minsky stated in 1967 that “within a generation... the problem of creating 'artificial intelligence' will substantially be solved” (Minsky, 1967). However, by the 1970s, these anticipated achievements had not materialized. While computers succeeded in specific narrow tasks, they failed to exhibit generalizable intelligence, leading to disappointment among both funders and the public. Notably, media reports in the late 1960s heralded imminent breakthroughs in machine translation and humanoid robots, which ultimately did not come to fruition. Consequently, in the 1970s, funding agencies became more cautious, criticizing AI projects for setting unrealistic goals.

5.2. Theoretical Criticisms – Dreyfus's Arguments

One of the most prominent philosophical critiques of AI came from philosopher Hubert Dreyfus, who began voicing his concerns in 1965. In his report “Alchemy and AI,” Dreyfus likened contemporary AI research to medieval alchemy, offering serious methodological criticisms (Dreyfus, 1965). His central argument was that digital computers operate based on symbolic rules and explicit representations, whereas human intelligence does not function in this manner. Humans often rely on implicit knowledge, contextual understanding, and embodied experience; thus, genuine intelligence cannot be achieved solely through symbolic manipulation. For example, understanding a simple sentence involves world knowledge, intuition, and often informally defined information. Dreyfus contended that AI programs could not replicate such implicit knowledge, rendering them prone to failure in complex situations. Initially, AI researchers dismissed Dreyfus's views, and he was even mocked at MIT's AI Lab. However, over time, some of the issues he highlighted, such as the “frame problem”—the difficulty programs have in handling unexpected situations—were acknowledged as legitimate technical challenges. In 1972, Dreyfus expanded his criticisms to a broader audience with his book “What Computers Can't

Do," which had a significant impact and underscored the need for AI researchers to adopt more cautious and theoretically grounded approaches (Dreyfus, 1972).

5.3. Practical Assessments – The Lighthill Report

In 1973, the UK government commissioned mathematician Sir James Lighthill to evaluate the state of AI research. His report, known as the Lighthill Report, offered a scathing critique of AI. It characterized AI research outcomes in the UK as a "complete failure" and claimed that most investments in the field had been wasted (Lighthill, 1973). The report emphasized that anticipated progress in areas like general problem-solving and machine translation had not been achieved, with successes limited to narrow, controlled domains. Lighthill noted that AI researchers frequently encountered the "combinatorial explosion" problem, where algorithmic complexity grew uncontrollably with problem size. Indeed, many programs developed post-Dartmouth Conference became impractical as problem dimensions increased. The report stated, "Most workers in AI research have been disappointed with what has been achieved in the past twenty-five years; the great hopes of the 1950s and 1960s have not been realized by 1973" (Lighthill, 1973). The report had a dramatic impact on the UK government, leading to a near-total withdrawal of public support for AI research, with only limited work continuing at two universities (Edinburgh and Sussex). This marked the onset of the AI winter in the UK. In response, a televised debate featuring AI pioneers like Minsky and McCarthy was held in 1973, but it failed to alter public perception of the report's findings.

5.4. Reduction of ARPA Support in the USA – The ALPAC Report

In the United States, support for AI was not limitless. A significant turning point came with the 1966 publication of the ALPAC Report (Automatic Language Processing Advisory Committee), which assessed the outcomes of long-term Russian-English translation projects. The report concluded that progress in automatic translation had been insufficient and that existing systems were inferior to human translators. It stated that fully automatic, high-quality translation was unlikely in the near future. As a result, the US government cut funding for machine translation projects, leading to a near-decade-long stagnation in the field. The collapse of machine translation efforts was one of the early signs of the AI winter and undermined confidence in symbolic AI approaches. In the early 1970s, ARPA (later DARPA) shifted its focus from general AI projects to narrower, more practical technologies, such as speech recognition, simple command-and-control systems, and expert system prototypes.

Projects aiming for "general intelligence," like general problem solvers, were deprioritized. This shift forced AI researchers to reframe their projects to secure funding.

5.5. The Second AI Winter (Late 1980s)

The stagnation of the 1970s gave way to a resurgence in the early 1980s with the advent of expert systems. These rule-based systems demonstrated that AI could be successfully applied in industrial contexts. Notable examples include MYCIN in medicine and DENDRAL in geology, which effectively solved specialized problems. This momentum peaked with Japan's announcement of the Fifth Generation Computer Systems project in 1982, aiming to revolutionize computing with AI. In response, similar initiatives emerged in the US and Europe. However, this second wave was unsustainable. By the late 1980s, the expert systems boom collapsed due to economic and practical issues: these systems were difficult to maintain, had limited adaptability, and failed to achieve widespread applicability, disappointing investors. Consequently, around 1987–1988, many AI companies closed or pivoted, and university programs saw declining interest. This period is referred to as the second AI winter.

The technical and socio-economic lessons from these AI winters influenced the direction of AI research. After the first winter, researchers learned not to underestimate problem complexity and began developing more robust theoretical foundations and mathematical tools. For instance, the gap between AI and related fields started to narrow in the 1970s: logic and computational theory were increasingly utilized to strengthen AI's foundations, and statistics and probability theory were reintegrated into AI in the 1980s, leading to the emergence of Bayesian networks (Pearl, 1988). Following the second winter, the AI community rediscovered the importance of generalizable problem-solving and learning capabilities. By the 1990s, alongside symbolic methods, machine learning and neural networks (revitalized after 1986 with the backpropagation algorithm) regained prominence.

In summary, while the first decade following the Dartmouth Conference saw significant progress, subsequent decades required reevaluation. Criticisms and winters prompted a reassessment of oversimplified aspects of human intelligence in AI research. For example, the lack of common sense knowledge in AI systems became a distinct research area from the 1980s onward (e.g., Lenat's Cyc project). Similarly, the need to integrate symbolic and connectionist approaches led to the development of hybrid systems in the 1990s. These critiques have been integral to AI's maturation, helping the field better understand its limitations. The symbolic logic and expert system approaches developed during the era beginning with the Dartmouth Conference laid the foundation for the use of artificial intelligence in complex decision support processes; these foundations have enabled the development and widespread adoption of AI technologies in many application areas, especially in healthcare services.

6. HISTORICAL DEVELOPMENT OF ARTIFICIAL INTELLIGENCE IN HEALTHCARE (FROM THE 1950S TO PRESENT)

The development of artificial intelligence (AI) technologies has not only transformed fields such as engineering and computer science but has also profoundly reshaped critical sectors like healthcare, which directly affect human well-being. From its early stages, healthcare has been influenced by AI-driven innovations. Initially focused on general decision support systems, AI applications in medicine gradually evolved to support clinical functions such as diagnosis, treatment planning, and medical data analysis. Beginning in the 1970s, expert systems emerged as one of the earliest functional applications of AI in healthcare, using knowledge bases and inference engines to systematically support physicians' decisions. These advancements were not limited to clinical or hospital environments; over time, they expanded into home healthcare settings, providing a technological foundation for remote monitoring, early risk detection, and the coordination of care, particularly for elderly and chronically ill patients. This section examines the historical trajectory of AI from the 1950s to the present, focusing on its evolution in home healthcare through technological milestones, application areas, and turning points.

6.1. Expert Systems and Clinical AI (1970s–1990s)

In the 1970s and 1980s, the **knowledge-engineering** paradigm dominated AI research. Large-scale initiatives (e.g. Stanford's SUMEX-AIM project and Rutgers AI workshops) promoted development of "expert systems" – computerized decision tools encoding expert knowledge in rules (Kulikovski, 2019). In medicine and nursing, these expert systems aimed at diagnoses and care planning. Notable projects included *INTERNIST-1* (Pittsburgh) and *DXplain* (UMass, 1986), an "electronic textbook" and diagnostic consultant. *DXplain* used patient symptoms to generate differential diagnoses, supporting physicians in complex cases (Dailah, 2024). By 1986 it covered 500 conditions (later 2,600) and was an early form of AI-based clinical assistant. During this era, digital patient records and decision-support grew as well. Electronic health record (EHR) systems began to appear, providing data infrastructure that later enabled AI. For instance, by the late 1980s some hospitals used computerized clinical notes and alerts, seeding later AI analytics.

However, progress was uneven. The so-called "AI winters" of the 1970s–early 2000s meant fluctuating funding and slow general progress. Even so, AI research persisted in healthcare. Clinical databases (e.g. MEDLARS) and early computer-assisted physician support created an infrastructure for later AI. In nursing, AI tools first took form as support systems and automation: for example, the HelpMate robot (circa 1980) was deployed in hospitals by 1991 to autonomously transport medications and equipment, improving workflow though not directly caring for patients. These technologies hinted at automation of simple tasks, a theme that would re-emerge in home care robotics years later.

6.2. Telehealth, Remote Sensing, and Early Home Care (1990s–2000s)

By the 1990s, home healthcare was recognized as a growing sector, especially for aging populations and chronic disease management. Advances in computing and communication enabled rudimentary remote monitoring and telehealth. Home visits by clinicians began to be supplemented by remote consultations via telephone and the emerging Internet. In parallel, consumer devices (blood pressure cuffs, glucometers) became digital and networked. Although academic AI still centered on hospitals, these trends shifted attention toward the home environment. Some large institutions (e.g. the U.S. Veterans Affairs) pioneered home telemonitoring programs, using early AI-like rule engines to flag patient alerts, though systematic AI integration was limited at first.

A major advance was the concept of Ambient Assisted Living (AAL) in the 2000s, particularly in Europe. AAL initiatives sought to use smart technology to support independent living for the elderly at home. The term "ambient assisted living" describes environments fitted with sensors and devices that monitor health and daily activities to help seniors live safely and autonomously. Typical AAL systems combined fall-detection sensors, movement and vital-sign monitors, and safety alarms. Early research demonstrated that these systems could analyze multimodal data (motion, vitals, activity patterns) to detect emergencies or health changes in a non-clinical setting. For example, wearable and ambient sensors were studied to predict falls, and AI-driven algorithms could recognize deviations in daily routines (Danielsen et al., 2016). Though many AAL projects remained prototypes, they established key ideas: embedding sensors in the home and using AI to interpret them for care.

Concurrently, telepresence robotics began to appear. The *Giraff* robot (a video-equipped mobile platform) enabled distant caregivers and family to "visit" homebound elders through video conferencing, while also carrying sensors for blood pressure, temperature and motion. Giraff exemplified how AI and robotics could connect home patients with remote providers: it collected vital signs and alerted caregivers if thresholds were crossed, effectively acting as a telemonitor with AI-driven decision logic. These innovations laid early groundwork for modern telehealth: they showed that technology could extend the care team's reach into the home, a critical principle for later AI systems.

6.3. Machine Learning and Data-Driven Home Care (2010s–present)

The 2010s saw a renaissance in AI, driven by machine learning (ML) and deep learning (DL) with large data. In healthcare, this ushered in new capabilities for analysis and prediction. Over the past half-century, AI in health has "experienced significant evolution, especially with the introduction of ML and DL". In practical terms, smart algorithms began to analyze continuous streams of home health data from wearables and IoT devices. For example, blood glucose sensors and wearable ECG monitors started to transmit data to ML models for anomaly detection. Reviews note that AI now enables personalized preventive care, disease prediction, and continuous monitoring to enhance outcomes (Sharma et al., 2025).

Remote Patient Monitoring (RPM) became a major application. Academic studies and reviews emphasize that integrating AI with Internet-of-Things (IoT) devices has "revolutionized remote patient monitoring" and home-based care. Wearable fitness trackers, smartwatches, and home medical IoT devices (wireless scales, connected pill dispensers, smart mattresses) began to feed data into AI systems for early warning. For instance, machine learning models have been developed to predict heart failure exacerbations or detect falls days before they happen, using data like gait, activity and vitals. These systems can alert clinicians to intervene before a crisis, reducing hospitalizations. Indeed, recent reviews highlight AI's role in enabling "continuous, real-time health assessments in home-based settings," and in reducing readmissions by supporting "early disease detection".

Meanwhile, consumer AI assistants also entered healthcare. Mobile health apps and chatbots (e.g. virtual symptom checkers) grew in the 2010s. The COVID-19 pandemic in 2020 notably accelerated telemedicine and AI-driven tools; one review observes that the pandemic "catalyzed" use of telemedicine and chatbots to enhance care accessibility. Thus, by the early 2020s, home healthcare began routinely leveraging AI: virtual visits, automated triage bots, and ML-driven home monitoring were integrated components of care delivery in many systems.

6.4. Robotics and Assistive Technologies for Home Care

Parallel to software advances, robotic and sensor technologies for the home matured. Modern social and assistive robots have been introduced to support daily living and provide companionship. For example, Paro (a robot seal developed in Japan in the early 2000s) was specifically designed as a therapeutic companion for elderly people with dementia. Paro's success inspired similar companion robots (some animal-like, some humanoid) that can engage users with speech, music or movement. Studies indicate older adults generally welcome robots for simple, non-intimate tasks (reminding medications, light chores). Robots like *Giraff* and *Matilda* (mentioned above) have demonstrated that telepresence and social engagement is feasible in home settings.

Other AI-driven robots have been created for practical assistance. For instance, Japan developed *RIBA* (Robot for Interactive Body Assistance) in 2009 to help lift and transfer patients. During the COVID era, hospitals deployed *Moxi* and *Pegasus* robots to transport supplies and handle materials, freeing staff for patient care. Although these were hospital robots, their development signals that the same principles (sensor-perception and navigation) can apply to home robotics. Some companies now market domestic helper robots (e.g. robotic vacuum cleaners like Roomba, emerging home-telehealth robots) that incorporate ML for navigation and monitoring. Human-centered AI research emphasizes that effective companion robots require speech, vision and context-awareness – for example, adapting to a user's preferences. Advances in ML (computer vision, voice recognition) are making it increasingly practical to build home robots that can remind, entertain, or even alert emergency responders.

A complementary trend is smart home technology. AI-powered voice assistants (e.g. Amazon Alexa, Google Home) have been adapted for health tasks: voice-activated medication reminders, symptom checkers, or integration with smart sensors. Smart sensors (e.g. motion detectors, smart smoke/CO alarms, bed sensors) are now often networked to home health platforms. Companies are integrating AI with environmental sensors to detect patterns of daily living – for instance, recognizing if a senior's nighttime movements change, which could indicate a health issue. Though outside strict "AI history," these developments reflect the wider adoption of AI-infused devices in the home care environment (Hirai et al., 2024).

Overall, robotics and smart-home AI systems have become part of an ecosystem for home healthcare. They illustrate how the field evolved from isolated lab projects to real-world deployments. A recent scoping review notes that AAL technologies and companion robots now focus on two main automated decision areas: health monitoring and activity recognition for older users. In effect, modern home healthcare often means a network of sensors, AI analytics, and sometimes robots, all aimed at keeping people safer and healthier in their own homes.

6.5. Global Perspectives

Advances in home healthcare AI have occurred worldwide. In Europe, government-supported Ambient Assisted Living programs and national pilot projects have spurred innovation. For example, in Italy's public health system, integrated digital tools including AI decision-support and care robots are being deployed in home care to meet the needs of an aging population (Cingolani, 2023).

A 2023 review reports that Italian health agencies see AI/robotics as key to more effective home services and better remote monitoring of chronic disease. The review also notes challenges (data infrastructure, privacy, cost), but underscores that many countries (Italy among them) are explicitly planning AI-enabled "Connected Care" models for home service.

In Asia, robotics has been particularly emphasized. Japan – facing one of the world's fastest-aging societies – has invested heavily in care robotics. The Japanese government has funded projects like Paro (introduced above), HAL (an exoskeleton to assist walking and lifting), and soft humanoid robots (such as *Pepper*) for eldercare support (Filipová et al, 2021). These robots supplement a shrinking workforce; as one report notes, robots in Japan's care facilities perform monitoring and assist with mobility while leaving more time for human caregivers. Similarly, South Korea and China have begun deploying AI-monitoring platforms and robots in senior homes and clinics, though peer-reviewed publications are still emerging (Soriano et al., 2022).

In North America, home health traditionally relied on nursing visits, but AI tools are now being introduced. The U.S. Veterans Health Administration has long led remote monitoring (for example, for diabetes management) using AI-driven alerts. More recently, home health agencies and insurers in the U.S. have started using predictive analytics to allocate home visits, and pilot home-assistant devices. Furthermore, the COVID-19 crisis sharply increased adoption of telehealth apps and remote-monitoring platforms in the United States and Canada. A 2024 analysis notes that enabling technologies for home care (wearable sensors, secure cloud data, ML algorithms) have matured enough that "AI for remote patient monitoring" is now a strategic priority for many providers.

Overall, the global trend is clear: as populations age, nations are turning to AI-augmented home care. The demand is evident in demographics – for instance, over 20% of Europe's population is 65+, and by 2030 an estimated 16.6% of people worldwide will be over 60. These pressures, plus labor shortages (as in Japan), drive innovation in AI and robotics for the home. Collaborative international research (through EU-AAL programs, WHO digital health initiatives, etc.) ensures that developments and lessons are shared across borders.

6.6. Integration and Future Directions

By 2025, AI in home healthcare has moved from concept to practice. Early expert systems like MYCIN and AAL prototypes have given way to machine learning pipelines and smart devices operating in real homes. Today's systems combine *data-driven* approaches (ML algorithms sifting big patient data) with *cyber-physical* technologies (robots and sensors in the environment). The integration of these AI technologies seeks to achieve multiple aims: improving patient safety, reducing caregiver workload, and personalizing care plans. For example, predictive models can identify which home-care patient is at highest risk of hospitalization, while companion robots can reduce loneliness and encourage compliance with treatment.

It is important to acknowledge challenges. Implementation of AI home care systems must address data privacy, user acceptance, and equitable access. Standards and regulations are still catching up: for instance, only in recent years have regulators begun approving AI-driven diagnostic devices (e.g. FDA clearance of imaging AI in 2017and guidelines for remote AI tools are evolving. Nevertheless, the trajectory is clear: home healthcare is increasingly "intelligent," leveraging decades of AI research. The application of AI from hospital decision-support systems of the 1970s to today's smart homes illustrates a century-long arc: early computing concepts matured through expert systems into modern ML, and robotics transitioned from factory floors into living rooms. As one recent review notes, AI in home care now "augments and complements" human expertise rather than replacing it, a sign that the field has moved into pragmatic collaboration. In sum, the historical development of AI in home healthcare is a tale of technological maturation: starting with abstract AI ideas in the 1950s, evolving through domain-specific expert systems, and culminating in today's integrated AI + IoT + robotics solutions that support health and independence in the home (Kulikovski, 2019).

REFERENCES

Abràmoff, M. D., Lavin, P. T., Birch, M., Shah, N., & Folk, J. C. (2018). Pivotal trial of an autonomous AI-based diagnostic system for detection of diabetic retinopathy in primary care offices. *NPJ Digital Medicine*, *1*(1), 39. DOI: 10.1038/s41746-018-0040-6 PMID: 31304320

Awotunde, J. B., Oluwabukonla, S., Chakraborty, C., Bhoi, A. K., & Ajamu, G. J. (2022). Application of artificial intelligence and big data for fighting COVID-19 pandemic. In Mishra, S., Suanpang, H. S., Wu, Y.-S., & Nagar, A. K. (Eds.), *Decision sciences for COVID-19: Learning through case studies* (pp. 3–26). Springer., DOI: 10.1007/978-3-030-87019-5_1

Brown, T. B., Mann, B., Ryder, N., Subbiah, M., Kaplan, J. D., Dhariwal, P., Neelakantan, A., Shyam, P., Sastry, G., Askell, A., Agarwal, S., Herbert-Voss, A., Krueger, G., Henighan, T., Child, R., Ramesh, A., Ziegler, D. M., Wu, J., Winter, C., & Amodei, D. (2020). Language models are few-shot learners. *Advances in Neural Information Processing Systems*, *33*, 1877–1901.

Buchanan, B., & Feigenbaum, E. (1993). DENDRAL and Meta-DENDRAL: Roots of knowledge systems and expert system applications. *Artificial Intelligence*, *59*(1–2), 233–240. DOI: 10.1016/0004-3702(93)90010-M

Char, D. S., Shah, N. H., & Magnus, D. (2018). Implementing machine learning in health care—Addressing ethical challenges. *The New England Journal of Medicine*, *378*(11), 981–983. DOI: 10.1056/NEJMp1714229 PMID: 29539284

Cingolani, M., Scendoni, R., Fedeli, P., & Cembrani, F. (2023). Artificial intelligence and digital medicine for integrated home care services in Italy: Opportunities and limits. *Frontiers in Public Health*, *10*, 1095001. DOI: 10.3389/fpubh.2022.1095001 PMID: 36684935

Clark, A. (2003). Artificial intelligence and the many faces of reason. In Stich, S., & Warfield, T. (Eds.), *The Blackwell guide to philosophy of mind* (pp. 309–321). Blackwell Publishing. DOI: 10.1002/9780470998762.ch13

Crevier, D. (1993). *AI: The tumultuous history of the search for artificial intelligence*. Basic Books.

Dailah, H. G., Koriri, M., Sabei, A., Kriry, T., & Zakri, M. (2024). Artificial intelligence in nursing: Technological benefits to nurse's mental health and patient care quality. *Health Care*, *12*(24), 2555. DOI: 10.3390/healthcare12242555 PMID: 39765983

Danielsen, A., Olofsen, H., & Bremdal, B. A. (2016). Increasing fall risk awareness using wearables: A fall risk awareness protocol. *Journal of Biomedical Informatics, 63*, 184–194. DOI: 10.1016/j.jbi.2016.08.016 PMID: 27544413

Dartmouth College. (n.d.). *The Dartmouth Summer Research Project on Artificial Intelligence*. https://home.dartmouth.edu

Davis, K., Biddulph, R., & Balashek, S. (1952). Automatic recognition of spoken digits. *The Journal of the Acoustical Society of America, 24*(6), 637–642. DOI: 10.1121/1.1906946

Doi, K. (2007). Computer-aided diagnosis in medical imaging: Historical review, current status and future potential. *Computerized Medical Imaging and Graphics, 31*(4–5), 198–211. DOI: 10.1016/j.compmedimag.2007.02.002 PMID: 17349778

Dreyfus, H. L. (1965). *Alchemy and artificial intelligence* (Report No. P-3244). RAND Corporation. https://www.rand.org/pubs/papers/P3244.html

Dreyfus, H. L. (1972). *What computers can't do: The limits of artificial intelligence*. Harper & Row.

Esteva, A., Kuprel, B., Novoa, R. A., Ko, J., Swetter, S. M., Blau, H. M., & Thrun, S. (2017). Dermatologist-level classification of skin cancer with deep neural networks. *Nature, 542*(7639), 115–118. DOI: 10.1038/nature21056 PMID: 28117445

Feigenbaum, E. A., & Feldman, J. (Eds.). (1963). *Computers and thought*. McGraw-Hill.

Fikes, R. E., & Nilsson, N. J. (1971). STRIPS: A new approach to the application of theorem proving to problem solving. *Artificial Intelligence, 2*(3–4), 189–208. DOI: 10.1016/0004-3702(71)90010-5

Filipová, I., Dulina, Ľ., Bigošová, E., & Plinta, D. (2021). Modern possibilities of patient transport aids. *Transportation Research Procedia, 55*, 510–517. DOI: 10.1016/j.trpro.2021.07.015

Freer, T. W., & Ulissey, M. J. (2001). Screening mammography with computer-aided detection: Prospective study of 12,860 patients in a community breast center. *Radiology, 220*(3), 781–786. DOI: 10.1148/radiol.2203001282 PMID: 11526282

French, R. M. (2000). The Turing Test: The first fifty years. *Trends in Cognitive Sciences, 4*(3), 115–122. DOI: 10.1016/S1364-6613(00)01453-4 PMID: 10689346

Gillies, R. J., Kinahan, P. E., & Hricak, H. (2016). Radiomics: Images are more than pictures, they are data. *Radiology, 278*(2), 563–577. DOI: 10.1148/radiol.2015151169 PMID: 26579733

Greenblatt, R. D., Eastlake, D. E.III, & Crocker, S. D. (1967). The Greenblatt chess program. *Proceedings of the* November 14–16, 1967, *Fall Joint Computer Conference*, 801–810. DOI: 10.1145/1465611.1465715

Hashimoto, D. A., Rosman, G., Rus, D., & Meireles, O. R. (2018). Artificial intelligence in surgery: Promises and perils. *Annals of Surgery*, *268*(1), 70–76. DOI: 10.1097/SLA.0000000000002693 PMID: 29389679

IBM. (n.d.). *The history of artificial intelligence.* https://www.ibm.com/artificial-intelligence/ai-history

Jaakkola, H., Henno, J., Mäkelä, J., & Thalheim, B. (2019). Artificial intelligence yesterday, today and tomorrow. In *2019 42nd International Convention on Information and Communication Technology, Electronics and Microelectronics (MIPRO)* (pp. 860–867). IEEE. DOI: 10.23919/MIPRO.2019.8756913

Jumper, J., Evans, R., Pritzel, A., Green, T., Figurnov, M., Ronneberger, O., Tunyasuvunakool, K., Bates, R., Žídek, A., Potapenko, A., Bridgland, A., Meyer, C., Kohl, S. A. A., Ballard, A. J., Cowie, A., Romera-Paredes, B., Nikolov, S., Jain, R., Adler, J., & Hassabis, D. (2021). Highly accurate protein structure prediction with AlphaFold. *Nature*, *596*(7873), 583–589. DOI: 10.1038/s41586-021-03819-2 PMID: 34265844

Kulikowski, C. A. (2019). Beginnings of artificial intelligence in medicine (AIM): Computational artifice assisting scientific inquiry and clinical art—With reflections on present AIM challenges. *Yearbook of Medical Informatics*, *28*(1), 249–256. DOI: 10.1055/s-0039-1677895 PMID: 31022744

Kutlusoy, Z. (2019). Felsefe açısından yapay zeka. [Artificial intelligence from a philosophical perspective] In Telli, G. (Ed.), *Yapay zeka ve gelecek* (pp. 25–43). Doğu Kitapevi.

LeCun, Y., Bengio, Y., & Hinton, G. (2015). Deep learning. *Nature*, *521*(7553), 436–444. DOI: 10.1038/nature14539 PMID: 26017442

Ledley, R. S., & Lusted, L. B. (1959). Reasoning foundations of medical diagnosis. *Science*, *130*(3366), 9–21. DOI: 10.1126/science.130.3366.9 PMID: 13668531

Levesque, H. J. (2017). *Common sense, the Turing Test, and the quest for real AI.* MIT Press. DOI: 10.7551/mitpress/10909.001.0001

Lighthill, J. (1973). Artificial intelligence: A general survey. In *Artificial intelligence: A paper symposium* (pp. 1–20). Science Research Council.

Lodwick, G. S., Haun, C. L., Smith, W. E., Keller, R. F., & Robertson, E. D. (1963). Computer diagnosis of primary bone tumors: A preliminary report. *Radiology, 80*(2), 273–275. DOI: 10.1148/80.2.273

Marcus, G., Rossi, F., & Veloso, M. (2016). Beyond the Turing Test. *AI Magazine, 37*(1), 3–4. DOI: 10.1609/aimag.v37i1.2650

McCarthy, J. (1959). Programs with common sense. In *Mechanisation of thought processes* (Vol. 2, pp. 77–84). Her Majesty's Stationery Office.

McCarthy, J., Minsky, M. L., Rochester, N., & Shannon, C. E. (1955). *A proposal for the Dartmouth Summer Research Project on Artificial Intelligence* Dartmouth College.

McCulloch, W. S., & Pitts, W. (1943). A logical calculus of the ideas immanent in nervous activity. *The Bulletin of Mathematical Biophysics, 5*(4), 115–133. DOI: 10.1007/BF02478259

Mei, C., Zhang, Y., Liu, H., & Wang, Z. (2024). Understanding versus imitation: Evaluating AI chatbots against human-like dialogue. *Journal of Artificial Intelligence Research*. Advance online publication.

Miller, R. A., Pople, H. E.Jr, & Myers, J. D. (1982). INTERNIST-1, an experimental computer-based diagnostic consultant for general internal medicine. *The New England Journal of Medicine, 307*(8), 468–476. DOI: 10.1056/NEJM198208193070803 PMID: 7048091

Minsky, M. (1961). Steps toward artificial intelligence. *Proceedings of the IRE, 49*(1), 8–30. DOI: 10.1109/JRPROC.1961.287775

Minsky, M., & Papert, S. (1969). *Perceptrons: An introduction to computational geometry*. MIT Press.

Moor, J. H. (2001). The status and future of the Turing Test. *Minds and Machines, 11*(1), 77–93. DOI: 10.1023/A:1011218925467

Newell, A., Shaw, J. C., & Simon, H. A. (1959). Report on a general problem-solving program. In *Proceedings of the International Conference on Information Processing* (pp. 256–264). UNESCO.

Newell, A., & Simon, H. A. (1956). The logic theory machine: A complex information processing system. *IEEE Transactions on Information Theory, 2*(3), 61–79. DOI: 10.1109/TIT.1956.1056797

Newell, A., & Simon, H. A. (1976). Computer science as empirical inquiry: Symbols and search. *Communications of the ACM*, *19*(3), 113–126. DOI: 10.1145/360018.360022

Nilsson, N. J. (1984). *Shakey the Robot* (Technical Note 323). SRI International.

Pearl, J. (1988). *Probabilistic reasoning in intelligent systems: Networks of plausible inference*. Morgan Kaufmann.

Rochester, N., Holland, J. H., Haibt, L. H., & Duda, W. L. (1956). Tests on a cell assembly theory of the action of the brain, using a large digital computer. *IEEE Transactions on Information Theory*, *2*(3), 80–93. DOI: 10.1109/TIT.1956.1056810

Rosenblatt, F. (1958). The perceptron: A probabilistic model for information storage and organization in the brain. *Psychological Review*, *65*(6), 386–408. DOI: 10.1037/h0042519 PMID: 13602029

Samuel, A. L. (1959). Some studies in machine learning using the game of checkers. *IBM Journal of Research and Development*, *3*(3), 210–229. DOI: 10.1147/rd.33.0210

Selfridge, O. G. (1959). Pandemonium: A paradigm for learning. In *Mechanisation of thought processes* (pp. 511–529). Her Majesty's Stationery Office.

Shannon, C. E. (1950). Programming a computer for playing chess. *The London, Edinburgh and Dublin Philosophical Magazine and Journal of Science*, *41*(314), 256–275. DOI: 10.1080/14786445008521796

Shapiro, S. C. (1992). Artificial intelligence. In Shapiro, S. C. (Ed.), *Encyclopedia of artificial intelligence* (Vol. 1, pp. 54–57). Wiley.

Sharma, A., Pesarlanka, D. B., & Sharma, S. (2025). Integrating machine learning, artificial intelligence, deep learning, and IoT in remote patient monitoring. In Tyagi, A. K., & Rajest, S. S. (Eds.), *Future innovations in the convergence of AI and Internet of Things in medicine* (pp. 285–318). IGI Global., DOI: 10.4018/979-8-3693-7703-1.ch011

Shortliffe, E. H. (1976). *Computer-based medical consultations: MYCIN*. Elsevier.

Simon, H. A. (1965). *The shape of automation for men and management*. Harper & Row.

Solomonoff, R. J. (1964). A formal theory of inductive inference. *Information and Control*, *7*(1), 1–22. DOI: 10.1016/S0019-9958(64)90223-2

Soriano, G. P., Yasuhara, Y., Ito, H., Matsumoto, K., Osaka, K., Kai, Y., Locsin, R., Shoenhofer, S., & Tanioka, T. (2022). Robots and robotics in nursing. *Health Care, 10*(8), 1571. DOI: 10.3390/healthcare10081571 PMID: 36011228

Topol, E. J. (2019). *Deep medicine: How artificial intelligence can make healthcare human again.* Basic Books.

Turing, A. M. (1936). On computable numbers, with an application to the Entscheidungsproblem. *Proceedings of the London Mathematical Society, 2*(42), 230–265. DOI: 10.1112/plms/s2-42.1.230

Turing, A. M. (1950). Computing machinery and intelligence. *Mind, 59*(236), 433–460. DOI: 10.1093/mind/LIX.236.433

Weizenbaum, J. (1966). ELIZA—A computer program for the study of natural language communication between man and machine. *Communications of the ACM, 9*(1), 36–45. DOI: 10.1145/365153.365168

Wiener, N. (1948). *Cybernetics: Or control and communication in the animal and the machine.* MIT Press.

Wiener, N. (1960). Some moral and technical consequences of automation. *Science, 131*(3410), 1355–1358. DOI: 10.1126/science.131.3410.1355 PMID: 17841602

Winograd, T. (1972). *Understanding natural language.* Academic Press. DOI: 10.1016/0010-0285(72)90002-3

Yampolskiy, R. V. (2013). Turing Test as a defining feature of AI-completeness. In Duch, W., & Mańdziuk, J. (Eds.), *Artificial intelligence, evolutionary computing and metaheuristics* (pp. 3–17). Springer., DOI: 10.1007/978-3-642-29694-9_1

Chapter 2
Transforming Home Healthcare:
A Business Ecosystem Approach to Digital Health Solutions

Mohammad Nabil Almunawar
https://orcid.org/0000-0001-5296-2576
Universiti Brunei Darussalam, Brunei

Mustafa Zeedan Younis
https://orcid.org/0000-0001-8448-808X
Jackson State University, USA

ABSTRACT

The widespread adoption of cloud computing and a variety of affordable client devices such as smartphones, sensors, wearable technology, and the Internet of Things (IoT) has transformed the way we collect data. The constant connectivity of these devices enables remote and continuous data access, making data-driven healthcare not only highly feasible but also executable from a distance. Data gathered from these devices enhances remote diagnostics and can be leveraged to deliver healthcare value in homecare settings, particularly for families and senior citizens. Health consultations can now be conducted remotely, and through coordinated collaboration within the healthcare business ecosystem, integrated healthcare solutions will improve well-being, especially for families and seniors. This chapter explores advancements in digital health, digital solutions for family and senior care, healthcare value creation, the digital healthcare business ecosystem, and recent case studies on digital healthcare innovations.

DOI: 10.4018/979-8-3373-3099-0.ch002

INTRODUCTION

In general, healthcare is a knowledge-intensive and data-driven service. Health professionals, such as doctors and nurses, have to undergo thorough and standardized education and training. They also need to obtain health-related certifications before they can provide healthcare services. The first step for a health professional in delivering care is to gather patient data, both personal and medical data, for health assessment. This data typically comes from existing medical/health records (historical data), diagnostic instruments, and patient interviews.

For example, in a simple or outpatient consultation setting, a doctor normally performs a basic health diagnosis through an interview, physical or visual examination, and checking important indications such as heartbeats (using a stethoscope) and blood pressure. By integrating the data gathered during a consultation with the medical record of the patient available in the system (such as stored in an Electronic Health Record or EHR), the doctor diagnoses the patient's condition and determines a suitable treatment, which may include professional advice and the prescription of medication. All data gathered during consultation, advice or recommendation, and prescriptions given are recorded in the system.

If the health-related data collected during a consultation is insufficient to come up with a solid decision in giving treatment, the doctor will ask the patient to undergo further checks (more data collection), such as blood and urine tests, X-ray, EEG (electroencephalogram) or even MRI (magnetic resonance imaging) at a different location or organization. If the doctor finds the problem and is unable to perform treatment due to limited knowledge, they will refer the patient to a specialist. Now, a collaborative effort within a healthcare ecosystem needs to be performed to solve the patient's problem.

The above describes conventional healthcare practices, where a patient needs to visit a doctor to have a face-to-face consultation. Observe that to come up with a decision for treatment, a doctor needs the patient's health-related data and a health ecosystem to gather more data and address more difficult problems. If the data can be collected through information and communication technology (ICT), the patient can schedule a virtual consultation via ICT means and, hence, may not need to see the doctor physically. This will save the patient time and money. Through a good healthcare ecosystem, a prescription given to the patient can be forwarded directly to a pharmacy, and a delivery agent can deliver the medicine to the patient's home. All related charges will be sent to the patient's insurance provider.

ICT-assisted healthcare is normally known as telemedicine, telehealth, or e-health (WHO Global Observatory for eHealth, 2010). The three terminologies are normally used interchangeably, although they may be defined differently. Telemedicine is a healthcare service that is delivered via ICT with much more concern for the clinical aspect of the care. Telehealth is more general than telemedicine, as it also delivers non-clinical aspects of healthcare, such as awareness programs and training. E-health is even more general, as it covers all healthcare, both remote and onsite services delivered via ICT, the EHR system, and the administrative system of healthcare. The advancement of ICT, or digital technology, in general, has ignited the healthcare industry to undertake digital transformation, enabling quality delivery of healthcare through digital technology-assisted home-based care. Telehealth is no longer a supplementary service of traditional healthcare; it is becoming the edge of modern healthcare, particularly enabling quality homecare (Monaghesh & Hajizadeh, 2020).

This chapter focuses on telehealth for homecare settings. Recent telehealth utilizes affordable digital devices such as smartphones, wearable devices, IoT, and specialized healthcare devices like digital stethoscopes, fall detection sensors, digital blood pressure monitors, smart insulin pens, and many more. These devices are enablers for remote diagnostics for homecare settings. They generate vast amounts of real-time data, which is useful for remote health consultations, early disease detection, and personalized care plans. They can provide snapshot or periodical data for a doctor or health provider to effectively diagnose a patient and deliver healthcare remotely. In addition, a dedicated mobile application (app) can be developed to constantly monitor a patient's well-being and collect medical-related data and personal records on emotional condition through written expression and various grievances. All data will help to provide better and more accurate remote diagnoses.

By providing snapshots or longitudinal health data, these tools empower doctors to diagnose and treat patients remotely with greater accuracy (Morita et al., 2023; Talal et al., 2019). Furthermore, dedicated mobile applications can be developed to continuously monitor patient well-being, collecting not only medical data but also personal records. These apps not only have the ability to track medical information, but they can also capture how patients are feeling emotionally and any symptoms they are experiencing in their own words. When we combine all this information, doctors can make better decisions from afar and provide care that truly focuses on each patient's unique needs.

However, the benefits of telehealth are not only remote diagnosis and care delivery. This happens when everyone in healthcare works together (Edirippulige & Armfield, 2017). For example, if doctors, tech companies, insurance providers, government leaders, patients, and all parts of a healthcare ecosystem collaborate and smoothly exchange information for the patient's well-being, the patient will receive great care through telehealth.

Imagine that you are a patient. Your smartwatch tracks your heart rate and sends the data to your family doctor, who notices an unusual pattern and initiates a video consultation with a specialist. Together, they update your treatment plan and keep your family caregivers in the loop—all without you leaving home. This kind of connected care makes healthcare faster to access, easier to use, and of better quality, especially for people receiving care at home.

The remainder of this chapter is organized as follows. The next section highlights the evolution of home healthcare, followed by a discussion on digital solutions in the healthcare sector. Subsequently, the chapter introduces the foundation of ecosystem thinking in healthcare and presents a framework for mapping and constructing healthcare business ecosystems. This is followed by an application of the framework to a multi-sided network healthcare business ecosystem. The chapter then discusses case examples of existing telehealth or homecare applications through the lens of business ecosystems. It concludes with a summary of key insights.

EVOLUTION OF HOME HEALTHCARE

Traditional healthcare is hospital-centric healthcare, where patients need to travel to visit hospitals or clinics physically for consultation, tests, and treatments. In contrast, home-based healthcare relies on technology for remote diagnosis and care of patients in their homes, freeing them from the hassle of transportation and being away from their families and reducing overall costs of care.

In the early 20th century, the healthcare paradigm was hospital-centric care, when hospitals were the center of the medical treatment of patients (Bodenheimer & Grumbach, 2020). With the advancements in medical technology, the Internet, and mobile technologies coupled with the increase in the costs of healthcare, there is a tendency for a gradual transition to decentralize healthcare, including home-based healthcare (homecare for short), especially with the advancement of IoT, mobile communications, and wearable devices (Güdük, 2025; Hamblin et al., 2025; Sockolow et al., 2021).

In tandem with the advancement of digital technologies, several digital health innovations, such as telehealth and remote health monitoring systems, have enabled healthcare delivery beyond hospitals. The COVID-19 pandemic necessitated care to avoid physical contact and reduce the risks of deadly infections (Bashshur et al., 2020; Seivert & Badowski, 2021). Nowadays, homecare not only handles post-acute recovery but also manages chronic disease, palliative care, and even hospital-at-home programs (Federman et al., 2018).

Besides the technology factor mentioned above, several other factors influence the adoption of homecare, such as aging populations, the rise of chronic diseases, and the skyrocketing cost of traditional healthcare. In terms of the aging population, more than 15% of the world's population (approximately 1 in 6 people) will be over 60 years old (WHO, 2024), making homecare a viable alternative to managing age-related diseases such as dementia and mobility impairments (Szanton et al., 2016). Traditional healthcare has struggled in managing chronic diseases (such as heart disease and diabetes), making homecare a viable and cheaper alternative. The advancement of wearable technologies and remote patient monitoring (RPM) allows constant monitoring and tracking and provides early detection of problems (Kvedar et al., 2016). In addition, the cost of hospital-based healthcare is expensive. For example, the cost for U.S. inpatient stays averages over $3,025 per day (McAllister, 2024). Homecare is a viable alternative as it provides cost-effective care. For example, a systematic review of cost-effective homecare services suggested that homecare interventions are cost-saving and as effective as hospitals (Curioni et al., 2023), and in general, homecare is cost-effective compared to hospital care (Ultimate Care, 2025). Nowadays, homecare is delivered through digital health solutions, as they are affordable, convenient, and effective.

DIGITAL HEALTH SOLUTIONS IN HEALTHCARE

Advancements in digital technology and myriad related innovations have driven digital transformation in the healthcare industry. For example, the utilization of wearable devices, remote patient monitoring (RPM), and IoT, as well as the incorporation of artificial intelligence (AI) in diagnostics, enables remote delivery of affordable and quality care, making telehealth and homecare great solutions for convenient and cost-effective quality healthcare.

IoT for Healthcare

IoT is the term that refers to smart gadgets or common objects that are connected to the Internet, which are normally used to collect data automatically. There are many kinds of IoT depending on the usage, such as IoT for smart cities, IoT for agriculture, IoT for industry, internet-enabled consumer electronics, IoT for healthcare, and wearable devices. Since many things can now be connected to the Internet, they are called the Internet of Things, or IoT for short.

Besides wearable devices used in healthcare, some commonly used IoT in telehealth and homecare are digital otoscopes/stethoscopes like Eko DUO, HD medical exam cameras like TytoCare, AI-powered symptom checkers like Symptomate or Ada, IoT-enabled dialysis machines like Tablo, and behavioral monitoring systems like CarePredict, to name a few. These IoT devices are designed for medical-related data of patients who are staying at home or remotely from doctors who observe or diagnose them. IoT devices are very handy for observing and monitoring patients at homes or community centers. They are affordable and effective data capture devices that can constantly collect data for diagnostic analysis (Iqubal et al., 2025; Islam et al., 2015; Talal et al., 2019).

Wearable Devices

Wearable devices are IoT devices that can be worn. These devices can capture data and perform some intended tasks. Some examples of wearable devices are biosensors, fitness trackers, medical-grade wearables, and smartwatches. Most wearable devices can be controlled remotely through wireless data communication, which normally can be connected to the Internet; hence, they can be used to collect data in real-time, which in turn can be used to perform analysis for healthcare purposes.

Wearable devices can be utilized to perform chronic disease management, elderly care, and monitoring. For example, ECG patches like Zio Patch assist patients in tracking the status of patients with cardiovascular diseases (Dunn, 2019), whereas glucose meters and continuous glucose monitors such as Signos CGM and Dexcom G6 support patients with diabetes in controlling their blood sugar levels. A dedicated RPM can be used to monitor the recovery of post-surgical patients, avoiding frequent hospital readmissions (Steinhubl et al., 2018). Apple Watch or similar devices can be used as fall detection sensors for elderly care. Similarly, activity trackers like Fitbit help monitor elderly patients. This reduces hospitalization rates (Gillespie et al., 2012). GPS-enabled wearable devices can be used to track dementia patients prone to wandering.

AI for Healthcare

The adoption of AI in healthcare is not new. It can be traced back to MYCIN, an expert system developed at Stanford University in the 1970s (Shortliffe, 1976). MYCIN was developed to help doctors in diagnosing and recommending treatments for bacterial infections. Since then, there have been many applications of AI in healthcare, from helping to diagnose, recommending treatments, and monitoring patients remotely to personal care.

Probably, there are four areas where the AI role is significant. Namely, *diagnostic and imaging*, *predictive analytics and early disease detection*, *drug discovery*, and *personalized medicine*. In addition, AI also significantly helps in robot surgery. For homecare, AI can be integrated into IoT or wearable devices to make them perform smarter. AI can also be handy in helping communicate with patients through chatbots and managing chronic diseases.

Medical imaging has utilized AI to increase precision in diagnosis. AI diagnostic tools for medical images have proven to be highly accurate in detecting diseases such as tumors or cancers, cardiovascular status, and neurological disorders (Ardila et al., 2019; Lim et al., 2020; McKinney et al., 2020). Deep learning algorithms in AI have performed on par with dermatologists for the accurate identification of skin cancers from images (Esteva et al., 2017). Gulshan et al. (2016) found that a deep-learning algorithm can detect referable diabetic retinopathy with high sensitivity and specificity.

With abundant data stored in EHRs and huge amounts of data captured from IoT and wearable devices, medical and health-related data are big data. Big data analytics or machine learning algorithms can be applied for knowledge discoveries that can be used for making predictions, such as outbreak prediction and patient health tendencies and risks. For example, the use of AI for machine learning predictive analytics to manage chronic diseases and the AI-powered system's ability to perform early detection of at-risk patients for cardiovascular disease, hypertension, and diabetes (Jiang et al., 2017; Weng et al., 2017).

By analyzing large datasets, AI can perform knowledge discovery to identify potential drugs for a particular disease and assess or predict their efficacy. This AI capability has been incorporated for fast and cost-effective drug development by some companies like BenevolentAI and Insilico Medicine (Topol, 2019). AI enables precision medicine using genetic, lifestyle, and environmental factors for AI to come up with precision medicine (Ashley, 2015).

For homecare, AI-powered devices and agents can perform many handy and cost-effective healthcare tasks, like AI-powered wearable devices and IoT sensors for monitoring purposes, AI-driven chatbots for medication reminders and symptom assessments, AI-assisted robots for elderly care, and AI applications for chronic disease management for chronically ill patients.

The Internet and Cloud Computing

The Internet, as a worldwide data communication, has revolutionized the connection of people and devices alike. Nowadays, affordable real-time data exchange can be done seamlessly regardless of location. The advancement of digital technology has made telehealth and homecare highly practical and cost-effective. As a matter of fact, they become a viable alternative to costly traditional healthcare.

The advancement of communication technology has significantly improved bandwidth capabilities over the Internet. High-speed communication media such as fiber optics, along with 4G and more recently 5G wireless technologies, have made the Internet a primary and cost-effective communication platform. The introduction of IPv6, with its 128-bit address space, can virtually accommodate an unlimited number of IP addresses, enabling anything to be assigned an IP address—and thus be connected to the Internet. It is no surprise, then, that a myriad of devices, including healthcare-related devices, are now connected to the Internet.

The ubiquitous and broadband connectivity of the Internet enables a new business model of computing resources like cloud computing. Cloud computing eliminates the investment and maintenance costs of computing resources, leaving only manageable and predictable operating costs (Armbrust et al., 2010; Marston et al., 2011). Consequently, like its predecessor, the Internet, cloud computing is also globally adopted. IPv6 and broadband connections enable cloud services to support the ever-growing digital ecosystem of connected devices. This model eliminates the need for substantial capital investment and ongoing maintenance of local computing infrastructure, replacing them with predictable and manageable operational costs. Much like a utility service, cloud computing offers on-demand scalability across a range of resources, including processing power, storage, platforms, and applications, without the burden of deploying local infrastructure, which can be prohibitively expensive. As such, healthcare devices can routinely transmit real-time data to cloud storage, where AI-powered analytics can perform diagnostics and make predictions. These AI-generated insights can then be shared with doctors, who may use them to support and enhance their clinical decision-making.

The combination of IPv6 and cloud computing is powerful (Ashraf et al., 2019; Kane, 2025). The enormous pool of IP addresses in IPv6 removes the need for complicated solutions offered previously, such as Network Address Translation (NAT), making it easier and faster for devices to communicate directly with the cloud. In addition, the low latency of 5G networks allows cloud-based applications, including applications in telehealth, to provide instant responses.

HEALTHCARE BUSINESS ECOSYSTEM

Telehealth is no longer a supplementary service of traditional healthcare; with the advancement of digital technologies, as discussed in the previous section, it is becoming the edge of modern healthcare, particularly enabling quality homecare. However, to enable quality homecare, a healthcare business ecosystem that provides seamless collaboration among relevant parties needs to be present.

The concept of a business ecosystem is a metaphor derived from the concept of an ecosystem in ecology. A business ecosystem is a constellation of entities that collaboratively work for the existence of the ecosystem. Normally, there is a central entity known as the keystone or ecosystem leader that controls the ecosystem. This entity oversees how other entities interact with one another; it ensures that all interactions benefit the ecosystem as a whole (Anggraeni et al., 2007; Iansiti & Levien, 2004; Moore, 2006; Senyo et al., 2019).

Jacobides et al. (2018) explain that a business ecosystem consists of various diverse yet complementary organizations working together to generate value at the system level. Adner and Kapoor (2010) provide a more detailed perspective, stating that a business ecosystem is a network focused on value where different stakeholders typically partner through transactions to facilitate value capture.

A business ecosystem can be defined as a value exchange network (VEN) among entities in the ecosystem (Almunawar et al., 2025; Almunawar & Anshari, 2020, 2022). Essentially, when two entities or individuals interact and carry out transactions, they are involved in a value exchange. Consequently, a business ecosystem can be viewed as a network made up of these exchanges of value. Value can take several forms, such as products, services, and information. A tool called Value Exchange Network Diagram (VEND) was developed to map an existing business ecosystem or to plan for its future.

A healthcare business ecosystem (HCBE) suggests that all healthcare stakeholders, including patients, are organized through coordinated and collaborative efforts to address the health issues of patients. The conventional HCBE is focused on a healthcare organization, where the majority of healthcare services are coordinated via resources belonging to that organization. While there are collaborations with entities outside the organization, they tend to be infrequent or lacking in depth, aside from financial interactions involving third parties or insurance, which are not related to healthcare. As noted by Viswanadham (2021), an HCBE describes a network of independent firms or organizations working together to gain competitive benefits through mutually advantageous relationships that are beneficial for all parties involved. Given that the modularity of services in a traditional healthcare business ecosystem is quite low, the typical HCBE is straightforward, as collaborations among independent organizations in solving patients' issues are restricted.

HCBE is a cooperative network made up of independent participants, including both primary and supplementary actors (Viswanadham, 2021). The primary participants encompass the healthcare platform, healthcare providers (such as doctors, hospitals, and clinics), and the customers or patients. Supplementary participants could include insurance firms, laboratories, government organizations, medical institutions, pharmacies, therapy facilities, and more.

The advancement of ICT, particularly the rise of the Internet and the availability of cost-effective smartphones with reliable Internet access, has changed the way individuals connect and conduct transactions (Almunawar et al., 2015). Consequently, digital transformation presents organizations, including healthcare facilities, with the chance to take advantage of these innovations and digitally engage with customers. As digital partnerships have become more practical, we have observed an increase in collaborations via digital platforms (Tsai et al., 2020). This indicates that a digital business ecosystem (DBE) serves as a beneficial framework for comprehending how value is generated and exchanged, aiming not only to enhance services but also to improve the customer experience. This concept is equally applicable to the healthcare digital business ecosystem (Götz et al., 2022).

Various digital technologies, including cloud computing, artificial intelligence (AI), blockchain, and big data analytics, have the potential to improve healthcare processes and delivery (Chang et al., 2009; Viswanadham, 2021). These technologies facilitate efficient collaboration among stakeholders in healthcare delivery and business ecosystems, leading to increased value for customers or patients.

Notable prominent examples of telehealth platforms are Teladoc Health[1] and Philips' Hospital-to-Home[2]. Both of them are digital healthcare business ecosystems that link their ecosystem members in a collaborative digital network to care for patients. The platform of the Teladoc Health business ecosystem coordinates all participants, such as healthcare providers, insurance providers, and technology partners, to deliver care to patients. For example, a diabetes patient uses a glucose monitor connected to the Teladoc, sends the reading data, and then interprets it. If the reading is abnormal, the Teladoc system immediately alerts a doctor, who then performs a video consultation to adjust treatment if necessary, and the insurer processes the claim from the doctor automatically.

In the case of Philips' Hospital-to-Home program, a digital business ecosystem manages the use of IoT and AI for post-acute and chronic care from hospitals to homes. For example, a patient with heart failure is sent home with a wireless wearable device that monitors vital signs. Information is transmitted to a care team that takes action if any irregularities are detected.

A FRAMEWORK FOR CONSTRUCTING HEALTH BUSINESS ECOSYSTEMS

How can we grasp a business ecosystem and understand what it looks like? According to Almunawar et al. (Almunawar et al., 2025), a business ecosystem is a network comprised of diverse and interrelated actors or entities that exchange value for mutual benefit. As such, a business ecosystem can be represented as a connected directed graph, denoted as $G(N, V)$, where N represents a finite and non-empty collection of symbols representing the actors and V consists of a set of edges labeled by a set of values. A directed and named edge going from actor X to actor Y shows that value has been transferred from A to B from B's point of view. In response, B reciprocates by transferring its value back to A, resulting in an exchange of values between A and B.

Different forms of values are identified by Allee (2000, 2008) in her value network model. Three separate groupings are used to classify these values: *hard value* stands for tangible value, such as goods and services; *soft value* stands for value in the form of data, information, or knowledge; and *intangible value* stands for value in the form of benefits.

A visual representation of a business ecosystem, including the healthcare business ecosystem, is called a Value Exchange Network Diagram (VEND). The development of a VEND uses the graph theory mentioned above. Think of a curved rectangular shape, with the letters *A, B, C*, and so on, standing for different actors in the business ecosystem. Values like products, services, data/information/knowledge, benefits, and revenue are all represented by the lowercase letters *p, s, i, b*, and *r*, respectively.

Figure 1 illustrates an exchange of value between *A* and *B*. A transfers a set of values, including *services* (*s*) and *information* (*i*) to *B*. In response, *B* reciprocates by exchanging its own set of values, which includes revenue (*r*) and information (i), with *A*.

Figure 1. Value exchange between A and B

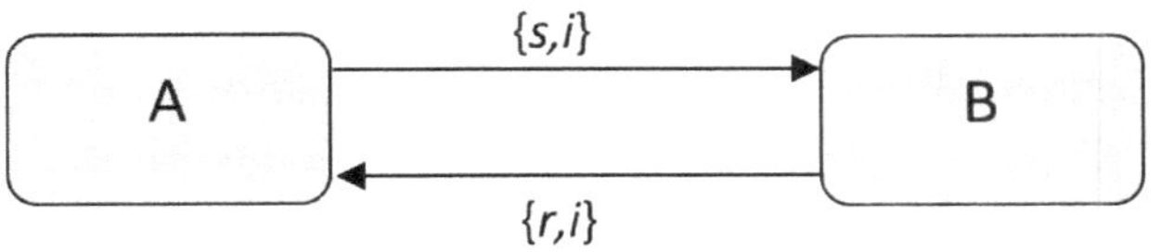

In the actual world, *A* might stand in for a doctor who examines and treats patient *B*. *B* receives high-quality service from *A*. Using his knowledge and the information gathered from *B* through instruments and interviews, *A* gives *B* advice and may even prescribe medication to treat *B*'s health problems.

A value exchange network, or VEN as previously highlighted, is formed when three or more actors engage in value exchanges. It is important to note that a business ecosystem itself is a VEN. Within this network, a specific actor, represented by a rectangular symbol and potentially responsible for overseeing the value exchanges within the ecosystem, assumes the role of the ecosystem's keystone. Figure 3 displays a simplified VEND with three actors, one of whom acts as the keystone. Among these actors, we have *Doctors* and *Patients*, while the keystone actor is a *Clinic*.

In VEN, the keystone of the ecosystem is a particular player, symbolized by a rectangle, who is in charge of managing the value exchanges in the ecosystem. A simplified VEND with three actors—one of whom serves as the keystone—is shown in Figure 2. A clinic is the main actor among these actors, together with doctors and patients.

Figure 2. The VEND of a simple healthcare business ecosystem

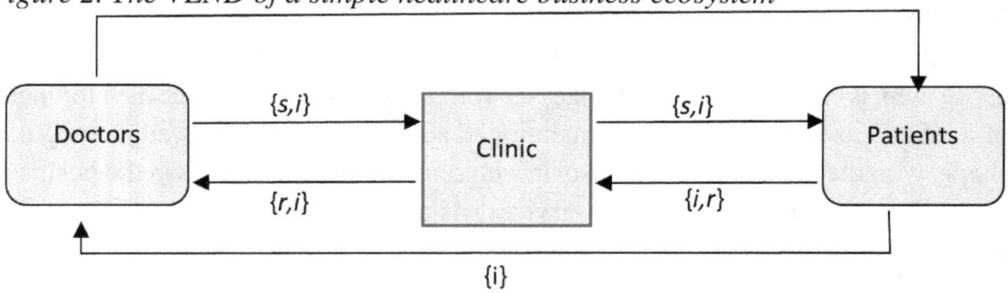

Doctors are employed by a clinic. They regularly deliver medical services (*s*) on behalf of the clinic while also documenting data (*i*) regarding patients' health (patient health records). In exchange, the clinic provides patients with health records (*i*) and remunerates them for their services, which constitutes the physicians' revenue (*r*). A patient arrives at the clinic seeking to resolve health concerns. The clinic presents high-quality services to patients, including a comfortable and enjoyable waiting area as well as friendly, compassionate reception staff (*s*). It also offers details about available services, the doctors, and their respective specialties (*i*). The patient registers for an appointment with a doctor and submits information such as height, weight, body temperature, and other necessary data (*i*). The patient pays for the medical services rendered by the clinic (*r*), which becomes the clinic's revenue. The doctor gathers health-related information from the patient through an interview and medical tools (*i*), while delivering friendly care that helps to put the patient at ease. Once the physician feels they have collected enough information from the patient, they advise the patient (*i*) using their expertise, on how to tackle the health issue and, if necessary, prescribe for the patient.

DIGITAL MULTI-SIDED NETWORK BUSINESS ECOSYSTEM FOR HEALTHCARE

Digital multi-sided networks are digital platforms that operate based on multi-sided market mechanisms on the Internet. They are currently expanding rapidly and transforming future enterprises (Akter et al., 2020; Almunawar et al., 2021; Almunawar & Anshari, 2022).

The primary role of a digital platform of multi-sided networks is to align supply with demand, even though the back end of the platform is more complex (Fradkin, 2017). In a conventional healthcare platform, patients and doctors or healthcare professionals meet in a clinic or hospital for consultations or treatments, resulting in place and time limitations, as value exchange needs to be done during operating hours at a particular place. In contrast to a conventional platform, a digital platform is free from spatial and temporal limitations since the meeting can be in a digital space that virtually functions around the clock, every day of the week. Patients and healthcare professionals can engage in exchange value on a digital platform virtually, independent of time and location.

In any digital multi-sided platform, there are three main components. In the case of a healthcare platform, these components are patients, healthcare professionals, and the platform itself, forming a two-sided network (patients and healthcare professionals) mediated by the platform. In this setting, a patient can use the platform to find healthcare professionals for remote healthcare services.

The platform manages the interactions that enable convenient and productive sessions between the patient and the healthcare professional. The VEND of the two-sided network in the above scenario is similar to Figure 2, with the clinic replaced by the healthcare digital platform (HDF). Assuming that the HDF provides all the necessary tools for both patients and healthcare professionals, along with large data storage to maintain all health-related records in an electronic health record (EHR) system and other relevant data, such as patient activity logs, dietary habits, and lifestyle information, the platform can utilize data analytics, big data, and AI to generate diagnostic or predictive reports. Healthcare professionals can also perform online diagnostic or predictive analyses using tools provided by the platform.

To enhance its operations, an HDF needs to collaborate with insurers for resolving health insurance claims and with tech firms for supporting data management and applications such as data analytics and AI. Figure 3 below is the VEND for the HDF, with insurers and tech firms becoming parts of its business ecosystem.

Figure 3 can be elaborated upon in detail; nonetheless, a comprehensive explanation would be excessively verbose. Presented here are two instances of value exchange: one occurring between *HDF* and *Patients*, and the other between *HDF* and *Tech Firms*.

Figure 3. The VEND of a digital healthcare business ecosystem

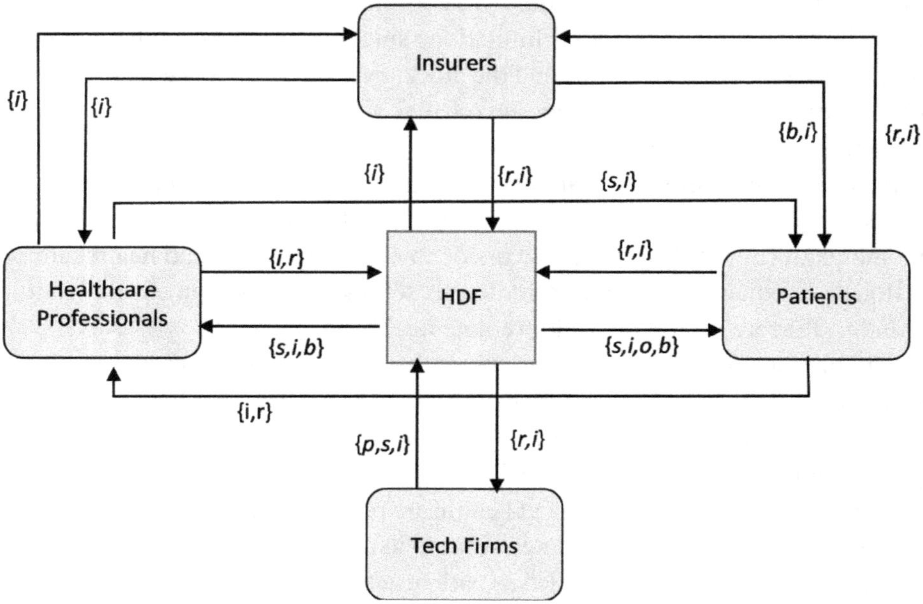

HDF provides a set of values to patients consisting of services (*s*), information (*i*)—such as details about healthcare professionals—options (*o*) for choosing among healthcare professionals, and benefits (*b*), which include the convenience of user-friendly digital services accessible from home or anywhere, at any time. In return, patients provide *HDF* with the required personal and medical data. Medical data can be captured when patients use available data acquisition tools such as smartphones or wearable devices connected to the *HDF* system. *HDF* also receives revenue from patients, typically through their insurers. In relation to *tech firms*, *HDF* received products, services, and related information to help improve its remote services to both patients and health professionals. Tech firms received revenue and related information from *HDF*.

An HDF business ecosystem shown in Figure 3 can be represented in a matrix, as shown in Table 1.

Table 1. The matrix representation of the HDF business ecosystem in Figure 3

	HDF	Patients	HF	Insurers	TF
HDF	-	{s,i,o,b}	{s,i,b}	{i}	{r,i}
Patients	{r,i}	-	{i,r}	{r,i}	{}
Health Professionals (HF)	{i,r}	{s,i}	-	{i}	{}
Insurers	{r,i}	{b,i}	{i}	-	{}
Tech Firms (TF)	{p,s,i}	{}	{}	{}	-

The matrix representation should be chosen if the ecosystem is complex and involves many entities. As the ecosystem expands, more entities, such as pharmacies, delivery agents, banks, regulators, clinics, hospitals, and integrated laboratories, can be easily incorporated into the matrix representation.

SELECTED CASES OF EXISTING IMPLEMENTATIONS

Teladoc Health

Established in 2002, Teladoc Health is among the most prominent telehealth platforms worldwide. The services that it provides cover primary care, mental health, chronic disease management, and specialty medicine. Its services cover 175 nations and cater to millions of patients each year. To start, patients need to register on the Teladoc website or app and select scheduled or on-demand service. Consultations are carried out through video, phone, or app messaging. After the consultations, doctors normally provide advice, give prescriptions if needed, and schedule follow-ups if necessary. All patients' records are stored in an EHR system, which can be accessed by registered health professionals.

Teladoc Health operates within its business ecosystem consisting of health insurance providers as payers, individual customers, employers, pharmacies, pharmaceutical companies, and technology partners, which are quite similar to the healthcare business ecosystem in the previous sections, where the Teladoc Health platform is the keystone of its ecosystem, like HDF in the previous section. As such, mapping the business ecosystem using VEND or a matrix is not necessary. However, we will describe the collaborative works or exchange value between some entities. Note that words written in italics are entities or their instances in the ecosystem.

A registered individual customer or *patient* needs to request consultations through the *Teladoc Health platform (THP);* they can select on-demand or scheduled consultations. During this process, a *patient* provides necessary information such as the health problems that need to be addressed. During this process, the system should provide the *patient* with information on available *doctors* or *health professionals* who can handle the problems. Once the matching is done, the *patient* will have a consultation session with the chosen *doctor* (health professional). More information from the *patient* will be tapped by the *doctor*. The *doctor* then advises the *patient* and gives them a prescription (if needed). The *doctor* can set a follow-up session if necessary. Next, the doctor will issue a claim to the *payer* (insurance) by completing a digital form and sending the claim to the patient's *payer*. Upon receiving a claim for payment, the *payer* will make payment to the *doctor* by transferring money to the doctor's *bank* account (becoming the doctor's revenue). A commission fee will also be transferred to *THP* (THP revenue).

Employers or *enterprises* can integrate Teladoc into their employees' benefits. *Employers* register their employees with Teledoc and pay Teledoc a monthly fee for each of their employees. This will make their employees get free or low-cost virtual care, which will provide good health protection to their workforce.

If a *doctor* issues a prescription after a consultation, the prescription will be sent to a *pharmacy* by *THP*, and the patient can collect the prescription or request delivery to their home. The pharmacy will acknowledge to the platform that the prescription has been dispatched to the patient.

Teladoc collaborates with *hospitals* or *clinics* to provide on-site care in *hospitals* or *clinics* and also allows *hospitals* or *clinics* to extend their services virtually via *THP*. This means selected *clinics* or *hospitals* become part of the *THP* healthcare business ecosystem. This is a win-win solution for Teladoc and hospitals/clinics. There are many cases where virtual consultations are not enough, as on-site physical examinations are needed. Similarly, follow-up from hospitals/clinics may not need to be physical, so *THP* is a cost-effective solution. To improve services and care, Teledoc integrates its EHR with the EHRs of the collaborated hospitals/clinics.

Teledoc collaborates with *tech firms* to enhance remote diagnostics, personal care, and data analytics. Data from healthcare devices such as IoT and wearable devices provided by *tech firms* (such as Apple HealthKit, Fitbit, Dexcom, and TytoCare) will be fed to Teladoc's chronic care programs. This will allow remote care of chronic diseases with data analytics or AI-driven personal care capability.

The above illustrates the healthcare business ecosystem of Teladoc Health, though it is not exhaustive. It demonstrates how Teladoc Health collaborates to enhance its virtual care services for its main customers—patients, either individually or through their employers, seamlessly.

TytoCare

TytoCare offers a home-smart clinic platform accessible via smart mobile devices. It provides devices approved by the U.S. Food and Drug Administration (FDA) for remote physical examinations. These devices enable patients to perform physical examinations at home for both acute and chronic conditions using digital tools that communicate with their smartphones through a dedicated app. The app transmits the collected data to the platform, where an AI system, in collaboration with healthcare professionals, analyzes the information and provides medical advice to patients. TytoCare also collaborates with other telecare providers, such as Teladoc Health, to support clinical examinations at home.

To operate, TytoCare provides the TytoHome Kit, a handheld digital medical examination device capable of performing multiple functions. The TytoHome Kit must be connected to the patient's smartphone or tablet. It includes a *digital stethoscope* for examining heart, lung, and abdominal sounds; an *otoscope* for ear examinations; a *tongue depressor and throat scope* for examining the throat and oral cavity; a *thermometer* for instant temperature readings; and an *HD camera* for imaging the skin, eyes, nose, and throat. TytoCare also offers a clinic-grade version of the TytoHome Kit for healthcare providers. This version enables healthcare professionals to perform remote patient monitoring (RPM) and provides high-precision tools for specialties such as cardiology, pulmonology, and pediatrics.

TytoCare's business ecosystem is simpler than that of Teladoc Health. It can be considered a two-sided network healthcare platform. The main components of the ecosystem include the TytoApp, which functions as a digital platform connecting two key stakeholders: doctors or healthcare providers (such as Teladoc Health) and patients—similar to the structure illustrated in Figure 2, where the clinic is represented by the TytoApp. The TytoApp can also be integrated with providers' Electronic Health Records (EHRs) to enable real-time transmission of data collected by the TytoHome Kit devices.

For homecare, the platform can be connected to patients' insurers to facilitate payment for services, including the interpretation of data collected from the Kit and professional advice from doctors. From a business ecosystem perspective, TytoCare is not only a device manufacturer but also a healthcare platform that provides homecare solutions and can function as part of a larger healthcare business ecosystem.

CONCLUSION

Healthcare is a knowledge-intensive and data-driven service. The first step in delivering medical treatment is the collection of patient data, both personal and medical, for health assessment. Once the necessary data has been gathered, doctors apply their knowledge and skills to advise the patient or administer appropriate treatments. If this data can be collected through digital technology, the patient may be able to schedule a virtual consultation and avoid the need for an in-person visit. This can save both time and money.

The advancement of digital technologies has driven the healthcare industry to embrace digital transformation, enabling the quality delivery of care through technology-assisted, home-based services. As a result, telehealth and homecare are no longer merely supplementary to traditional healthcare; they are becoming central components of modern healthcare, particularly in enabling high-quality homecare.

However, the benefits of telehealth go beyond remote diagnosis and care delivery. These benefits are realized when all stakeholders in the healthcare system work collaboratively to provide high-quality, accessible, and affordable care. To achieve this, a well-designed healthcare business ecosystem (HBE) is essential for delivering seamless healthcare solutions remotely.

An HBE brings together all healthcare stakeholders, including patients, through coordinated and collaborative efforts to address health challenges effectively. This indicates that a digital business ecosystem (DBE) provides a valuable framework for understanding how value is created and exchanged. It not only enhances service delivery but also improves the overall patient experience. This concept is directly applicable to the digital healthcare business ecosystem.

The healthcare business ecosystem framework we propose enables the mapping of existing healthcare ecosystems by connecting all elements or entities through value exchange to form a Value Exchange Network (VEN). It is a straightforward framework, easy to understand and apply. In addition to mapping existing ecosystems, it can also provide strategic insights for ecosystem expansion and allow observation of its growth. The VEN can also serve as a strategic tool for designing healthcare business ecosystems.

LIMITATION AND FUTURE WORK

The business ecosystem framework, VEN, currently models only the structural aspect of a business ecosystem and does not address its behavioral aspect. Our future work will focus on this limitation by incorporating ways to observe the behavior of each element or entity and how they interact with others. In its current form, the model captures only a snapshot of the ecosystem; the dynamic nature of business ecosystems is not considered. This presents another opportunity for future work: to develop a dynamic model of business ecosystems by introducing a time dimension.

This chapter also does not address how to measure a business ecosystem, particularly in the healthcare context. It would be valuable to explore how effectively an existing ecosystem functions and identify its critical aspects for problem detection.

Finally, this paper presents only two case studies. Future research can explore more cases in greater depth. With a behavioral model in place, such case studies would become even more insightful and meaningful.

REFERENCES

Adner, R., & Kapoor, R. (2010). Value creation in innovation ecosystems: How the structure of technological interdependence affects firm performance in new technology generations. *Strategic Management Journal, 31*(3), 306–333. DOI: 10.1002/smj.821

Akter, S., Motamarri, S., Hani, U., Shams, R., Fernando, M., Mohiuddin Babu, M., & Shen, K. N. (2020). Building dynamic service analytics capabilities for the digital marketplace. *Journal of Business Research, 118*, 177–188. DOI: 10.1016/j.jbusres.2020.06.016

Allee, V. (2000). Reconfiguring the value network. *The Journal of Business Strategy, 21*(4), 36–39. DOI: 10.1108/eb040103

Allee, V. (2008). Value network analysis and value conversion of tangible and intangible assets. *Journal of Intellectual Capital, 9*(1), 5–24. DOI: 10.1108/14691930810845777

Almunawar, M. N., & Anshari, M. (2020). Multi-sided networks of digital platform ecosystem: The case of ride-hailing in Indonesia. *Asia Pacific Journal of Information Systems, 30*(4), 803–825. DOI: 10.14329/apjis.2020.30.4.808

Almunawar, M. N., & Anshari, M. (2022). Digital enabler and value integration: Revealing the expansion engine of digital marketplace. *Technology Analysis and Strategic Management, 34*(7), 847–857. DOI: 10.1080/09537325.2021.1926967

Almunawar, M. N., Anshari, M., de Pablos, P. O., & Fauzi, A. M. (2025). Embracing digital business ecosystem: Transforming traditional marketplaces. *Journal of Science and Technology Policy Management*. DOI: 10.1108/JSTPM-09-2022-0144

Almunawar, M. N., Anshari, M., & Lim, S. A. (2021). Value network view on digital marketplace. In Khosrow-Pour, M. (Ed.), *Encyclopedia of organizational knowledge, administration, and technology* (pp. 1349–1363). IGI Global., DOI: 10.4018/978-1-7998-3473-1.ch091

Almunawar, M. N., Anshari, M., Susanto, H., & Chen, C. K. (2015). Revealing customer behavior on smartphones. *International Journal of Asian Business and Information Management, 6*(2), 33–49. DOI: 10.4018/IJABIM.2015040103

Anggraeni, E., den Hartigh, E., & Zegveld, M. (2007). Business ecosystem as a perspective for studying the relations between firms and their business networks. In *ECCON 2007 Annual meeting* (pp. 1–21). Netherlands Organisation for Scientific Research.

Ardila, D., Kiraly, A. P., Bharadwaj, S., Choi, B., Reicher, J. J., Peng, L., Tse, D., Etemadi, M., Ye, W., Corrado, G., Naidich, D. P., & Shetty, S. (2019). End-to-end lung cancer screening with three-dimensional deep learning on low-dose chest computed tomography. *Nature Medicine*, *25*(6), 954–961. DOI: 10.1038/s41591-019-0447-x PMID: 31110349

Armbrust, M., Stoica, I., Zaharia, M., Fox, A., Griffith, R., Joseph, A. D., Katz, R., Konwinski, A., Lee, G., Patterson, D., & Rabkin, A. (2010). A view of cloud computing. *Communications of the ACM*, *53*(4), 50–58. DOI: 10.1145/1721654.1721672

Ashley, E. A. (2015). The precision medicine initiative: A new national effort. *Journal of the American Medical Association*, *313*(21), 2119–2120. DOI: 10.1001/jama.2015.3595 PMID: 25928209

Ashraf, Z., Sohail, A., & Yousaf, M. (2019). Performance analysis of network applications on IPv6 cloud connected virtual machine. *International Journal of Computer Network and Information Security*, *11*(12), 1–9. DOI: 10.5815/ijcnis.2019.12.01

Bashshur, R., Doarn, C. R., Frenk, J. M., Kvedar, J. C., & Woolliscroft, J. O. (2020). Telemedicine and the COVID-19 pandemic, lessons for the future. *Telemedicine Journal and e-Health*, *26*(5), 571–573. DOI: 10.1089/tmj.2020.29040.rb PMID: 32275485

Bodenheimer, T. S., & Grumbach, K. (2020). *Understanding health policy: A clinical approach* (8th ed.). McGraw Hill.

Chang, H. H., Chou, P. B., & Ramakrishnan, S. (2009). An ecosystem approach for healthcare services cloud. In *2009 IEEE International Conference on e-Business Engineering* (pp. 608–612). IEEE. DOI: 10.1109/ICEBE.2009.98

Curioni, C., Silva, A. C., Damião, J., Castro, A., Huang, M., Barroso, T., Araujo, D., & Guerra, R. (2023). The cost-effectiveness of homecare services for adults and older adults: A systematic review. *International Journal of Environmental Research and Public Health*, *20*(4), 3373. DOI: 10.3390/ijerph20043373 PMID: 36834068

Dunn, R. (2019, January 15). 4 promising IoT use cases in agriculture. *IoT For All*. https://www.iotforall.com/4-iot-use-cases-agriculture/

Edirippulige, S., & Armfield, N. R. (2017). Education and training to support the use of clinical telehealth: A review of the literature. *Journal of Telemedicine and Telecare*, *23*(2), 273–282. DOI: 10.1177/1357633X16632968 PMID: 26892005

Esteva, A., Kuprel, B., Novoa, R. A., Ko, J., Swetter, S. M., Blau, H. M., & Thrun, S. (2017). Dermatologist-level classification of skin cancer with deep neural networks. *Nature*, *542*(7639), 115–118. DOI: 10.1038/nature21056 PMID: 28117445

Federman, A. D., Soones, T., DeCherrie, L. V., Leff, B., & Siu, A. L. (2018). Association of a bundled hospital-at-home and 30-day postacute transitional care program with clinical outcomes and patient experiences. *JAMA Internal Medicine*, *178*(8), 1033–1040. DOI: 10.1001/jamainternmed.2018.2562 PMID: 29946693

Fradkin, A. (2017). *Search, matching, and the role of digital marketplace design in enabling trade: Evidence from Airbnb* (SSRN Scholarly Paper ID 2939084). Social Science Research Network. DOI: 10.2139/ssrn.2939084

Gillespie, L. D., Robertson, M. C., Gillespie, W. J., Sherrington, C., Gates, S., Clemson, L., & Lamb, S. E. (2012). Interventions for preventing falls in older people living in the community. *Cochrane Database of Systematic Reviews*, *9*(6), CD007146. DOI: 10.1002/14651858.CD007146.pub3 PMID: 22972103

Götz, F., Reelitz, C., Buck, C., Eymann, T., & Meckl, R. (2022). Potentials of digital business ecosystems in the healthcare market. In Mehdi Khosrow-Pour, D. B. A. (Ed.), *Handbook on digital business ecosystems* (pp. 662–679). Edward Elgar Publishing., DOI: 10.4337/9781839107191.00051

Güdük, Ö. (2025). Telehealth applications in home health services: A bibliometric analysis. *Türkiye Aile Hekimligi Dergisi*, *29*(1), 20–35. DOI: 10.54308/turkjfam-pract.2025.811

Gulshan, V., Peng, L., Coram, M., Stumpe, M. C., Wu, D., Narayanaswamy, A., Venugopalan, S., Widner, K., Madams, T., Cuadros, J., Kim, R., Raman, R., Nelson, P. C., Mega, J. L., & Webster, D. R. (2016). Development and validation of a deep learning algorithm for detection of diabetic retinopathy in retinal fundus photographs. *Journal of the American Medical Association*, *316*(22), 2402–2410. DOI: 10.1001/jama.2016.17216 PMID: 27898976

Hamblin, K., Burns, D., & Goodlad, C. (2025). Technology and homecare in the UK: Policy, storylines and practice. *Journal of Social Policy*, *54*(2), 412–428. DOI: 10.1017/S0047279423000156

Iansiti, M., & Levien, R. (2004). Strategy as ecology. *Harvard Business Review*, *82*(3), 68–78. PMID: 15029791

Iqubal, S., Khan, S., Pant, N., Sarkar, S., Rey, T., & Mohapatra, H. (2025). A study on IoT-enabled smart bed with brain-computer interface for elderly and paralyzed individuals. In Sarveshwaran, V., Periyaswami, K., & Yu, K. (Eds.), *Future innovations in the convergence of AI and Internet of Things in medicine* (pp. 61–88). IGI Global., DOI: 10.4018/979-8-3693-7703-1.ch004

Islam, S. M. R., Kwak, D., Kabir, M. H., Hossain, M., & Kwak, K.-S. (2015). The Internet of Things for health care: A comprehensive survey. *IEEE Access : Practical Innovations, Open Solutions*, *3*, 678–708. DOI: 10.1109/ACCESS.2015.2437951

Jacobides, M. G., Cennamo, C., & Gawer, A. (2018). Towards a theory of ecosystems. *Strategic Management Journal*, *39*(8), 2255–2276. DOI: 10.1002/smj.2904

Jiang, F., Jiang, Y., Zhi, H., Dong, Y., Li, H., Ma, S., Wang, Y., Dong, Q., Shen, H., & Wang, Y. (2017). Artificial intelligence in healthcare: Past, present and future. *Stroke and Vascular Neurology*, *2*(4), 230–243. DOI: 10.1136/svn-2017-000101 PMID: 29507784

Kane, A. (2025). Navigating the transition: Challenges and benefits of shifting from IPv4 to IPv6 in a rapidly evolving internet landscape. *International Journal of Internet and Distributed Systems*, *7*(2), 15–26. DOI: 10.4236/ijids.2025.72002

Kvedar, J. C., Fogel, A. L., Elenko, E., & Zohar, D. (2016). Digital medicine's march on chronic disease. *Nature Biotechnology*, *34*(3), 239–246. DOI: 10.1038/nbt.3495 PMID: 26963544

Lim, L. J., Tison, G. H., & Delling, F. N. (2020). Artificial intelligence in cardiovascular imaging. *Methodist DeBakey Cardiovascular Journal*, *16*(2), 138–145. DOI: 10.14797/mdcj-16-2-138 PMID: 32670474

Marston, S., Li, Z., Bandyopadhyay, S., Zhang, J., & Ghalsasi, A. (2011). Cloud computing—The business perspective. *Decision Support Systems*, *51*(1), 176–189. DOI: 10.1016/j.dss.2010.12.006

McAllister, R. (2024, November 22). *State-by-state breakdown—Average cost of hospital stays in the U.S.* North American Community Hub. https://nchstats.com/average-cost-of-hospital-stays-in-us/

McKinney, S. M., Sieniek, M., Godbole, V., Godwin, J., Antropova, N., Ashrafian, H., Back, T., Chesus, M., Corrado, G. S., Darzi, A., Etemadi, M., Garcia-Vicente, F., Gilbert, F. J., Halling-Brown, M., Hassabis, D., Jansen, S., Karthikesalingam, A., Kelly, C. J., King, D., & Shetty, S. (2020). International evaluation of an AI system for breast cancer screening. *Nature*, *577*(7788), 89–94. DOI: 10.1038/s41586-019-1799-6 PMID: 31894144

Moore, J. F. (2006). Business ecosystems and the view from the firm. *Antitrust Bulletin*, *51*(1), 31–75. DOI: 10.1177/0003603X0605100103

Seivert, S., & Badowski, M. E. (2021). The rise of telemedicine: Lessons from a global pandemic. *European Medical Journal. Innovations*, *5*(1), 64–69. DOI: 10.33590/emjinnov/20-00239

Senyo, P. K., Liu, K., & Effah, J. (2019). Digital business ecosystem: Literature review and a framework for future research. *International Journal of Information Management, 47*, 52–64. DOI: 10.1016/j.ijinfomgt.2019.01.002

Shortliffe, E. H. (1976). *Computer-based medical consultations: MYCIN*. Elsevier.

Sockolow, P. S., Bowles, K. H., Topaz, M., Koru, G., Hellesø, R., O'Connor, M., & Bass, E. J. (2021). The time is now: Informatics research opportunities in home health care. *Applied Clinical Informatics, 12*(1), 100–106. DOI: 10.1055/s-0040-1722222 PMID: 33598906

Steinhubl, S. R., Waalen, J., Edwards, A. M., Ariniello, L. M., Mehta, R. R., Ebner, G. S., Carter, C., Baca-Motes, K., Felicione, E., Sarich, T., & Topol, E. J. (2018). Effect of a home-based wearable continuous ECG monitoring patch on detection of undiagnosed atrial fibrillation: The mSToPS randomized clinical trial. *Journal of the American Medical Association, 320*(2), 146–155. DOI: 10.1001/jama.2018.8102 PMID: 29998336

Szanton, S. L., Leff, B., Wolff, J. L., Roberts, L., & Gitlin, L. N. (2016). Home-based care program reduces disability and promotes aging in place. *Health Affairs, 35*(9), 1558–1563. DOI: 10.1377/hlthaff.2016.0140 PMID: 27605633

Talal, M., Zaidan, A. A., Zaidan, B. B., Albahri, A. S., Alamoodi, A. H., Albahri, O. S., Alsalem, M. A., Lim, C. K., Tan, K. L., Shir, W. L., & Mohammed, K. I. (2019). Smart home-based IoT for real-time and secure remote health monitoring of triage and priority system using body sensors: Multi-driven systematic review. *Journal of Medical Systems, 43*(3), 42. DOI: 10.1007/s10916-019-1158-z PMID: 30648217

Topol, E. J. (2019). *Deep medicine: How artificial intelligence can make healthcare human again*. Basic Books.

Tsai, C.-H., Zdravkovic, J., & Stirna, J. (2020). Capability management of digital business ecosystems—A case of resilience modeling in the healthcare domain. In Herbaut, N., & La Rosa, M. (Eds.), *Advanced information systems engineering* (pp. 126–137). Springer., DOI: 10.1007/978-3-030-58135-0_11

Ultimate Care. (2025). *The impact of home care on reducing healthcare costs*. https://www.ultimatecareny.com/resources/the-impact-of-home-care-on-reducing-healthcare-costs

Viswanadham, N. (2021). Ecosystem model for healthcare platform. *Sadhana, 46*(4), 188. DOI: 10.1007/s12046-021-01708-y

Weng, S. F., Reps, J., Kai, J., Garibaldi, J. M., & Qureshi, N. (2017). Can machine-learning improve cardiovascular risk prediction using routine clinical data? *PLoS One*, *12*(4), e0174944. DOI: 10.1371/journal.pone.0174944 PMID: 28376093

World Health Organization. (2024, October 1). *Ageing and health*. https://www.who.int/news-room/fact-sheets/detail/ageing-and-health

ENDNOTES

1 https://www.teladochealth.com/

2 https://www.philips.com/a-w/about/news/archive/standard/news/articles/2021/20210921-hospital-at-home-the-future-of-care-is-anywhere-anytime.html

Chapter 3
Human-Machine Interaction in Home Healthcare

Yasin Aras
https://orcid.org/0000-0002-5171-7779
Aksaray University, Turkey

ABSTRACT

Human-Machine Interaction (HMI) is the interaction of patients, families and healthcare staff with technologies such as sensors, software and robots in home healthcare. It offers elderly and chronic patients the opportunity to live independently at home. Due to the aging population and the increase in chronic diseases, the desire of individuals to live independently in their own homes has stimulated the development of these technologies. In this context, HMI should be designed in accordance with the physical and cognitive capacities of the users, as well as to improve health outcomes. HMI consists of physical devices, social relationships and data layer. User-centered design and accessibility are important. Home care is supported by monitoring systems, security solutions and emergency assistance technologies.

INTRODUCTION

In recent years, the convergence of technology and healthcare has catalyzed profound transformations in the way medical services are delivered, accessed, and experienced. Among the most significant developments in this domain is the rise of Human-machine Interaction (HMI) in home healthcare. This advancement has not only redefined the landscape of patient care but also opened new frontiers for research, innovation, and policy-making. As societies worldwide grapple with

DOI: 10.4018/979-8-3373-3099-0.ch003

aging populations, rising healthcare costs, and the persistent need for accessible, high-quality care, the integration of intelligent machines into home environments emerges as a compelling solution. This chapter explores the evolution, significance, challenges, and future directions of HMI in home healthcare, emphasizing its potential to reshape the fabric of modern medicine (Thacharodi et al., 2024).

The demographic shifts occurring globally are both striking and consequential. According to the World Health Organization (WHO), the proportion of the global population aged 60 and above is expected to nearly double by 2050, reaching over 2 billion people. This demographic trend is accompanied by an increase in chronic illnesses such as diabetes, cardiovascular disease, and neurodegenerative disorders, which often require long-term management rather than acute intervention (World Health Organization [WHO], 2024). Traditional healthcare systems, primarily hospital-centric and reactive in nature, are increasingly inadequate to meet the evolving needs of this demographic. Consequently, there is a growing impetus to develop home-based care models that are proactive, patient-centered, and technology-enabled.

Human–machine Interaction, as applied to home healthcare, encompasses a wide range of technologies and systems designed to support individuals in maintaining their health, managing chronic conditions, and accessing medical services without leaving their homes. These systems include but are not limited to wearable health monitors, telepresence robots, intelligent voice assistants, automated medication dispensers, and AI-driven diagnostic tools. The common thread linking these innovations is the interface between the human user and the machine—an interface that must be intuitive, responsive, and adaptive to individual needs. The success of HMI in this context hinges on its ability to foster trust, ensure safety, and enhance the user experience, particularly among populations that may be less technologically literate (Demiris & Olson, 2010).

The home setting presents unique opportunities and challenges for HMI. Unlike clinical environments, which are controlled, standardized, and staffed by trained professionals, home environments are heterogeneous, dynamic, and populated by individuals with varying degrees of health literacy and physical ability. Designing HMI systems that can function effectively in such contexts requires a multidisciplinary approach, drawing on insights from computer science, engineering, medicine, psychology, and design. Moreover, these systems must be sensitive to cultural, socioeconomic, and linguistic differences that influence how users interact with technology. Inclusivity and accessibility are not optional features but essential components of effective HMI in home healthcare.

One of the most promising aspects of HMI in home healthcare is its capacity to enable continuous monitoring and early intervention. For example, wearable sensors can track vital signs such as heart rate, blood pressure, and oxygen saturation in real-time, transmitting this data to healthcare providers who can intervene promptly if abnormalities are detected (Vo & Trinh, 2024). Similarly, AI-powered analytics can identify patterns and trends that may indicate a deteriorating condition, prompting preventive measures before a crisis occurs. Such capabilities represent a paradigm shift from episodic care to continuous, data-driven health management. By integrating HMI systems into daily routines, individuals can receive personalized care that evolves with their needs, thereby improving outcomes and reducing the burden on formal healthcare institutions.

Another critical benefit of HMI in home healthcare is the potential for enhanced autonomy and quality of life among elderly and chronically ill individuals. Technologies such as robotic assistants can help with activities of daily living, including mobility, hygiene, and meal preparation, while voice-activated systems can provide reminders for medication, appointments, and hydration. These tools empower individuals to live independently for longer periods, preserving dignity and reducing the need for institutional care. Furthermore, remote communication tools facilitate social interaction and mental stimulation, which are vital for emotional well-being and cognitive health (Padhan et al., 2023). In this way, HMI not only supports physical health but also addresses the holistic needs of users.

Despite these promising developments, the implementation of HMI in home healthcare is not without its challenges. Privacy and data security are paramount concerns, particularly given the sensitive nature of health information and the potential for cyber threats. Ensuring robust encryption, user consent, and ethical data governance is essential to maintaining trust and compliance with regulations such as the General Data Protection Regulation (GDPR). Moreover, the effectiveness of HMI systems depends on their usability; interfaces must be designed with the end-user in mind, incorporating feedback from diverse populations to avoid alienating those who stand to benefit the most (Dubey & Kumar, 2025).

Technical reliability and interoperability also pose significant hurdles. Home healthcare systems often involve multiple devices and platforms that must communicate seamlessly to function effectively. A malfunction in one component can compromise the entire system, potentially endangering the user (Torab-Miandoab et al., 2023). Therefore, standards for interoperability, rigorous testing protocols, and mechanisms for real-time technical support are critical to the success of HMI applications. Additionally, considerations around affordability and access must be addressed to prevent the digital divide from exacerbating health disparities. Policymakers and stakeholders must work collaboratively to ensure that these technologies are equitably distributed and supported by adequate infrastructure.

Ethical considerations are equally important in the context of HMI in home healthcare. As machines assume roles traditionally held by human caregivers, questions arise about the nature of care, empathy, and human connection. While technology can augment and extend the reach of human care, it cannot replicate the emotional intelligence, moral reasoning, and cultural sensitivity of human providers. Designers and developers must therefore strike a balance between automation and human oversight, ensuring that machines enhance rather than replace the human touch. Ethical frameworks must guide the development and deployment of HMI systems, safeguarding the dignity, autonomy, and rights of users (Mennella et al., 2024).

Furthermore, the successful integration of HMI in home healthcare depends on systemic changes within healthcare delivery models. Clinicians must be trained to interpret data from remote monitoring systems and integrate it into their decision-making processes. Health systems must adapt their workflows, reimbursement models, and care coordination strategies to accommodate the unique dynamics of home-based care. Collaboration across sectors—healthcare, technology, academia, and government—is essential to building the ecosystems needed to support HMI innovations. Research and development must be adequately funded, and pilot programs should be rigorously evaluated to inform best practices and scale-up strategies (Tsvetanov, 2024).

The COVID-19 pandemic has accelerated the adoption of telehealth and remote care solutions, highlighting the potential of HMI to enhance resilience and continuity in healthcare delivery. As lockdowns and social distancing measures limited access to traditional care settings, home-based technologies emerged as lifelines for patients and providers alike. This experience has underscored the importance of investing in HMI infrastructure, ensuring digital literacy, and fostering public acceptance of new modes of care. Moving forward, the lessons learned from the pandemic can inform the design of more robust, responsive, and inclusive HMI systems that are prepared to meet both everyday needs and future crises (Bouabida et al., 2022).

Looking ahead, the future of HMI in home healthcare is both exciting and complex. Advances in artificial intelligence, machine learning, natural language processing, and robotics promise to make machines more intuitive, empathetic, and capable. Emerging technologies such as augmented reality, brain–computer interfaces, and ambient intelligence hold the potential to further personalize and contextualize care. However, realizing this vision requires a concerted effort to address existing limitations, bridge knowledge gaps, and align technological innovation with human values. The development of HMI must be guided by a clear understanding of user needs, clinical efficacy, ethical standards, and societal implications (Mourtzis et al., 2023).

In conclusion, HMI in home healthcare represents a transformative approach to managing health and well-being in the 21st century. By enabling personalized, continuous, and context-sensitive care, HMI has the potential to improve outcomes, reduce costs, and enhance the quality of life for millions of people worldwide. However, its successful implementation depends on careful attention to design, ethics, policy, and inclusivity. This chapter sets the stage for an in-depth exploration of the key components, applications, and considerations surrounding HMI in home healthcare, offering insights that are both timely and essential for researchers, practitioners, and policymakers navigating the future of digital health.

1. HUMAN-MACHINE INTERACTION (HMI): CONCEPT & HISTORY

Human-machine Interaction (HMI) represents a dynamic field of interdisciplinary inquiry focused on understanding, designing, and evaluating the ways in which humans and machines communicate and collaborate. The conceptualization of HMI must encompass a broader, more integrated understanding of human behavior, technological capacity, and socio-environmental contexts.

The term *Human–machine Interaction* (HMI) is used in a broad and inclusive manner, encompassing synonymous concepts such as *Human–machine Interface*, *Man–machine Interface* (MMI), and *Human–computer Interaction* (HCI). While these terms have been used interchangeably across different domains, HMI is adopted here as the most comprehensive descriptor. It refers to the dynamic processes through which humans engage with machines—defined broadly as mechanical or electronic systems designed to transmit or transform energy in order to execute or support human tasks (Cannan & Hu, 2011).

Many computer-executed tasks today rely on collaboration between humans and machines. This collaboration requires effective communication between the two, a process known as human-computer interaction (Figure 1). In Figure 1 HMI is an intersection of the software and hardware interfaces (Li & Xu, 2022).

Figure 1. Schematic diagram of human-machine interaction

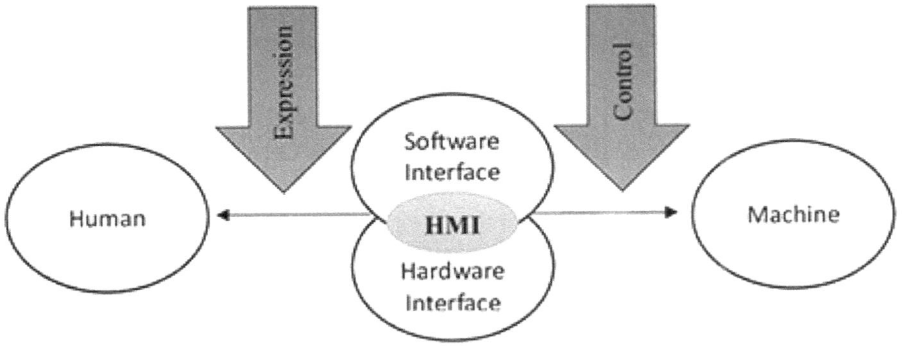

HMI is a science that seeks to understand, evaluate and improve the interactions between 'human' and 'machine'. In the narrowest sense, this interaction usually takes place through tools such as keyboards, mice and screens, but today, more advanced interfaces such as touch screens, voice command systems, virtual reality (VR) and augmented reality (AR) have diversified this interaction. The quality of this communication between the user and the system directly affects the success of the system. UI is not only concerned with the design of user interfaces, but also with various fields such as modeling user behavior, user experience (UX), cognitive psychology, ergonomics, software engineering and artificial intelligence. This interdisciplinary approach makes it possible to design systems not only technically but also user-centered (Mourtzis et al., 2023).

Human-computer Interaction (HCI) is an interdisciplinary field dedicated to enhancing the interaction between users and computer systems by developing interfaces that are both efficient and user-centered. Drawing upon disciplines such as computer science, cognitive psychology, ergonomics, behavioral sciences, and design, HMI aims to ensure that technological systems align with human capabilities and expectations. The origins of HCI date back to the early era of computing, when machines were large, technically complex, and accessible only to trained specialists. With the rapid advancement and democratization of computing technologies, the focus of HCI shifted toward creating more intuitive, accessible, and user-friendly interfaces that support a wider range of users and contexts (Mourtzis et al., 2023).

The primary objective of HMI is to facilitate smooth, intuitive, and efficient communication between humans and technological systems. By enhancing usability and responsiveness, HMI plays a pivotal role in ensuring that systems are not only functional but also safe, accessible, and supportive of user needs. Effective human–computer interaction transforms complex technologies into user-friendly tools, minimizing confusion and frustration while promoting a positive and engaging user experience. Ultimately, well-designed HMI systems contribute to making technology more understandable, predictable, and aligned with human expectations (McFarlane & Latorella, 2002).

The origin of HMI dates back to the 1940s and 1950s, when computers first began to interact directly with users. However, it took until the 1980s for the field to take shape as a scientific discipline. Early computers appealed to a limited user base due to their large size and the fact that they could only be used by experts. Over time, as computer technology became smaller and less expensive, individual users were introduced to computers. This transformation necessitated the development of user-friendly interfaces (Grudin, 2018).

The mouse, introduced by Douglas Engelbart in his presentation "The Mother of All Demos" in the 1960s, revolutionized graphical user interfaces (GUIs) and greatly facilitated interaction. The widespread adoption of GUI in the 1980s with

Xerox PARC and later with Apple's Macintosh computer became one of the basic building blocks of HMI. With this period, UX has evolved from being a sub-branch of computer science to a field that interacts with different fields such as psychology, design and engineering. In particular, user experience and usability testing have helped to systematize this field (Grudin, 2018; Mourtzis et al., 2023).

In the last century, rapid advances in computing power, artificial intelligence (AI), robotics, and connectivity reshaped the landscape of HMI. Devices evolved from being tools operated by users to intelligent agents capable of sensing, reasoning, and acting autonomously. In parallel, the proliferation of smartphones, wearable devices, and ambient sensors enabled continuous, context-aware interactions between humans and machines (Solanes et al., 2024).

The conceptualization of HMI in home healthcare is a multifaceted endeavor that draws upon decades of research and a wide array of disciplines. From its historical roots in human factors engineering to its current applications in intelligent, connected care systems, HMI has evolved into a cornerstone of modern healthcare innovation.

2. CONCEPTUAL FRAMEWORK OF HUMAN–MACHINE INTERACTION IN HOME HEALTHCARE SERVICES

Home healthcare services refer to the delivery of healthcare and support in a patient's home environment, an approach growing in importance as populations age. Many older adults face increased frailty, chronic illness, and difficulty with daily activities, yet most express a strong preference to "age in place" (remain in their own homes rather than move to institutional care) (Tian et al., 2024; Morita et al., 2023). This demographic reality creates a demand for technological solutions that enable safe and effective care at home. In this context, human-machine interaction (HMI) in home health involves the interplay between people (patients, caregivers, clinicians) and technological systems (devices, software, sensors, robots) designed to support health and well-being in the home setting. Developing a conceptual framework for HMI in home health requires understanding both the human factors (needs, behaviors, capabilities) and the machine factors (technologies, interfaces, intelligence) that must work together harmoniously (Czaja et al., 2006; Nielsen, 1994).

A useful starting point is defining what constitutes a "smart" home health environment. One classic definition describes a smart home for health as "a residence wired with technology features that monitor the well-being and activities of residents to improve quality of life, increase independence and prevent emergencies" (Kang et al., 2019; Morita et al., 2023). This emphasizes that the goal of home health technology is not merely to introduce gadgets, but to support human health outcomes such as safety, independence, and quality of life. The conceptual framework, therefore, centers on how humans interact with such technologies to achieve these outcomes. Key stakeholders include the patient (who may be an older adult or someone with chronic needs), informal caregivers (such as family members), formal caregivers or clinicians (nurses, doctors monitoring remotely), and the technology designers. All these actors form a socio-technical system within the home environment (Tenner, 2015; Antona & Stephanidis, 2020).

One can conceptualize HMI in home health from an ecological systems perspective, considering multiple layers of the environment. Kang et al. (2019) proposed a "Smart Servicescape Wheel" framework that divides the smart home healthcare system into perceptible and imperceptible elements. The perceptible layer includes the physical scape (hardware devices, sensors, and environmental cues in the home) as well as the social scape (the interactions and relationships between the user, family, and care providers). The imperceptible layer is the datascape, encompassing computing intelligence, data-processing algorithms, and communication networks operating behind the scenes (Kang et al., 2019; Morita et al., 2023). Such a framework highlights that human–machine interaction is influenced by physical context (e.g., where a device is placed, how it is accessed), social context (e.g., whether a caregiver is present to assist, or how a patient perceives the technology's role in their care relationships), and digital context (e.g., how data flows and how intelligent the system is). A comprehensive conceptual model thus accounts for the holistic environment: technology does not operate in isolation, but within a living space and social setting (Czaja et al., 2006; Antona & Stephanidis, 2020).

Central to the conceptual framework is the recognition that user-centered design and human factors are critical in healthcare technology. Decades of human-computer interaction (HCI) research have shown that focusing on users' needs, limitations, and experiences is essential for successful technology adoption (Czaja et al., 2006; Nielsen, 1994). In the home health context, this means devices and interfaces must be designed to be usable, accessible, and acceptable to patients who may not be tech-savvy or who might have physical/cognitive limitations. For instance, an older adult with arthritis or poor eyesight will require different interface considerations (larger buttons, voice interaction options, etc.) than a younger user (Antona & Stephanidis, 2020; Tenner, 2015). The conceptual framework of HMI therefore incorporates principles like usability, learnability, and feedback—ensuring that the patient can easily operate devices and understand the information they provide.

Another component of the framework is understanding the roles of the human and the machine in home care. Unlike in clinical settings where professionals operate complex equipment, home health technologies are often used directly by patients or lay caregivers. Thus, the machine (whether a sensor, app, or robot) often takes on tasks of monitoring, reminding, or even decision support, while the human user remains in control of their care routines. Effective HMI means the technology augments human capabilities. For example, by continuously tracking health indicators that a person could not feasibly monitor on their own-without undermining the person's autonomy or comfort (Davis, 1989; Venkatesh et al., 2003). In essence, if the technology is helpful and simple to use, and if it aligns with the user's values and needs, the interaction is more likely to succeed. Conversely, if the technology is confusing or intrusive, the human–machine interaction may break down, leading to non-use or misuse (Davis, 1989; Venkatesh et al., 2003).

In summary, the conceptual framework for human-machine interaction in home-based healthcare can be seen as a socio-technical ecosystem. It involves understanding the user's health goals and daily routines, the technological tools available (and their design), and the surrounding context (physical home setting, social support, and data infrastructure). By framing HMI in home health as a partnership between humans and supportive machines within a living environment, we set the stage for exploring specific technologies, their practical applications, and the broader implications on care—all of which are detailed in the subsequent sections of this chapter.

3. TECHNOLOGIES USED IN HOME HEALTHCARE SERVICES

A wide range of technologies are employed in home healthcare services today, enabling remote monitoring, assistance, and intervention. These technologies span from simple sensors and mobile apps to sophisticated robots and AI-driven systems (Morita et al., 2023; Tian et al., 2024). It is useful to categorize the main types of home health technologies and their functions (Figure 2).

Figure 2. Types of technologies in home healthcare

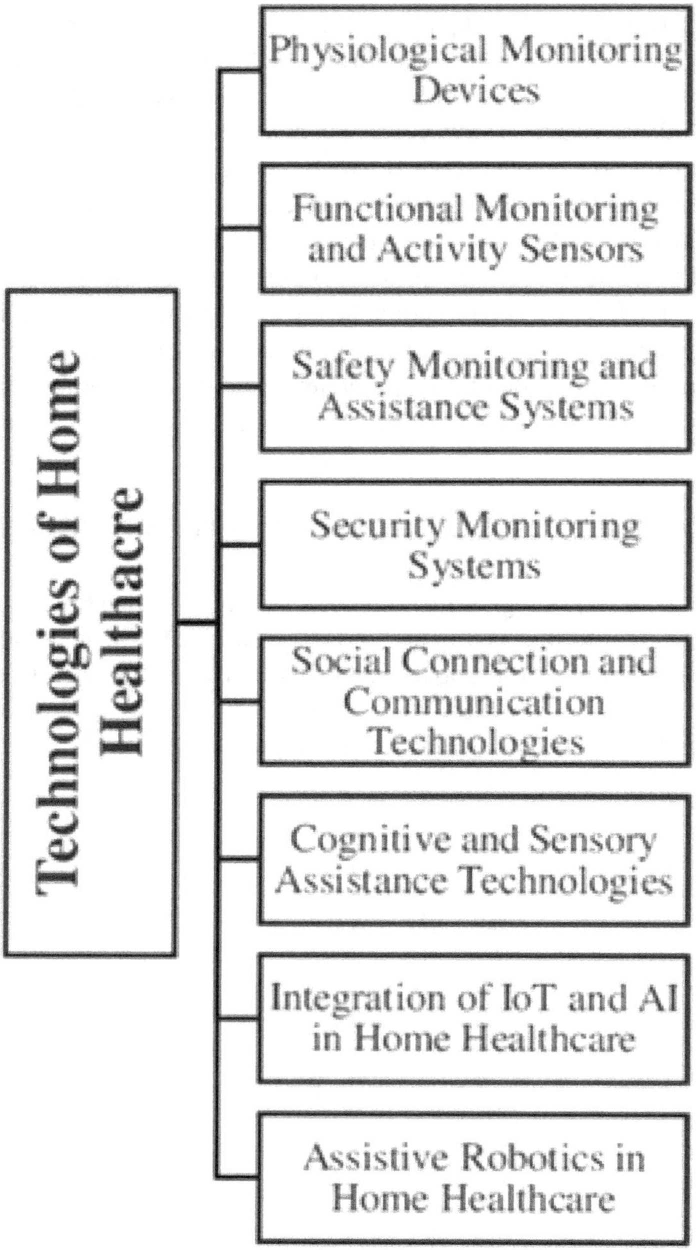

3.1. Physiological Monitoring Devices

Physiological monitoring technologies play a pivotal role in home-based healthcare by enabling continuous or periodic assessment of vital health parameters. These devices, including digital blood pressure monitors, glucometers, pulse oximeters, smart scales, and electrocardiogram (ECG) patches, are designed to collect critical health metrics such as heart rate, blood oxygen saturation, blood pressure, respiratory rate, body temperature, and weight. The integration of wireless connectivity options like Bluetooth and Wi-fi allows these devices to transmit collected data seamlessly to smartphone applications or cloud-based platforms, facilitating remote monitoring by healthcare professionals. The adoption of these technologies empowers patients, particularly those managing chronic conditions, to actively participate in their health management. By providing real-time feedback and alerts for abnormal readings, these devices enable timely interventions, potentially reducing hospital admissions and improving overall health outcomes. Moreover, the data collected can be analyzed over time to identify trends and inform personalized treatment plans, enhancing the quality of care delivered in home settings (Morita et al., 2023; Vargemidis et al., 2020).

3.2. Functional Monitoring and Activity Sensors

Functional monitoring technologies are essential for assessing the daily activities and functional status of individuals, especially older adults and those with mobility challenges. Devices such as passive infrared motion sensors, bed occupancy detectors, wearable activity trackers (e.g., fitness bands and smartwatches), and gait analysis mats are employed to monitor movement patterns, sleep quality, and physical activity levels. These sensors provide valuable insights into an individual's routine behaviors, enabling the detection of deviations that may indicate health issues or functional decline. For instance, a significant reduction in daily steps or changes in sleep patterns could signal the onset of health problems, prompting early intervention. Furthermore, the data collected supports personalized care planning and can be shared with caregivers and healthcare providers to coordinate support effectively (Morita et al., 2023; Vargemidis et al., 2020).

3.3. Safety Monitoring and Assistance Systems

Ensuring safety within the home environment is a critical aspect of home healthcare, particularly for older adults at risk of accidents and injuries. Safety monitoring and assistance systems encompass a range of technologies designed to prevent incidents such as falls, fires, and flooding. Wearable fall detectors, which may include pendants or devices with integrated accelerometers, can automatically detect falls and alert emergency contacts or services. Additional safety measures include automatic stove shut-off devices that prevent kitchen fires by turning off appliances after a period of inactivity, flood sensors in bathrooms that detect water leaks to prevent slips and water damage, and motion-activated night lights that enhance visibility during nighttime movements. These technologies collectively contribute to creating a safer living environment, reducing the risk of accidents, and promoting independent living among vulnerable populations (Tian et al., 2024; Liu et al., 2016).

3.4. Security Monitoring Systems

Beyond health and safety, security monitoring systems are integral to protecting individuals from external threats and emergencies. Smart doorbells equipped with cameras and intercom systems allow residents to see and communicate with visitors remotely, enhancing control over home access. Surveillance cameras provide continuous monitoring of the premises, deterring potential intruders and recording incidents for review. Panic buttons offer a quick means to summon help during emergencies, while integrated smoke and carbon monoxide detectors provide early warnings of fire or gas leaks. These systems often connect to alert services or emergency responders, ensuring timely assistance. By incorporating these technologies, individuals can feel more secure in their homes, which is particularly important for those living alone or in areas with higher security concerns (Liu et al., 2016; Rai et al., 2020).

3.5. Social Connection and Communication Technologies

Maintaining social connections is vital for mental health and well-being, especially for older adults who may experience isolation. Communication technologies such as video-calling platforms facilitate regular interactions with family, friends, and healthcare providers, supporting social engagement and telehealth services. Telepresence robots represent an advanced form of communication technology, enabling remote visits through mobile robots equipped with cameras and screens. These robots allow users to navigate through a home environment, providing a more immersive interaction experience. Voice-activated smart speakers serve as companions, offering conversational interactions, reminders, and access to information, thereby reducing feelings of loneliness and promoting cognitive stimulation (Wong et al., 2023; Rai et al., 2020).

3.6. Cognitive and Sensory Assistance Technologies

For individuals with cognitive impairments or sensory limitations, specialized technologies provide essential support to manage daily tasks and maintain independence. Automated medication dispensers ensure timely and accurate medication intake, reducing the risk of missed doses or overdoses. Reminder applications assist with scheduling and task management, supporting individuals with memory challenges. Object locators help users find misplaced items, while amplified phones and captioning devices enhance communication for those with hearing impairments. Screen readers and magnification tools assist individuals with visual impairments in accessing digital content. These technologies are crucial in enabling users to perform daily activities, engage with their environment, and maintain a sense of autonomy (Deusdad, 2024; Haanes, 2023).

3.7. Integration of IoT and AI in Home Healthcare

The integration of Internet of Things (IoT) and Artificial Intelligence (AI) technologies underpins the functionality of many home healthcare devices. IoT enables the interconnection of various devices, allowing for seamless data sharing and system coordination. For example, physiological monitors can transmit data to centralized platforms where AI algorithms analyze the information to detect anomalies, predict health trends, and provide decision support AI-driven personalization enhances the user experience by adapting system responses to individual behaviors and preferences. For instance, smart home systems can learn a user's routine and adjust environmental controls accordingly, or provide tailored health recommendations based on collected data. This level of customization improves the relevance and effectiveness of home healthcare interventions (Shet et al., 2018; Bender & Sartipi, 2013).

3.8. Assistive Robotics in Home Healthcare

Assistive robotics represents a significant advancement in supporting individuals with physical and social needs within the home setting. Physically assistive robots, such as exoskeletons and robotic lifting aids, assist with mobility and daily activities, reducing the physical strain on users and caregivers. These technologies enable individuals with mobility impairments to perform tasks that would otherwise require assistance, promoting independence. Socially assistive robots, including devices like Paro (a robotic seal) and humanoid robots, provide companionship and emotional support. Studies have shown that regular interaction with these robots can alleviate feelings of loneliness, improve mood, and enhance the overall quality of life for older adults (Wong et al., 2023; Broadbent et al., 2009). These robots can engage users in conversations, play music, provide reminders, and offer information, serving as interactive companions that enrich daily routines.

4. THE ROLE OF HUMAN-MACHINE INTERACTION IN PRACTICE

Implementing HMI in home health transforms patient experience and outcomes when effectively executed. One major role is remote chronic disease management. Telehealth systems integrating home monitoring devices (for glucose, blood pressure, weight) with clinician oversight allow patients active participation in their care. Patients report valuing in-home monitoring's convenience and increased health awareness, though they note gaps in device functionality (Jalil et al., 2019; Paré, et al., 2007).

HMI also modifies patient behavior. Immediate feedback from fitness trackers or diet apps serves as a coach, increasing engagement. Family members often join the loop-helping with device setup, interpreting data, or responding to alerts-which creates a network of patient–device–caregiver interactions (Jalil et al., 2019; Robinson et al., 2014).

Medication adherence benefits from smart dispensers with auditory reminders and lock features. These interactions reduce missed doses and errors, crucial for users with memory challenges (Morita et al., 2023; Tian et al., 2024).

Socially assistive robots in elder care supplement human contact. Older adults living alone interacted daily with robots, reporting reduced loneliness, diversified activities, and improved family engagement (Wong et al., 2023; Robinson et al., 2014).

During the COVID-19 pandemic, telepresence and virtual visits became mainstream. Older patients appreciated convenience, safety, and the comfort of home during consultations, reporting high satisfaction when technology was reliable and interfaces were simple (Hays & Skootsky, 2022; Kruse et al., 2022).

Home healthcare HMI also fosters proactive interventions via caregiver portals. For example, weight alerts from a wireless scale can prompt a nurse's follow-up call, enhancing patients' sense of security (Wang et al., 2024; Jalil et al., 2019).

Finally, successful HMI often requires human facilitation. Public health nurses or care coordinators introduce and train users on new technologies, acting as intermediaries until users become comfortable (Morita et al., 2023; Antona & Stephanidis, 2020).

5. ETHICAL, SAFETY, AND PRIVACY ISSUES

As healthcare technologies become increasingly embedded in home environments, their integration raises complex ethical, safety, and privacy challenges that must be addressed to ensure patient-centered, secure, and equitable care. These concerns are especially pressing as smart systems, AI, robotics, and IoT devices play a growing role in supporting patients with chronic illnesses, cognitive decline, or physical impairments.

One of the foremost ethical concerns in home healthcare is the protection of patient data. These technologies often collect highly sensitive and personal information from biometric indicators like blood pressure and heart rate to behavioral patterns, location data, and even private conversations. Without robust safeguards, this intimate data is at risk of being exposed, misused, or accessed without consent (Hall & McGraw, 2014; Robles et al., 2020). Data breaches can have devastating effects, particularly when information is used by third parties such as insurers or advertisers to discriminate or exploit vulnerable populations.

Moreover, the issue of security is deeply entwined with privacy. IoT-based home healthcare devices are especially vulnerable to cyberattacks. Many of these systems lack proper encryption protocols, making them attractive targets for malicious actors (Robles et al., 2020). Hall and McGraw (2014) emphasize that a comprehensive data security strategy must go beyond encryption, requiring continuous monitoring, authentication protocols, and timely patching of system vulnerabilities. As patients and families become reliant on these systems, any breach of security not only violates privacy but also threatens patient safety and trust.

Respecting patient autonomy is a foundational principle of medical ethics. Yet, integrating monitoring systems into the home environment can infringe upon personal freedoms. Sensors that track movement, cameras that capture activity, and AI systems that interpret behavior can intrude into private spaces, making individuals feel watched or controlled. While these technologies may enhance safety such as through fall detection or medication reminders they must be implemented in ways that are transparent and consent-driven.

Consent becomes particularly problematic in the context of cognitive impairments, such as dementia. Patients with diminished decision-making capacity may not be able to provide informed consent. In these situations, families or legal proxies often act on behalf of the patient. However, this can create ethical tensions between beneficence (acting in the patient's best interests) and respect for autonomy (Sharkey & Sharkey, 2012; Deusdad, 2024). These dilemmas are compounded when the technology in question has far-reaching implications for privacy and lifestyle. Ensuring ongoing, revisable consent and prioritizing the patient's dignity are crucial in these scenarios.

Another critical ethical consideration is the impact of healthcare technologies on emotional well-being and human relationships. While robotic companions and virtual assistants may offer stimulation, reminders, or conversation, they cannot replicate genuine human empathy. Over-reliance on machines may lead to emotional isolation, particularly among older adults who may already experience loneliness. Technology, therefore, must serve to complement rather than replace compassionate human caregiving (Sharkey & Sharkey, 2012; Broadbent et al., 2009).

Broadbent and colleagues (2009) found that while some patients benefit from robotic assistance, many still crave meaningful human interaction. Ethical deployment of such systems requires striking a balance-where robots assist with routine tasks, enabling human caregivers to focus on emotional support and complex care rather than being supplanted entirely.

A growing reliance on healthcare technologies can also lead to unintended forms of dependence. For patients, this may manifest as "learned helplessness," where they become passive recipients of care and lose confidence in their ability to manage their health independently. For caregivers-particularly informal caregivers such as family members-there may be a heightened burden, especially when systems generate false alarms or require constant monitoring and maintenance (Ferlito et al., 2024; Jh et al., 2025).

Ferlito et al. (2024) highlight the mental toll on caregivers when alarm fatigue sets in-caused by frequent, non-critical alerts that can desensitize them to actual emergencies. Jh et al. (2025) further argue that such technologies should be co-designed with caregivers to ensure usability, reduce stress, and offer training and support infrastructure. A holistic approach to design is necessary-one that empowers users without creating new dependencies or exacerbating caregiver strain.

The physical and operational safety of home healthcare technologies is non-negotiable. Devices must undergo rigorous testing to ensure they do not pose hazards-whether through electrical faults, improper installation, or software glitches. More subtly, algorithmic systems such as AI tools that predict health deterioration or deliver medical advice must be evaluated for accuracy and reliability. False positives (e.g., detecting a fall where none occurred) or false negatives (e.g., missing a real health emergency) can have dire consequences (Procter et al., 2023; Tenner, 2015).

Moreover, algorithmic errors are not solely technical issues; they also raise ethical questions about responsibility and accountability. If a device gives incorrect advice or fails to detect a critical incident, who bears the blame the developer, the healthcare provider, or the user? Procter et al. (2023) emphasize that clear accountability frameworks are essential to address such issues and prevent the undue burden from falling on patients or their families.

Another dimension of concern is algorithmic bias. AI systems used in home healthcare are often trained on datasets that may not represent diverse populations.

As Obermeyer et al. (2019) demonstrate, even widely used algorithms can exhibit racial or socioeconomic biases that systematically disadvantage certain groups. Anderson and Visweswaran (2025) also point out that poorly trained algorithms can lead to inequitable care delivery, especially if developers fail to include inclusive and representative training data.

To mitigate bias, developers must commit to transparency in algorithm design, continuously audit system performance, and actively involve diverse stakeholders in the development process. This not only improves fairness but also enhances public trust in the technology.

Transparency in how technologies operate is central to ethical implementation. Users should be able to understand, at least at a basic level, how systems collect data, make decisions, and trigger interventions. Black-box systems, where algorithmic decision-making is opaque, can alienate users and undermine their trust (Procter et al., 2023; Hall & McGraw, 2014). Ensuring that patients, families, and caregivers are informed participants rather than passive subjects helps uphold autonomy and responsibility.

Equally important is accountability. When errors ocur whether due to software bugs, hardware failures, or user misuse there must be clear mechanisms to address and remediate harm. Developers and providers, not patients, should carry the responsibility for ensuring that systems are safe, accurate, and responsive.

Finally, the ethical integration of machines in home healthcare must confront issues of equity. Advanced technologies are often expensive, placing them out of reach for low-income individuals or under-resourced communities. Additionally, the digital divide formulated by limited digital literacy or lack of internet Access can exclude already marginalized groups from benefiting from these innovations (Voigt & Von dem Bussche, 2017; Deusdad, 2024).

To ensure fairness, policies must support inclusive design, subsidized access, and widespread digital education. Community-based training programs and public health outreach can play a critical role in bridging this divide and making technology-supported home healthcare a reality for all.

6. USER EXPERIENCE AND SATISFACTION

User experience (UX) plays a central role in determining the effectiveness, adoption, and sustained use of human–machine interaction (HMI) technologies in home healthcare environments. For aging populations and individuals managing chronic conditions, the integration of health-monitoring systems, smart assistants, and wearable devices depends heavily on how users interact with these technologies. A well-designed UX-encompassing usability, emotional comfort, perceived value, and support structures-not only fosters acceptance but also enhances safety, satisfaction, and overall health outcomes.

Ease to use remains one of the most critical UX factors for older adults, who represent a significant portion of the home healthcare demographic. Devices with complex or unintuitive interfaces can become sources of frustration, leading to abandonment or non-compliance. Conversely, interfaces that align with users' mental models and expectations promote adoption and sustained engagement (Tian et al., 2024; Morita et al., 2023).

Aging-related physical and cognitive limitations such as declining vision, memory lapses, and reduced dexterity necessitate the development of systems that are simple, clear, and forgiving of errors. Morita et al. (2023) emphasize that systems designed without considering age-related impairments often create barriers, even if they are functionally robust. Simple navigation structures, clear labeling, large buttons, and audible confirmations are among the features that significantly improve the usability of home healthcare systems for older users.

The Technology Acceptance Model (TAM) offers a robust framework for understanding how users come to accept and use technology. According to TAM, two core beliefs-perceived usefulness and perceived ease of use strongly influence a user's intention to engage with a system (Venkatesh et al., 2003). In the context of home healthcare, these beliefs translate into the user's perception that the technology will help manage health more effectively and that it will be easy enough to use without expert assistance.

Wang et al. (2024) demonstrated that users are more likely to embrace home health technologies when they believe the systems will lead to tangible health benefits, such as better medication adherence or early detection of symptoms. However, the perceived benefits must outweigh the perceived effort required to learn or operate the system. Thus, developers must prioritize both functionality and usability, ensuring that every feature contributes to a seamless and purposeful user experience.

Human-centered design extends beyond the interface itself; it encompasses the environment and social context in which technology is used. Social and community support particularly from family members, caregivers, and health professionals greatly influences user experience. Training programs, tutorials, and one-on-one coaching are effective strategies to build digital confidence and reduce the psychological barriers to initial use (Antona & Stephanidis, 2020; Wang et al., 2024).

Older adults who feel supported by caregivers or community networks are more likely to persist through initial challenges and develop trust in the technology. Robinson et al. (2014) found that when users received consistent feedback from clinicians based on the data collected by their home systems, they were more engaged and confident in using those systems. Feedback not only validates the utility of the technology but also reinforces the connection between device use and meaningful health outcomes, thereby closing the loop between interaction and care delivery.

Despite technological advances, the digital divide continues to hinder equitable access to home healthcare HMI. Many older adults remain unfamiliar with digital tools or lack access to high-speed internet, particularly those with lower levels of income or education (Wang et al., 2024; Venkatesh et al., 2003). These disparities limit their ability to adopt and benefit from health technologies, potentially exacerbating existing health inequities.

Responsive support systems such as helplines, remote technical assistance, and in-person orientation can alleviate early frustrations and build user competence. Kruse et al. (2022) highlight that such interventions are particularly effective when tailored to the individual's technological baseline and learning preferences. For instance, older users may prefer printed guides with step-by-step instructions over app-based tutorials. Ensuring access to culturally sensitive, language-appropriate, and personalized support mechanisms can mitigate many of the barriers posed by the digital divide.

Beyond functionality and usability, emotional design significantly shapes user experience in home healthcare HMI. Devices that appear sterile, mechanical, or clinical may evoke discomfort or stigma, especially when used in social or communal living environments. In contrast, technologies with friendly aesthetics, warm tones, and customizable features can foster emotional connection and reduce resistance (Broadbent et al., 2009; Tenner, 2015).

Personalization options such as naming a digital assistant, choosing alert sounds, or selecting interface themes allow users to humanize and emotionally invest in their devices. Tenner (2015) suggests that such design elements create a sense of familiarity and comfort, which is particularly important for long-term engagement. Broadbent et al. (2009) found that users who perceived their robotic assistants as friendly and approachable were more likely to accept their presence in the home and follow their health prompts.

Emotional engagement also involves reducing fear and anxiety associated with new technologies. For first-time users, especially those managing serious illnesses, emotional reassurance can be as vital as technical reliability. Designers should strive to create systems that feel supportive and empowering, not intimidating or intrusive.

To optimize UX, it is essential to embed human–computer interaction (HCI) evaluation methods within the clinical deployment of these technologies. Tools such as contextual inquiry, usability testing, and semi-structured interviews enable developers and healthcare providers to uncover subtle user needs, frustrations, and behaviors that may not be evident through quantitative usage metrics alone (Jalil et al., 2019; Czaja et al., 2006).

Czaja et al. (2006) emphasize that UX evaluation must be iterative and ongoing. User needs often evolve over time, particularly as patients' health conditions change or as caregivers rotate. Jalil et al. (2019) advocate for a co-design approach, where users-patients and caregivers alike-are directly involved in the development and refinement of technologies. This participatory process ensures that design choices reflect real-world use patterns and user priorities, rather than assumptions made in laboratory settings.

By incorporating feedback loops and agile development cycles, developers can iteratively enhance usability and satisfaction, leading to better health outcomes and reduced technology abandonment.

Optimizing user experience in home healthcare HMI is a multifaceted challenge that requires careful attention to usability, emotional engagement, social support, and equitable access. Ease of use is particularly vital for older adults, whose ability to engage with technology can be impaired by physical, cognitive, or socio-economic barriers. The Technology Acceptance Model provides valuable insights into the psychological factors influencing technology adoption, while emotional design and personalized support help foster trust and sustained engagement.

Community support structures, responsive training, and clinician involvement reinforce the perceived usefulness of these systems. At the same time, bridging the digital divide through accessible design and targeted interventions ensures that no group is left behind. Finally, the integration of robust HCI evaluation methods allows for the continuous refinement of user experience, making home healthcare technologies more responsive, humane, and effective for all.

7. POLICY AND REGULATIONS

A robust policy and regulatory framework is essential in home healthcare because it provides the legal and ethical infrastructure necessary to ensure patient safety, protect privacy, and maintain quality standards in a decentralized care environment. As home healthcare increasingly relies on digital technologies, such as remote monitoring devices, telemedicine platforms, and AI-driven decision support systems, clear regulations help define responsibilities, data governance protocols, and clinical accountability. Without appropriate oversight, patients may be exposed to risks such as data breaches, misuse of personal health information, or the deployment of untested or biased technologies. Furthermore, regulatory frameworks guide reimbursement structures, standardize interoperability between systems, and ensure equitable access to care across diverse populations. By aligning innovation with compliance and ethical practice, policy frameworks create trust among patients, caregivers, and providers, which is fundamental for the sustainable integration of technology in home-based healthcare services.

The expansion of home health HMI demands robust policy and regulation. In the United States, Health Insurance Portability and Accountability Act (HIPAA) governs health information privacy but does not cover consumer-purchased devices unless integrated with providers; the Food and Drug Administartion (FDA) regulates medical devices and software as a medical device (SaMD), though many health apps remain outside its purview (Hall & McGraw, 2014; Voigt & Von dem Bussche, 2017).

In the European Union, General Data Protection Regulation (GDPR) enshrines "Privacy by Design and by Default," requiring explicit consent, data minimization, and breach notifications for health data (Lyapina & Kisselova-Yaneva, 2017; Voigt & Von dem Bussche, 2017). The EU Medical Device Regulation (MDR) now includes software, mandating CE marking for health apps (Lyapina & Kisselova-Yaneva, 2017; U.S. FDA, 2022).

Telehealth policy has evolved post-COVID: U.S. states and Medicare extended cross-state licensure and reimbursement, making home an authorized origin site (Trout et al., 2020; CMS, 2020). Professional boards stipulate that telehealth care must meet in-person standards, with protocols for emergencies and privacy measures (Trout et al., 2020; CMS, 2020).

AI governance is emerging: the proposed European Union (EU) AI Act classifies healthcare AI as high-risk, requiring transparency, risk management, and conformity assessments (European Commission, 2021; Procter et al., 2023). Soft law, such as WHO guidances on digital health and industry standards (IEC 62366 on usability, cybersecurity guidance), further shape ethical and safe deployment (WHO, 2022; Jha et al., 2025).

Liability frameworks for device malfunctions or AI errors are under development, emphasizing a "human in the loop" and clear accountability for vendors and providers (Procter et al., 2023; Avis, 2018).

Infrastructure and reimbursement policies such as Medicare's remote patient monitoring codes and broadband subsidies drive adoption and address equity, recognizing that without connectivity, home HMI cannot reach underserved areas (Avis, 2018; WHO, 2022).

Internationally, approaches vary: Japan's Society 5.0 supports eldercare robotics via regulatory sandboxes and public engagement, while some developing countries adopt mobile health platforms under simpler regulations, often guided by international standards to ensure quality (WHO, 2022; Yuksel, 2024).

8. CHALLENGES AND FUTURE DIRECTIONS

Despite progress, key challenges remain, pointing to future research and policy directions.

- Fragmented apps and devices hinder a unified user experience. Adopting standards and developing secure, open platforms will enable seamless data sharing and holistic care dashboards (Bender & Sartipi, 2013; Mandel et al., 2016).
- Distinguishing data from multiple residents requires advanced context-aware sensing-using wearable identifiers or AI vision-to respect individual privacy and data integrity (Ciuffreda et al, 2023; Benmansour et al., 2015).
- Addressing the digital divide at scale necessitates age-friendly training programs and roles like "digital health navigators" who assist older adults in setup and use (Nichols et al., 2020; Antona & Stephanidis, 2020).
- Preventing novelty fade-out may leverage gamification and behavioral science to create respectful, motivating routines (Hamari et al., 2014; Lister et al., 2014).
- Co-design processes and continuous ethical oversight ensure fairness, transparency, and respect for persons are integral from ideation to deployment (Ferlito et al.,, 2024; Jha et al., 2025).
- Future systems may detect mood from voice or expressions, offering empathetic responses; however, simulating empathy raises complex ethical debates (Picard, 2000; Broadbent et al., 2009).
- Developing user-friendly explanations for AI decisions and instituting "algorithm audits" will bolster trust and allow recourse in case of errors (Procter et al., 2023; Obermeyer et al., 2019).
- Infrastructure scalability. Universal broadband access (5G, satellite), power resilience, and robust cloud platforms are prerequisites for widespread HMI adoption (WHO, 2022; Bender & Sartipi, 2013).
- Clinician training in telehealth communication and data interpretation must expand, while AI-driven alert filtering prevents clinician overload (Nichols et al., 2020; Avis, 2018).
- Demonstrating value in reduced hospitalizations and aligning incentives under value-based care will sustain investment in home HMI (Hays & Skootsky, 2022; Kruse et al., 2022).
- As consumer tech raises user expectations, systems must adapt to individual preferences and behaviors, balancing personalization with privacy (Shet et al., 2018; Picard, 2000).

- Industry 5.0/Society 5.0 envisions humans and machines collaborating-machines handling routine tasks while humans focus on empathy and complex decisions (Yuksel, 2024; Avis, 2018).
- Post-market surveillance and learning health system approaches, potentially driven by AI, will monitor device performance and user outcomes, ensuring iterative improvements (Morita et al., 2023; WHO, 2022).

The horizon of home health human–machine interaction promises more intelligent, empathetic, and integrated systems centering on human needs. Addressing challenges in interoperability, usability, ethics, and equity through interdisciplinary collaboration, evolving regulation, and user-centered design will enable truly transformative care at home in the years to come.

9. CONCLUSION AND RECOMMENDATIONS

The integration of human–machine interaction (HMI) into home healthcare marks a transformative shift in how medical services are delivered, especially for aging populations and individuals managing chronic conditions. As societies grapple with rising healthcare demands, workforce shortages, and a growing preference for "aging in place," HMI technologies offer scalable solutions that promote independence, monitor well-being, and facilitate timely interventions. However, for these systems to deliver on their promise, they must be conceptualized not merely as isolated devices, but as components of a dynamic socio-technical ecosystem—one that bridges physical, digital, and social domains.

This ecosystem spans both visible components, such as wearable sensors, voice assistants, digital interfaces, and robotic aids, and invisible layers, including machine learning algorithms, cloud-based data processing, predictive analytics, and AI-driven decision-making. Successful integration hinges on the alignment of these elements with users' daily routines, physical environments, cognitive abilities, and social support networks. HMI systems that harmonize with home contexts responding to real-life needs and variations are more likely to be adopted, trusted, and sustained over time.

Current technologies illustrate the broad spectrum of HMI applications in the home. Physiological monitoring devices track metrics like heart rate, glucose levels, or blood pressure, enabling real-time health insights and reducing the need for frequent in-person checkups. Activity sensors and fall detectors provide safety assurance, particularly for those with mobility impairments. AI-powered assistants and social robots offer reminders, companionship, and cognitive engagement, enhancing emotional well-being. Together, these systems enable self-management, early detection of health deterioration, and continuity of care all within the comfort and familiarity of one's home.

However, the technological potential of HMI in home healthcare is only fully realized when paired with user-centered design, personalized training, and human facilitation. Without attention to accessibility, literacy levels, and intuitive design, even the most sophisticated tools may be rejected or misused. Training programs delivered through in-person coaching, remote support, or interactive tutorials build digital confidence and reduce anxiety, especially among older adults. Ongoing human facilitation, whether through family caregivers, visiting nurses, or community health workers, serves as a bridge between machine capabilities and patient experience, ensuring that individuals remain empowered and not sidelined by automation.

At the same time, the integration of machines into domestic healthcare environments introduces a host of ethical, safety, and privacy challenges. These concerns are not secondary they are foundational to building public trust and ensuring equitable outcomes. Data privacy is paramount, as devices collect intimate, continuous streams of information ranging from sleep patterns to medication intake to interpersonal conversations. Strong cybersecurity protocols, such as end-to-end encryption, secure authentication, and regular updates, are essential to prevent breaches.

Moreover, existing legal and regulatory frameworks must evolve to accommodate new realities. As software becomes classified as a medical device, oversight should include mechanisms for auditing algorithms, ensuring explainability, and holding developers accountable for harmful or biased outcomes. Systems must also offer transparent user interfaces, with clearly stated data practices and opt-in mechanisms for consent.

Looking ahead, several key challenges and priorities must be addressed to ensure the ethical, inclusive, and sustainable integration of HMI in home healthcare:

- Developers must prioritize inclusive design principles that account for variations in age, education, language, vision, hearing, and mobility. Co-design with users-especially older adults and caregivers-should be standard practice.
- To avoid fragmented systems, manufacturers and software developers should adopt open standards that allow data to be shared securely across platforms, providers, and devices, supporting continuity of care.
- Governments and insurers must broaden reimbursement schemes to include HMI-enabled home care, recognizing the clinical value of remote monitoring and virtual care interventions.
- Public health agencies and care organizations should invest in training, digital helplines, and in-person assistance to reduce the digital divide and increase engagement with HMI technologies.

- All home healthcare technologies should undergo regular performance reviews, incorporating both clinical efficacy and user experience feedback. Explainable AI frameworks must be adopted to ensure transparency and accountability.
- Ethical impact assessments-focusing on autonomy, equity, and informed consent-should be conducted during product development. Technologies should augment rather than replace human compassion and connection.

By viewing HMI as a socio-technical system and embedding ethics, usability, and inclusiveness into every phase of design and deployment, we can move toward a future where high-quality, personalized, and compassionate care is not limited to institutions but extended into the most vital healthcare setting of all the patient's own home.

REFERENCES

Anderson, J. W., & Visweswaran, S. (2025). Algorithmic individual fairness and healthcare: A scoping review. *JAMIA Open*, *8*(1), ooae149. DOI: 10.1093/jamiaopen/ooae149 PMID: 39737346

Antona, M., & Stephanidis, C. (Eds.). (2020). *Universal access in human-computer interaction. Design approaches and supporting technologies: 14th International Conference, UAHCI 2020, Held as Part of the 22nd HCI International Conference, HCII 2020, Copenhagen, Denmark, July 19–24, 2020, Proceedings, Part I* (Vol. 12188). Springer. DOI: 10.1007/978-3-030-49282-3

Avis, J. (2018). Socio-technical imaginary of the fourth industrial revolution and its implications for vocational education and training: A literature review. *Journal of Vocational Education and Training*, *70*(3), 337–363. DOI: 10.1080/13636820.2018.1498907

Bender, D., & Sartipi, K. (2013). HL7 FHIR: An agile and RESTful approach to healthcare information exchange. In *2013 IEEE 26th International Symposium on Computer-Based Medical Systems (CBMS)* (pp. 326–331). IEEE. DOI: 10.1109/CBMS.2013.6627810

Benmansour, A., Bouchachia, A., & Feham, M. (2016). Multioccupant activity recognition in pervasive smart home environments. *ACM Computing Surveys*, *48*(3), 34. DOI: 10.1145/2835372

Bouabida, K., Lebouché, B., & Pomey, M.-P. (2022). Telehealth and COVID-19 pandemic: An overview of the telehealth use, advantages, challenges, and opportunities during COVID-19 pandemic. *Health Care*, *10*(11), 2293. DOI: 10.3390/healthcare10112293 PMID: 36421617

Broadbent, E., Stafford, R., & MacDonald, B. (2009). Acceptance of healthcare robots for the older population: Review and future directions. *International Journal of Social Robotics*, *1*(4), 319–330. DOI: 10.1007/s12369-009-0030-6

Cannan, J., & Hu, H. (2011). *Human-machine interaction (HMI): A survey* (Technical Report CES-508). University of Essex.

Centers for Medicare & Medicaid Services. (2020, March 17). *Medicare telemedicine health care provider fact sheet.* https://www.cms.gov/newsroom/fact-sheets/medicare-telemedicine-health-care-provider-fact-sheet

Ciuffreda, I., Casaccia, S., & Revel, G. M. (2023). A multi-sensor fusion approach based on PIR and ultrasonic sensors installed on a robot to localise people in indoor environments. *Sensors (Basel)*, *23*(15), 6963. DOI: 10.3390/s23156963 PMID: 37571746

Czaja, S. J., Charness, N., Fisk, A. D., Hertzog, C., Nair, S. N., Rogers, W. A., & Sharit, J. (2006). Factors predicting the use of technology: Findings from the Center for Research and Education on Aging and Technology Enhancement (CREATE). *Psychology and Aging*, *21*(2), 333–352. DOI: 10.1037/0882-7974.21.2.333 PMID: 16768579

Davis, F. D. (1989). Perceived usefulness, perceived ease of use, and user acceptance of information technology. *Management Information Systems Quarterly*, *13*(3), 319–340. DOI: 10.2307/249008

Demiris, G., & Olson, S. (2010). Information technology and systems in home health care. In *The role of human factors in home health care: Workshop summary* (pp. 173–200). National Academies Press., DOI: 10.17226/12927

Deusdad, B. (2024). Ethical implications in using robots among older adults living with dementia. *Frontiers in Psychiatry*, *15*, 1436273. DOI: 10.3389/fpsyt.2024.1436273 PMID: 39391087

Dubey, P., & Kumar, M. (2025). Integrating explainable AI with federated learning for next-generation IoT: A comprehensive review and prospective insights. *Computer Science Review*, *56*, 100697. DOI: 10.1016/j.cosrev.2024.100697

European Commission. (2021). *Proposal for a regulation of the European Parliament and of the Council laying down harmonised rules on artificial intelligence (Artificial Intelligence Act)*. https://eur-lex.europa.eu/legal-content/EN/TXT/?uri=CELEX%3A52021PC0206

Ferlito, B., Segers, S., De Proost, M., & Mertes, H. (2024). Responsibility gap(s) due to the introduction of AI in healthcare: An Ubuntu-inspired approach. *Science and Engineering Ethics*, *30*(4), 34. DOI: 10.1007/s11948-024-00501-4 PMID: 39090479

Grudin, J. (2018). From tool to partner: The evolution of human-computer interaction. In *Extended Abstracts of the 2018 CHI Conference on Human Factors in Computing Systems* (pp. 1–3). ACM. DOI: 10.1145/3170427.3174358

Haanes, G. G. (2023). Multidisciplinary approaches and community-based interventions: Adaptable strategies for managing sensory impairments in older adults. *Journal of Multidisciplinary Healthcare*, *16*, 2701–2705. DOI: 10.2147/JMDH.S416762 PMID: 37724317

Hall, J. L., & McGraw, D. (2014). For telehealth to succeed, privacy and security risks must be identified and addressed. *Health Affairs*, *33*(2), 216–221. DOI: 10.1377/hlthaff.2013.0997 PMID: 24493763

Hamari, J., Koivisto, J., & Sarsa, H. (2014). Does gamification work? A literature review of empirical studies on gamification. In *2014 47th Hawaii International Conference on System Sciences* (pp. 3025–3034). IEEE. DOI: 10.1109/HICSS.2014.377

Hays, R. D., & Skootsky, S. A. (2022). Patient experience with in-person and telehealth visits before and during the COVID-19 pandemic at a large integrated health system in the United States. *Journal of General Internal Medicine*, *37*(4), 847–852. DOI: 10.1007/s11606-021-07196-4 PMID: 34982370

Jalil, S., Bache, S., & Lin, X. (2019). Complementing a clinical trial with human–computer interaction: Patients' user experience with telehealth. *JMIR Human Factors*, *6*(2), e11458. DOI: 10.2196/humanfactors.9481 PMID: 31172958

Jha, D., Durak, G., Sharma, V., Keles, E., Cicek, V., Zhang, Z., & Bagci, U. (2025). A conceptual framework for applying ethical principles of AI to medical practice. *Bioengineering (Basel, Switzerland)*, *12*(2), 180. DOI: 10.3390/bioengineering12020180 PMID: 40001699

Kang, H. J., Kim, S., & Lee, H. (2019). An ecological approach to smart homes for healthcare services: Conceptual framework of a smart servicescape wheel. *JMIR mHealth and uHealth*, *7*(2), e12425. DOI: 10.2196/12425 PMID: 30735145

Kruse, C. S., Krowski, N., Rodriguez, B., Tran, L., Vela, J., & Brooks, M. (2017). Telehealth and patient satisfaction: A systematic review and narrative analysis. *BMJ Open*, *7*(8), e016242. DOI: 10.1136/bmjopen-2017-016242 PMID: 28775188

Li, X., & Xu, Y. (2022). Role of human-computer interaction healthcare system in the teaching of physiology and medicine. *Computational Intelligence and Neuroscience, 2022*, Article 5849736. (Retraction published *Computational Intelligence and Neuroscience, 2023*, Article 9812579. https://doi.org/)DOI: 10.1155/2022/5849736

Lister, C., West, J. H., Cannon, B., Sax, T., & Brodegard, D. (2014). Just a fad? Gamification in health and fitness: A systematic review. *JMIR Serious Games*, *2*(2), e9. DOI: 10.2196/games.3413 PMID: 25654660

Liu, L., Stroulia, E., Nikolaidis, I., Miguel-Cruz, A., & Rios Rincon, A. (2016). Smart homes and home health monitoring technologies for older adults: A systematic review. *International Journal of Medical Informatics*, *91*, 44–59. DOI: 10.1016/j.ijmedinf.2016.04.007 PMID: 27185508

Lyapina, M., & Kisselova-Yaneva, A. (2017). Why new regulations of the European Parliament on medical devices are needed. *Medical Informatics*, *4*(1), 591–596. DOI: 10.18044/Medinform.201741.591

Mandel, J. C., Kreda, D. A., Mandl, K. D., Kohane, I. S., & Ramoni, R. B. (2016). SMART on FHIR: A standards-based, interoperable apps platform for electronic health records. *Journal of the American Medical Informatics Association : JAMIA*, *23*(5), 899–908. DOI: 10.1093/jamia/ocv189 PMID: 26911829

McFarlane, D. C., & Latorella, K. A. (2002). The scope and importance of human interruption in human-computer interaction design. *Human-Computer Interaction*, *17*(1), 1–61. DOI: 10.1207/S15327051HCI1701_1

Mennella, C., Maniscalco, U., De Pietro, G., & Esposito, M. (2024). Ethical and regulatory challenges of AI technologies in healthcare: A narrative review. *Heliyon*, *10*(4), e26297. DOI: 10.1016/j.heliyon.2024.e26297 PMID: 38384518

Morita, P. P., West, R., Da Costa, D., Michalski, A., Kalesnikava, V., Kuziemsky, C., & St-Amant, O. (2023). Health monitoring using smart home technologies: Scoping review. *JMIR mHealth and uHealth*, *11*, e37347. DOI: 10.2196/37347 PMID: 37052984

Mourtzis, D., Angelopoulos, J., & Panopoulos, N. (2023). The future of the human–machine interface (HMI) in society 5.0. *Future Internet*, *15*(5), 162. DOI: 10.3390/fi15050162

Nichols, T., Calder, R., Morgan, M., Lawn, S., Beauchamp, A., Trezona, A., & Klepac Pogrmilovic, B. (2020). *Self-care for health: A national policy blueprint* (Policy Paper 2020-01). Mitchell Institute, Victoria University. https://www.vu.edu.au/sites/default/files/self-care-for-health-national-policy-blueprint-mitchell-institute.pdf

Nielsen, J. (1994). *Usability engineering*. Morgan Kaufmann.

Obermeyer, Z., Powers, B., Vogeli, C., & Mullainathan, S. (2019). Dissecting racial bias in an algorithm used to manage the health of populations. *Science*, *366*(6464), 447–453. DOI: 10.1126/science.aax2342 PMID: 31649194

Padhan, S., Mohapatra, A., Ramasamy, S. K., & Agrawal, S. (2023). Artificial intelligence (AI) and robotics in elderly healthcare: Enabling independence and quality of life. *Cureus*, *15*(8), e42905. DOI: 10.7759/cureus.42905 PMID: 37664381

Paré, G., Jaana, M., & Sicotte, C. (2007). Systematic review of home telemonitoring for chronic diseases: The evidence base. *Journal of the American Medical Informatics Association : JAMIA*, *14*(3), 269–277. DOI: 10.1197/jamia.M2270 PMID: 17329725

Picard, R. W. (2000). *Affective computing*. MIT Press. DOI: 10.7551/mit-press/1140.003.0008

Procter, R., Tolmie, P., & Rouncefield, M. (2023). Holding AI to account: Challenges for the delivery of trustworthy AI in healthcare. *ACM Transactions on Computer-Human Interaction, 30*(2), 26. DOI: 10.1145/3577009

Rai, H. K., Cavalcanti Barroso, A., Yates, L., Schneider, J., & Orrell, M. (2020). Involvement of people with dementia in the development of technology-based interventions: Narrative synthesis review and best practice guidelines. *Journal of Medical Internet Research, 22*(12), e17531. DOI: 10.2196/17531 PMID: 33270034

Robinson, H., MacDonald, B., & Broadbent, E. (2014). The role of healthcare robots for older people at home: A review. *International Journal of Social Robotics, 6*(4), 575–591. DOI: 10.1007/s12369-014-0242-2

Robles, T., Bordel, B., Alcarria, R., & Sánchez-de-Rivera, D. (2020). Enabling trustworthy personal data protection in eHealth and well-being services through privacy-by-design. *International Journal of Distributed Sensor Networks, 16*(5), 1550147720912110. DOI: 10.1177/1550147720912110

Sharkey, A., & Sharkey, N. (2012). Granny and the robots: Ethical issues in robot care for the elderly. *Ethics and Information Technology, 14*(1), 27–40. DOI: 10.1007/s10676-010-9234-6

Sheth, A., Jaimini, U., & Yip, H. Y. (2018). How will the Internet of Things enable augmented personalized health? *IEEE Intelligent Systems, 33*(1), 89–97. DOI: 10.1109/MIS.2018.012001556 PMID: 29887765

Tenner, E. (2015). The design of everyday things by Donald Norman [Review of the book The design of everyday things, by D. A. Norman]. *Technology and Culture, 56*(3), 785–787. DOI: 10.1353/tech.2015.0104

Thacharodi, A., Singh, P., Meenatchi, R., Tawfeeq Ahmed, Z. H., Kumar, R. R. S., v, N., Kavish, S., Maqbool, M., & Hassan, S. (2024). Revolutionizing healthcare and medicine: The impact of modern technologies for a healthier future—A comprehensive review. *Health Care Science, 3*(5), 329–349. DOI: 10.1002/hcs2.115 PMID: 39479277

Tian, Y. J., Wong, T., Chen, Q., & Denver, L. (2024). Benefits and barriers associated with the use of smart home health technologies in the care of older persons: A systematic review. *BMC Geriatrics, 24*(1), 152. DOI: 10.1186/s12877-024-04702-1 PMID: 38355464

Torab-Miandoab, A., Samad-Soltani, T., Jodati, A., & Rezaei-Hachesu, P. (2023). Interoperability of heterogeneous health information systems: A systematic literature review. *BMC Medical Informatics and Decision Making*, *23*(1), 18. DOI: 10.1186/s12911-023-02115-5 PMID: 36694161

Trout, K. E., Rampa, S., Wilson, F. A., & Stimpson, J. P. (2017). Legal mapping analysis of state telehealth reimbursement policies. *Telemedicine Journal and e-Health*, *23*(10), 805–814. DOI: 10.1089/tmj.2017.0016 PMID: 28430029

Tsvetanov, F. (2024). Integrating AI technologies into remote monitoring patient systems. *Engineering Proceedings*, *70*(1), 54. DOI: 10.3390/engproc2024070054

Vargemidis, D., Gerling, K., Spiel, K., Vanden Abeele, V., & Geurts, L. (2020). Wearable physical activity tracking systems for older adults—A systematic review. *ACM Transactions on Computing for Healthcare*, *1*(4), 25. DOI: 10.1145/3402523

Venkatesh, V., Morris, M. G., Davis, G. B., & Davis, F. D. (2003). User acceptance of information technology: Toward a unified view. *Management Information Systems Quarterly*, *27*(3), 425–478. DOI: 10.2307/30036540

Vo, D. K., & Trinh, K. T. L. (2024). Advances in wearable biosensors for healthcare: Current trends, applications, and future perspectives. *Biosensors (Basel)*, *14*(11), 560. DOI: 10.3390/bios14110560 PMID: 39590019

Voigt, P., & von dem Bussche, A. (2017). *The EU General Data Protection Regulation (GDPR): A practical guide*. Springer., DOI: 10.1007/978-3-319-57959-7

Wang, N., Cao, Z., Zhang, J., & Fuh, Y.-C. (2024). Perceptions and satisfaction with the use of digital medical services in urban older adults of China: Mixed methods study. *Journal of Medical Internet Research*, *26*, e48654. DOI: 10.2196/48654 PMID: 39303282

World Health Organization. (2020). *Global strategy on digital health 2020–2025*. https://www.who.int/docs/default-source/documents/gs4dhdaa2a9f352b0445bafbc79ca799dce4d.pdf

World Health Organization. (2024, October 1). *Ageing and health*. https://www.who.int/news-room/fact-sheets/detail/ageing-and-health

Yuksel, O. (2024). An overview of health services in the Industry 5.0 era. *International Journal of Engineering and Innovative Research*, *6*(3), 222–237. DOI: 10.47933/ijeir.1537942

Chapter 4
Remote Healthcare

Murat Konca
https://orcid.org/0000-0002-6830-8090
Çankırı Karatekin University, Turkey

ABSTRACT

In this chapter, a comprehensive evaluation of remote healthcare is presented, beginning with the definition of the concept and a detailed explanation of the key terms associated with it. Subsequently, the historical background of remote healthcare is examined and then the major benefits and the potential risks of remote healthcare are discussed. Furthermore, the possible challenges that may arise during the integration of remote healthcare services into national healthcare systems are addressed, alongside proposed solutions to these challenges. Afterward, future trends in remote healthcare are analyzed, with a particular focus on emerging issues likely to become prominent in the near future. The chapter concludes with a general evaluation, summarizing the main interests and insights. It is intended that this chapter will serve as a valuable resource for policymakers involved in decision-making processes related to remote healthcare, researchers conducting academic studies in this field, and all stakeholders engaged in the provision, utilization, and financing of remote healthcare.

INTRODUCTION

Advances in remote control and monitoring technology such as wireless connectivity, sensors, and identification along with the Internet of Things (IoT) have changed the way to provide healthcare services enabling remote healthcare, that is e-healthcare, to emerge (Boric-Lubecke et al. 2014). Remote healthcare can be defined as provision and utilization of healthcare services through technology without the necessity of healthcare services providers and users to come together

DOI: 10.4018/979-8-3373-3099-0.ch004

physically, and it refers to a broad range of health care aspects including electronic medical records, electronic prescriptions, remote monitoring, and health knowledge management (Jordanova & Lievens, 2011).

Remote healthcare is poised to significantly transform healthcare delivery soon. The worldwide remote healthcare market was thought to value at about 69 billion United States of America (U.S.) dollars in 2024 and is expected to expand at a compound annual growth rate of 21.3% from the beginning of 2025 to the end of 2030. This growth is largely a result of the increasing use of tele-medicine and advancements in digital health tools (Acumen Research and Consulting, 2024; Grand View Research, 2025).

In addition to its expanding economic footprint, the growing role of remote healthcare services in the overall provision of healthcare services is increasingly significant. The proportion of remote healthcare services within total global healthcare delivery varies by region and medical specialty. Nevertheless, recent scientific literature suggests a steady rise in the adoption of these services. Key drivers of this growth include positive consumer attitudes and substantial investments in digital health infrastructure. Furthermore, the SARS-CoV-2 / COVID-19 pandemic has served as a major catalyst, dramatically accelerating the adoption of remote healthcare (Keesara et al. 2020). For instance, it is estimated that the use of remote healthcare increased by a factor of 38 during the pandemic compared to pre-pandemic levels (Bestsennyy et al., 2021a). While usage rates have stabilized in the post-pandemic period, remote healthcare is expected to remain a central element of national healthcare strategies. In light of its sustained relevance, policymakers are increasingly called upon to critically assess the benefits and limitations of remote healthcare. This chapter seeks to explore these dimensions and contribute to an informed understanding of remote healthcare's implications for future healthcare policy and practice.

This chapter provides a comprehensive exploration of issues related to remote healthcare. Initially, it offers a detailed definition of remote healthcare and presents key concepts that form the foundation of this emerging field. This is followed by a subsection that focuses on the historical development of remote healthcare, offering insights into how the concept has evolved over time and gained significance in contemporary health systems.

Subsequently, the chapter examines both the advantages and the challenges associated with the implementation of remote healthcare practices. The benefits are considered from various perspectives, including patient accessibility, cost-effectiveness, and healthcare system efficiency, while the challenges are discussed in terms of technological limitations, data security concerns, and the need for regulatory frameworks.

In the latter part of the chapter, attention is directed toward future trends in remote healthcare, with particular emphasis on developments that are likely to become prominent in the near future. These include technological advancements, shifts in policy, and the evolving expectations of healthcare consumers and providers.

The chapter concludes with a general evaluation of the topics discussed, synthesizing the key points and providing a summary of the insights gained. This structured approach aims to provide readers with a coherent understanding of the current landscape and potential trajectory of remote healthcare services.

DEFINITION AND KEY CONCEPTS OF REMOTE HEALTHCARE

There is no generally accepted definition of remote healthcare in literature, however, there are some common points in different definitions (Wakerman, 2004; Smith et al. 2008; Roy et al. 2022). These common points can be specified as healthcare providers' and users' being in physically different locations and communicating through technological communication tools. From this point of view, the concept of remote healthcare is defined as provision and utilization of healthcare services without the necessity of healthcare services providers and users to come together physically thanks to the technology (Jordanova & Lievens, 2011). In a similar definition by Health Resources & Services Administration (HRSA) (2022), remote healthcare is defined as "*the use of electronic information and telecommunication technologies to support long-distance clinical health care, patient and professional health-related education, health administration, and public health*".

Celdrán et al. (2019) state that "*remote healthcare refers to the idea of removing the hospital borders and allowing people to stay in their own homes, providing person-centered medical services and technologies to support their individual care*". According to another definition of remote healthcare, "*patient care interactions that are geographically disparate and enabled by telecommunications, information technology, and sensor technology*" can be treated as remote healthcare (Haselkorn et al. 2007).

Remote healthcare means to provide "*healthcare services and exchange medical information through electronic communication technologies*" (Almathami et al 2020) or "*the utilization of technology to provide healthcare services beyond the confines of traditional settings*" (Atluri & Thummisetti, 2022) in some simpler definitions.

In all these definitions, the "*physical distance*" and "*technology*" come to the fore, and therefore, remote healthcare can be considered as the use of technology to remove the problem of inability to benefit from healthcare due to the physical distance (Institute of Medicine, 1996; NEJM-Catalyst, 2018).

The concept of remote healthcare, also known as e-healthcare, clearly defines what is implied by the terms of "*tele-health*" and "*tele-medicine*" (Ganapathy, 2020) and these terms have different meanings (Bashshur et al. 2011); the term "*tele-health*" is the broader term and "*tele-medicine*" is the component of "tele-health" specific to clinical care according to the Rural Tele-health Evaluation Center (RTEC) (2022). In this point, tele-health can be defined as: "*an improvement in the way healthcare provision is conceived and delivered by healthcare providers through the use of information and communication technologies to monitor and improve the wellbeing and health of patients and to empower patients in the management of their health and that of their families*" (Iyawa et al. 2016). while "*tele-medicine specifically refers to remote medical administrations*" (Puri, 2021).

As can be seen from the above definitions, *tele-medicine* is dealt with only medical administrations while *tele-health* also includes distant nonclinical administrations, such as supplier training, administrative gatherings, and continuing clinical education, in addition to clinical administrations (Puri, 2021). In other words, although the terms *tele-health* and *tele-medicine* are frequently used interchangeably in various publications, books, and magazines, they represent distinct concepts. *Tele-medicine* is defined as "*the remote diagnosis and treatment of patients by means of telecommunications technology*" whereas *tele-health* is described as "*the delivery and facilitation of health and health-related services including medical care, provider and patient education, health information services, and self-care via telecommunications and digital communication technologies*" (NEJM Catalyst, 2018). Based on these definitions, it is evident that *tele-health* encompasses a broader scope, as it includes a wider range of digital healthcare activities and services.

In the literature, it is seen that some other concepts are frequently used instead of or together with the concept of remote healthcare. Especially remote monitoring and imaging (tele-radiology), remote consultation (tele-consultation) and remote surgery (tele-surgery) are among the most frequently used concepts with remote health care.

Remote monitoring and imaging are components of remote healthcare. Remote monitoring can be seen as a way of collecting health data (for instance, heart rate, blood pressure, body temperature, blood sugar, etc.) from individuals at a distance through digital technologies and transmitting the data to healthcare providers in a different location for assessment and recommendations (Vegesna et al. 2017), whereas, remote imaging, or tele-radiology in other word, is limited to medical imaging services only such as X-rays, computed tomography and magnetic resonance imaging scans (Conway, 2016).

Remote consultation also stands out among the first concepts that come to mind when it comes to remote healthcare. However, remote consultations are related to functionality of tele-medicine, which is conceptually considered under remote healthcare (Bashshur et al. 2011). Therefore, although remote consultations are considered to be equivalent to remote healthcare in daily life, they are considered under the heading of tele-medicine, which is considered under remote healthcare.

Remote surgery, which has been a focal point of discussions about remote healthcare since the beginning of the 2000s, refers to the performance of surgeries by surgeons using robotic systems across geographically distant locations (Marescaux et al., 2001). This definition suggests that remote surgery falls under the umbrella of remote healthcare and is exclusively associated with surgical procedures.

HISTORICAL BACKGROUND

Although the historical origins of remote healthcare can be traced back to ancient times and early civilizations (Bashshur & Shannon, 2009; Ryu, 2010), in the modern sense, delivering healthcare remotely —through applications such as tele-medicine and tele-health— was first discussed in the late nineteenth century thanks to the widespread use of telephone and telegraph systems (Shirzadfar & Lotfi, 2017). Therefore, it can be stated that remote healthcare has a history spanning approximately 150 years.

An 1879 article in the *Lancet*, one of the longest-running and most famous journals in the field of medicine, proposed to use the telephone to reduce unnecessary office visits (Gaydos, 2019). It took approximately a quarter century for this proposal to be realized, and in 1906, Willem Einthoven —recognized as the inventor of the electrocardiogram— utilized the telephone network to conduct remote medical consultations (Rinde & Balteskard, 2002).

During the 1920s, interest in remote healthcare grew significantly, and several early implementations were introduced in this context. The Seamen's Church Institute (SCI), established in 1843 to improve conditions for seafarers, developed a radio service in 1920 under the call sign KDKF, marking a significant innovation in maritime medicine. Designed to connect land-based physicians with ships at sea, the KDKF service was soon adopted by the U.S. federal government and inspired similar tele-medical initiatives worldwide (Thayer & Dreisbach-Williams, 2023). Moreover, a 1925 issue of *Science and Invention Magazine* featured a cover illustration of a physician diagnosing a patient remotely via radio communication (Nesbitt, 2012), reflecting early public expectations that remote healthcare services and applications would become more prevalent in everyday life in the future.

A significant milestone in the history of remote healthcare occurred in 1948, when some physicians sent radiology images 24 miles over a telephone line to discuss the results with another physician in the U.S., which was the first formal implementation of tele-health and remote patient monitoring (HealthSnap, 2024). Meanwhile, physicians at the University of Nebraska began utilizing television technology to deliver instructional content to medical students. This initiative later expanded into a dedicated television link between the university and Norfolk State Hospital —located over 100 miles away— enabling applications such as remote psychiatric evaluations, speech therapy sessions, and the transmission of research seminars (Peng, 2022).

In the beginning of 1960s, with the development of technology and increasing reliance on technology, remote healthcare was used much more for psychiatric consultations (Hwei & Octavius, 2021). In the 1960s, the studies by the Nebraska Psychiatric Institute using a two-way closed-circuit TV link for education and consultations between specialists and general practitioners (Allan, 2006) somewhat helped remote healthcare increase its popularity among the medical community and patients. Meanwhile, officials at the National Aeronautics and Space Administration (NASA) used physiologic monitoring over a distance as a "tele-diagnosis" (Nesbitt, 2012), and the use of remote healthcare by NASA made the doubt for remote healthcare partially clear up (Zundel, 1996). Another important event that occurred towards the end of the 1960s was the establishment of the 9-1-1 system in the U.S. and its use for emergencies, especially emergency healthcare services. This system helped to eliminate the public's reservations about using technological communication tools in remote healthcare (Shirzadfar & Lotfi, 2017). As a result of the increase in the level of trust in technology and remote healthcare in 1960s, remote consultations and diagnoses were becoming common, and hence, exchange of medical information, laboratory data, images, X-rays, and health records via technological tools became popular, which paved the way for remote healthcare's adoption by wider circles, particularly by governments (Pallotta, 2021).

The acceptance of remote healthcare by governments was an important issue as it increased the access to the financing and funding necessary for further development of remote healthcare in the early 1970s (Zundel, 1996). The project of *Space Technology Applied to Rural Papago Advanced Health Care* (STARPAHC), which was developed by the Lockheed Missiles and Space Corporation and sponsored by NASA, was put into practice in 1975, and this project delivered remote healthcare for patients with major health problems, and great difficulty in accessing healthcare in southern Arizona. The outcomes of this project provided sufficient evidence regarding the reliability of remote healthcare, particularly remote consultations, and therefore, some other countries along with the U.S. initiated their infrastructure works for remote healthcare (Pallotta, 2021).

The proliferation of the Internet in the late 1980s and early 1990s marked a turning point for remote healthcare. The rise of the Internet has had significant consequences for the provision of healthcare services. It has become possible to transmit the information required for remote healthcare to even very distant locations using Internet protocols. In particular, this has made it possible to access medical images such as X-rays and scans remotely, to provide real-time audio and video consultations, and to instantly transmit vital signs and measurements related to human health (Shirzadfar & Lotfi, 2017).

In parallel to the proliferation of the Internet, the establishment of the American Tele-medicine Association (ATA) in 1993 represented another major milestone. According to the National Consortium of Tele-health Resource Centers (NCTRC, 2021), ATA played a crucial role in promoting the adoption of tele-medicine both in the U.S. and internationally. As Krupinski and Bernard (2014) note, ATA's foundation significantly contributed to the development of standards, the institutionalization of remote healthcare services, and the formulation of corresponding legal frameworks. In addition, the MUMPS (Massachusetts General Hospital Utility Multi-Programming System) programming language, originally developed at Massachusetts General Hospital in the 1970s, began to be integrated into electronic health record systems during this period. This marked a foundational shift in the technological infrastructure supporting remote healthcare in the U.S. (Munnecke & Kuhn, 1989).

When it came to remote healthcare in the 1990s, developed countries, especially the U.S., came to mind, however, remote healthcare was also piloted in several countries with limited resources during the 1990s. Satel-Life, an international non-profit organization, utilized micro-satellite technology to deliver health communication and information services in developing countries. This initiative played a significant role in promoting the global adoption of remote healthcare (Beard, 1993).

The 2000s can be seen as the years when the development rate of remote healthcare was at its highest. Although many events occurred during this period that increased the popularity of remote healthcare, especially those experienced in 2001, 2008, 2009 and 2020 come to the fore.

The Medicare, Medicaid, and Children's Health Insurance Program (CHIP) — formerly known as the State Children's Health Insurance Program (SCHIP)— *Benefits Improvement and Protection Act* (BIPA), enacted in 2001, significantly contributed to the advancement of remote healthcare in the U.S. The legislation facilitated the implementation of payment parity between in-person and tele-medicine visits under Medicare, mandated a $24 facility fee payment to the originating site for each tele-health encounter, and expanded the scope of remote healthcare services reimbursed by Medicare (Mathews et al. 2023).

The year 2001 marked a significant milestone in the history of remote surgery. In that year, Professor Jacques Marescaux successfully performed the first long-distance tele-surgical procedure—known as the Lindbergh Operation—in Strasbourg, France. The laparoscopic cholecystectomy, conducted on a 68-year-old patient, was completed in 54 minutes without complications, and had a major global impact on the development of tele-surgery (Picozzi et al., 2023).

In 2008, the *Medicare Improvements for Patients and Providers Act* (MIPPA), which came into force in the U.S., further expanded the range of remote healthcare services covered under Medicare by broadening the categories of eligible providers, including community mental health centers (Mathews et al. 2023).

In 2009, the *American Recovery and Reinvestment Act*, which was passed to mitigate the negative effects of the 2008 financial crisis in the U.S., further promoted and facilitated remote healthcare and technology related to it (National Consortium of Tele-health Resource Centers [NCTRC], 2021). In the same year, the *Health Information Technology for Economic and Clinical Health* (HITECH) *Act* was put into effect to encourage widespread use of electronic health records (Menachemi & Collum, 2011). In 2010, however, the Center for Medicare and Medicaid Services limited use of electronic health records in some issues due to the privacy of patient records (NCTRC, 2021).

And finally, in 2020, when the COVID-19 outbreak broke out, remote healthcare began to experience its golden age because it became mandatory rather than preferred due to the outbreak. The COVID-19 pandemic significantly accelerated the adoption of remote healthcare services worldwide. Before the pandemic, remote healthcare primarily served as a supplementary method to traditional in-person healthcare. However, with the outbreak of COVID-19 in 2020, remote healthcare became an essential tool for continuing patient care while reducing the risk of infection. The rapid transition of remote healthcare from a complementary service to a primary mode of healthcare delivery marked its golden age during the pandemic (NCTRC, 2021).

This shift is evident in the statistical data. For instance, during the COVID-19 pandemic, 30.1% of all physician visits in the U.S. were conducted via remote healthcare, a significant increase compared to the pre-pandemic period (Patel et al., 2021). This transition underscores the pivotal role of remote healthcare during a time when face-to-face healthcare delivery faced unprecedented challenges.

It is understood from the historical journey of remote healthcare, for a certain period, remote healthcare had been seen a way to deliver a rapid solution for the emergency healthcare needs of physically far away staff such as military personnel and those involved in space studies, or for delivering healthcare to people residing in distance places, however, at present, it has been used in many fields (Ganapathy, 2020; Pallotta, 2021; Madsen et al. 2023). Today, along with delivering healthcare services to physically far away staff for emergencies and patients who cannot access healthcare services due to the distance or another reason, remote healthcare is also used for a wide variety of purposes such as ensuring time saving, realizing cost-efficiency, and reducing health expenditure.

BENEFITS OF REMOTE HEALTHCARE

Remote healthcare and its applications represent a promising solution to the challenges faced by rural populations who require medical care but are unable to access it due to physical distance (Pramanik et al., 2019). Hence, these technologies can help reduce barriers to healthcare access in rural areas stemming from geographic isolation, economic limitations, and shortages of healthcare personnel. Although the proportion of people living in rural areas varies across countries and is gradually declining worldwide, a substantial segment of the global population still resides in these regions and often lacks adequate healthcare services due to geographic constraints. At this point, remote healthcare plays a critical role by enabling individuals in rural areas to access at least primary healthcare services, and in some cases, even advanced medical care (Dorsey & Topol, 2020). In addition, it facilitates service delivery in domains requiring continuity, such as chronic disease management and mental health services (Totten et al., 2016) and also contributes to cost reduction by minimizing the need for travel and shortening the time required to access medical services for people living in rural areas (Shigekawa et al., 2018). Moreover, in rural areas with limited healthcare personnel, tele-consultations support local healthcare providers, which improves the quality of diagnosis and treatment processes (WHO, 2010).

Remote healthcare also represents a significant alternative for individuals who experience difficulties in accessing healthcare institutions due to old age or severe disabilities. Given the benefits that remote healthcare provides —particularly for elderly individuals— and the rapidly increasing global aging population, these services are expected to become central to health policies in the near future (Hussain et al., 2015).

The fact that remote healthcare eliminates distances provides significant benefits not only for those living in rural areas and having problems related to accessing healthcare services, but also for those travelling long distances to utilize health tourism activities, which are gaining popularity day by day (Doğramacı, 2020). Patients can confirm their medical fitness via tele-consultation before travel, thus preventing unnecessary travel; follow-ups after surgical operations can be done remotely, allowing health tourists to return to their countries early. All of these can reduce costs in health tourism and pave the way for patients to turn to health tourism (Gu et al. 2021).

In emergencies, remote healthcare can be life-saving —one of its most significant advantages (Göde, 2023). Remote healthcare technologies enable patients to be rapidly assessed and appropriately directed for immediate intervention in time-sensitive conditions such as heart attacks, strokes, and trauma (Shiferaw & Zolfo, 2012).

Another important benefit of remote healthcare is its association with relatively low costs and an acceptable level of clinical effectiveness, contributing to overall cost-efficiency (Kruse et al., 2017; Ahmad et al., 2022), which implies that remote healthcare offers significant advantages in terms of both time and financial savings (Hwei & Octavius, 2021). Remote healthcare can be used efficiently and effectively in secondary and tertiary healthcare services as well as primary healthcare services. With the help of remote healthcare in primary healthcare services, accessing healthcare services, especially for those with chronic diseases, can be facilitated, patients and physicians can save time, unnecessary health expenditures can be reduced, and workforce losses can be prevented (Ekinci, 2022).

Remote healthcare can also be considered crucial in enhancing patient safety by eliminating the need for physical presence in healthcare facilities, thereby reducing the risk of hospital-acquired infections (Garzotto et al., 2021). Furthermore, remote healthcare may help reduce hospital-acquired infections through shortening hospital stays via remote postoperative follow-ups, decreasing hospital admissions through regular remote monitoring of chronic diseases, and filtering hospital visits of patients with suspected infectious diseases using tele-medicine-based triage systems (Bestsennyy et al. 2021b).

Remote healthcare has enabled significant gains to be achieved in extraordinary times such as the COVID-19 pandemic (Smolić et al., 2022). It can be stated that remote healthcare was often the only possible way of providing care to patients during a certain period of the outbreak (Abdellatif & Mohamed, 2020). Moreover, it was possible to protect hospitals from being overwhelmed with cases that can be managed at home through remote healthcare and its applications (Rouidi et al. 2022).

Shortly, remote healthcare and its applications help people in rural areas access to healthcare, enables patients to manage their illness, can be life-saving in emergencies, enhance the quality of life among people receiving healthcare at home, make things easier for both receiving and providing home-based palliative care services, reduce unnecessary hospitalization along with the hospital care costs and hospital-acquired infections and enable uninterrupted provision of healthcare services during pandemics (Abdellatif & Mohamed, 2020; Garzotto et al., 2021; Steindal et al. 2023).

CHALLENGES IN THE IMPLEMENTATION OF REMOTE HEALTHCARE

Although the benefits of remote healthcare are indisputable, this mode of healthcare delivery also raises several concerns, particularly regarding ethical issues such as patient privacy and information confidentiality. Individuals who utilize remote healthcare services must place complete trust in their providers, as they often lack the means to verify whether regulatory standards for privacy and security are being upheld (Javed et al., 2021). This reliance on trust may cause individuals to hesitate in using remote healthcare services. The literature highlights that recurring security vulnerabilities in remote healthcare services undermine users' confidence and impede the widespread adoption of such services (Kruse et al., 2017).

Furthermore, fulfilling ethical responsibilities can be more challenging in remote settings, primarily due to the inherently limited nature of the doctor —patient relationship in virtual interactions. Consequently, scholars have emphasized the need to revisit fundamental ethical principles —such as patient privacy and informed consent— within the context of expanding remote healthcare practices (Shachar et al., 2020).

Concerns surrounding remote healthcare extend beyond ethical and privacy-related matters to include pricing and reimbursement mechanisms, inadequacies in the legal framework —particularly in handling malpractice lawsuits— the scope of services deliverable via remote platforms, and the availability of requisite technological infrastructure (Doğramacı, 2020; Arık, 2023). In many countries, regulatory and policy frameworks governing the reimbursement of remote healthcare services remain ambiguous. This uncertainty may erode the confidence of both healthcare providers and patients regarding the long-term viability of such services. To ensure sustainability and broader adoption, reimbursement mechanisms must be clearly defined and standardized.

Moreover, reimbursement rates for remote healthcare are often lower than those for traditional in-person services. While this cost reduction may be considered beneficial from a governmental budgeting perspective, it may simultaneously deter private sector investment in remote healthcare infrastructure. Therefore, it is essential to develop comprehensive policy mechanisms that incentivize private stakeholders to actively support and expand remote healthcare delivery systems (Wilson et al., 2017).

When it comes to remote healthcare, deficiencies in the legal framework —particularly the inadequacy of current structures in addressing malpractice cases— pose a significant concern. Countries intending to implement remote healthcare should thoroughly re-examine their legal nature. Legal ambiguity may arise especially regarding physicians' obligations to conduct in-person examinations and the alignment of remote healthcare practices with established medical standards. Furthermore, since patients are considered consumers under healthcare law, remote healthcare applications may fall under the category of distance contracts governed by consumer protection regulations. Without specific legal provisions in this area, uncertainties —particularly concerning malpractice liability— are likely to emerge. Therefore, tailored legal reforms are essential for countries planning to adopt remote healthcare systems (Doğramacı, 2020).

In addition to legal ambiguities, technological limitations pose another substantial barrier to the effectiveness of remote healthcare. Inadequate infrastructure compromises the efficiency and accessibility of services, particularly in underserved or rural areas, thereby exacerbating existing healthcare disparities (Bashshur et al., 2014). In addition, technical limitations —such as low-resolution image transfers or interrupted video conferences —may hinder diagnostic accuracy in image-based specialties (e.g., radiology or dermatology), potentially leading to misdiagnoses (Warshaw et al. 2009; Wootton et al., 2012).

Disparities in access to remote healthcare arise not only from regional technological inequalities but also from variations in patients' digital literacy levels. These disparities may be further compounded by generational gaps and socioeconomic status, making it more difficult for certain populations to benefit from digital health innovations. As such, future healthcare models may necessitate the integration of digital literacy training and technology access programs to ensure equitable service delivery (Norman & Skinner, 2006).

In the provision of remote healthcare, unauthorized or unlicensed service providers may exploit regulatory gaps or operate through unregulated platforms. This situation poses serious risks to patient safety and treatment quality (Akgün, 2021). Therefore, governments aiming to integrate remote healthcare into their national systems must implement strict regulatory measures and oversight mechanisms to prevent the involvement of illegitimate actors.

In summary, governments seeking to integrate remote healthcare into their national health systems must consider several critical factors. These include addressing ethical concerns such as patient privacy and informed consent, reforming legal frameworks —particularly regarding malpractice liability— and establishing clear reimbursement mechanisms. Additionally, investments in technological infrastructure, initiatives to enhance digital literacy among populations, and stringent measures to prevent unauthorized or unlicensed service provision are essential for sustainable implementation.

FUTURE TRENDS AND DEBATES IN REMOTE HEALTHCARE

Recent developments in remote healthcare have demonstrated a marked shift towards the use of mobile technologies and smart devices —including wearable, portable, and even implantable systems— for the provision of healthcare services. Alongside these physical technologies, mobile applications and cloud-based platforms are being actively investigated for their utility in remote healthcare. These evolving trends collectively suggest that remote healthcare will increasingly depend on mobile and internet-connected devices, a framework broadly encompassed by the concept of "*Mobile Health*" (mHealth).

mHealth refers to a subset of remote healthcare that involves the delivery and monitoring of medical services via mobile devices and wireless communication technologies. Core functionalities of mHealth include patient monitoring, real-time health data collection, and enhanced patient-provider communication through devices such as smartphones, tablets, and wearable technologies (Free et al., 2013).

The increasing relevance of mHealth is driven not only by technological advancement but also by global healthcare challenges. These include aging populations, the growing prevalence of chronic diseases, and escalating healthcare costs —all of which place substantial pressure on traditional health systems. In this context, mHealth emerges as a cost-effective and scalable solution that both facilitates individual access to care and contributes to the sustainability of healthcare infrastructures (Mangone et al. 2016; Tornvall et al. 2025).

Looking ahead, mHealth is expected to play a critical role in various domains, including chronic disease management, mental health tracking, prenatal care, and medication adherence. One of its most promising features is the capacity to collect patient health data in real time and integrate it into clinical decision support systems, thereby enabling timely and proactive medical interventions (Mosa et al., 2012).

The transformation in remote healthcare driven by mHealth is further accelerated by advancements in the IoT and Artificial Intelligence (AI). IoT-enabled devices ensure continuous monitoring by transmitting patient data to central systems, where AI-driven algorithms can analyze it for irregularities and generate alerts for healthcare professionals. This technological synergy not only enables early diagnosis but also facilitates the development of personalized treatment strategies, ultimately improving clinical outcomes (Islam et al., 2015).

mHealth represents a paradigm shift in healthcare delivery —one that is increasingly data-driven, patient-centered, and enabled by emerging technologies. Its integration with IoT and AI promises to redefine the landscape of remote healthcare in the near future.

Another crucial issue to be discussed in a near future regarding to the remote healthcare is the use of AI in remote mode of healthcare delivery. AI has increasingly become integrated into healthcare systems, particularly into diagnostic systems. The AI-assisted diagnostic tools utilize machine learning algorithms, deep neural networks and deep learning to analyze complex medical data, including radiographic images, pathology slides, and electronic health records, to support clinical decision-making processes (Topol, 2019). Their promise lies in improving diagnostic accuracy, reducing human error, and alleviating workload in overburdened health systems. When AI systems are integrated into remote healthcare systems, the promises of

AI systems will be felt more and therefore the use of both remote healthcare and AI systems will be almost inevitable in a near future.

Despite the above-mentioned advantages of AI, several key debates surround the deployment of AI in healthcare. One central concern is whether AI systems may eventually replace human physicians. While current consensus suggests that AI is more likely to help rather than replace human expertise, the possibility of deskilling among healthcare professionals and overreliance on algorithms remains a valid concern (Jiang et al., 2017). Another major topic is data bias. AI models trained on unrepresentative or biased datasets may produce inequitable outcomes, particularly disadvantaging minority populations (Obermeyer et al., 2019). Ensuring diversity in training datasets and transparency in model development is crucial to mitigate these issues.

Ethical considerations also come to the fore when it comes to AI in healthcare. Questions around accountability arise when errors occur in the diagnosis, prognosis and treatment processes —whether the blame lies with the AI developers, the healthcare institution, or the clinicians using the system. Additionally, the use of patient data to train AI models raises privacy and consent concerns. Though anonymization techniques are often employed, the potential for re-identification persists, necessitating stringent data governance frameworks (Morley et al., 2020).

Using AI-assisted systems in remote healthcare systems hold transformative potential in improving healthcare delivery and diagnostic precision. However, realizing this potential requires careful navigation of ethical, legal, and social implications. Collaborative efforts among technologists, clinicians, ethicists, and policymakers are essential to develop frameworks that ensure safety, fairness, and accountability while using AI in remote healthcare.

The digital divide while using remote healthcare services and unequal access to them are also thought to be among the debates expected to shape the near future of remote healthcare. Remote healthcare is now a pivotal component of the broader digital transformation in health systems. However, this evolution has not been uniformly experienced across all segments of the population. Individuals without reliable internet connectivity or adequate access to digital devices often find themselves unable to fully benefit from such services. Consequently, the concept of the "digital divide" has gained renewed attention within the context of remote healthcare delivery (Saeed & Masters, 2021).

The digital divide encompasses more than the mere absence of physical access and also reflects disparities in digital literacy, technological competence, and socioeconomic status. Vulnerable populations —including older adults, rural residents, and low-income groups—face disproportionately greater challenges in utilizing remote healthcare platforms (Nouri et al., 2020). These disparities exacerbate existing inequalities in healthcare access and contribute to broader social stratification.

In light of these challenges, targeted efforts aimed at enhancing digital literacy among both healthcare providers and patients will be essential. Addressing these barriers is likely to form a core element of future policy discussions on equitable access to remote healthcare.

A summary of what is stated above can be expressed as follows; AI, the IoT and wearable technologies have become the basic components of remote healthcare services within Health 4.0. Thanks to these technologies, patients' health data can be monitored instantly, and diagnosis and treatment processes can be carried out more quickly and effectively. Today, there is a transition towards Health 5.0, and this transformation highlights individual-focused, personalized and more human-centered healthcare services. In the near future, with the use of advanced virtual technologies such as the metaverse in remote healthcare services, innovative applications such as virtual clinics, avatar doctor examinations and simulation-based treatment methods will be implemented. These developments will increase the accessibility of healthcare services and radically transform the patients' experience.

Advancement in technology also brings risks, and these risks will be discussed more soon as using technology becomes more prevalent in healthcare provision. In the near future, it is quite possible to encounter a wide range of risks, such as confidentiality of information and private life, the complete elimination of human interaction, which is a requirement of human nature, in the healthcare provision process, and how and by which authority AI will be judged as a result of a wrong decision.

CONCLUSION

Remote healthcare holds considerable promise in improving the accessibility of healthcare services across diverse populations. This potential is particularly critical for individuals residing in geographically isolated or underserved rural areas, where physical proximity to healthcare facilities is limited or entirely lacking. Furthermore, remote healthcare offers practical solutions for people whose professional responsibilities hinder their ability to access conventional healthcare settings —examples include maritime workers who spend extended periods at sea, as well as individuals engaged in space missions where access to on-site medical care is virtually non-existent. Additionally, remote healthcare serves as a crucial enabler of healthcare access for individuals with limited mobility due to advanced age or severe physical disabilities, thereby fostering greater inclusivity within the healthcare system.

Another significant advantage of remote healthcare is its ability to facilitate the rapid assessment and triage of patients experiencing time-sensitive medical emergencies such as myocardial infarctions (heart attacks), cerebrovascular accidents (strokes), and various forms of traumatic injury. In such scenarios, the immediacy with which patients can be evaluated and appropriately directed toward necessary interventions through remote healthcare platforms can be life-saving. This function underscores the critical role that remote healthcare can play in emergency response systems.

In addition to enhancing accessibility and improving emergency response times, remote healthcare tends to be associated with relatively lower operational costs when compared to traditional, in-person healthcare delivery models. The reduction in costs stems from decreased infrastructure needs and the minimization of ancillary expenses, such as patient transportation or administrative overhead.

Moreover, from a public health perspective, remote healthcare also contributes significantly to infection control, as it minimizes the risk of nosocomial, or hospital-acquired, infections by reducing the number of patients who need to be physically present in clinical environments.

Remote healthcare is increasingly being recognized as a favorable alternative to traditional modes of care delivery, especially in crisis times such as pandemics. The advantages of remote healthcare become particularly pronounced during periods of widespread infectious disease outbreaks, as exemplified by the global COVID-19 pandemic. During such crises, remote healthcare has demonstrated a critical capacity to maintain continuity of care while simultaneously mitigating viral transmission risks associated with in-person medical visits.

It is obvious that remote healthcare will become a part of daily life in a near future. mHealth technologies and AI applications will radically transform the delivery of healthcare services in the digital environment probably in the next few decades. With smartphones, wearable devices and remote monitoring systems, individuals will be able to monitor their health status instantly, while artificial intelligence-supported applications will increase the effectiveness of healthcare services in many areas, from symptom analysis to early diagnosis, from personalized treatment recommendations to medication monitoring. In this way, the workload of healthcare professionals will be reduced, and individuals living in rural and disadvantaged areas will have easier access to qualified healthcare services.

In summary, remote healthcare not only expands access to medical services for hard-to-reach populations and individuals with mobility constraints but also enhances the healthcare system's ability to respond to emergencies efficiently, operates at lower costs, reduces infection risks, and proves especially advantageous during public health emergencies. Each of these attributes highlights the multifaceted value of remote healthcare in both routine and extraordinary healthcare contexts.

Owing to its numerous advantages, remote healthcare has attracted growing interest from policymakers worldwide. As a result, an increasing number of governments are actively exploring ways to incorporate remote healthcare solutions into their national health systems. This growing momentum places a set of critical responsibilities on policymakers to ensure effective and equitable implementation.

In this context, a key responsibility is the formulation of supportive regulatory frameworks that facilitate the widespread adoption of remote healthcare technologies. Equally important is the prioritization of investments in robust technical infrastructure, particularly in underserved and rural areas where digital connectivity remains limited. Additionally, providing targeted training for healthcare professionals to ensure effective use of remote care tools is vital for operational success.

As discussed in detail in this section, remote healthcare provides a wide range of benefits in many areas. However, these benefits do not necessitate ignoring the risks of remote healthcare. It is essential that governments preparing to integrate remote healthcare services into national healthcare systems are aware of the risks of data leakage, unauthorized access, eavesdropping on confidential conversations, recording video calls without consent, cyber-attacks, lack of informed consent, incorrect/incomplete diagnosis, and weakening of the doctor-patient relationship, and take precautions.

For remote healthcare to be sustainably integrated into existing health systems, policymakers must also address systemic factors such as reimbursement mechanisms. Incorporating remote healthcare services into insurance and public funding schemes will be essential in building a resilient and trustworthy remote healthcare ecosystem.

REFERENCES

Abdellatif, M. M., & Mohamed, W. (2020). Telemedicine: An IoT based remote healthcare system. *International Journal of Online and Biomedical Engineering*, *16*(6), 72–85. DOI: 10.3991/ijoe.v16i06.13651

Acumen Research and Consulting. (2024). *Remote healthcare market*. https://www.acumenresearchandconsulting.com/press-releases/remote-healthcare-market

Ahmad, I., Asghar, Z., Kumar, T., Li, G., Manzoor, A., Mikhaylov, K., Shah, S. A., Höyhtyä, M., Reponen, J., Huusko, J., & Harjula, E. (2022). Emerging technologies for next generation remote health care and assisted living. *IEEE Access : Practical Innovations, Open Solutions*, *10*, 56094–56132. DOI: 10.1109/ACCESS.2022.3177278

Akgün, Z. (2021). Evaluation of the regulation on providing remote healthcare services. *Türkiye Biyoetik Dergisi*, *8*(4), 194–198. DOI: 10.5505/tjob.2021.49344

Allan, R. (2006, June 15). *A brief history of telemedicine*. Electronic Design. https://www.electronicdesign.com/technologies/components/article/21770508/a-brief-history-of-telemedicine

Almathami, H. K. Y., Win, K. T., & Vlahu-Gjorgievska, E. (2020). Barriers and facilitators that influence telemedicine-based, real-time, online consultation at patients' homes: Systematic literature review. *Journal of Medical Internet Research*, *22*(2), e16407. DOI: 10.2196/16407 PMID: 32130131

Arık, Y. (2023). Evaluation of telemedicine applications within the scope of healthcare marketing. *Hacettepe Journal of Health Administration*, *26*(2), 511–534.

Atluri, H., & Thummisetti, B. S. P. (2022). A holistic examination of patient outcomes, healthcare accessibility, and technological integration in remote healthcare delivery. *Transactions on Latest Trends in Health Sector*, *14*(14), 1–14.

Bashshur, R. L., & Shannon, G. W. (2009). *History of telemedicine: Evolution, context, and transformation*. Mary Ann Liebert.

Bashshur, R. L., Shannon, G. W., Krupinski, E. A., & Grigsby, J. (2011). The taxonomy of telemedicine. *Telemedicine Journal and e-Health*, *17*(6), 484–494. DOI: 10.1089/tmj.2011.0103 PMID: 21718114

Bashshur, R. L., Shannon, G. W., Smith, B. R., Alverson, D. C., Antoniotti, N., Barsan, W. G., Bashshur, N., Brown, E. M., Coye, M. J., Doarn, C. R., Ferguson, S., Grigsby, J., Krupinski, E. A., Kvedar, J. C., Linkous, J., Merrell, R. C., Nesbitt, T., Poropatich, R., Rheuban, K. S., & Yellowlees, P. (2014). The empirical foundations of telemedicine interventions for chronic disease management. *Telemedicine Journal and e-Health*, *20*(9), 769–800. DOI: 10.1089/tmj.2014.9981 PMID: 24968105

Beard, N. (1993, March 1). *Wired doctors*. Wired. https://www.wired.com/1993/03/wired-doctors/

Bestsennyy, O., Gilbert, G., Harris, A., & Rost, J. (2021a). *Telehealth: A quarter-trillion-dollar post-COVID-19 reality?* McKinsey & Company. https://www.mckinsey.com/industries/healthcare/our-insights/telehealth-a-quarter-trillion-dollar-post-covid-19-reality

Bestsennyy, O., Gilbert, G., Harris, A., & Rost, J. (2021b). *Telehealth: A quarter-trillion-dollar post-COVID-19 reality?* Connect with Care. https://connectwithcare.org/wp-content/uploads/2021/07/telehealth-a-quarter-trillion-dollar-post-covid-19-reality.pdf

Boric-Lubecke, O., Gao, X., Yavari, E., Baboli, M., Singh, A., & Lubecke, V. M. (2014). E-healthcare: Remote monitoring, privacy, and security. In *2014 IEEE MTT-S International Microwave Symposium (IMS2014)* (pp. 1–3). IEEE. DOI: 10.1109/MWSYM.2014.6848595

Celdrán, A. H., Pérez, M. G., Clemente, F. J. G., Ippoliti, F., & Pérez, G. M. (2019). Dynamic network slicing management of multimedia scenarios for future remote healthcare. *Multimedia Tools and Applications*, *78*(17), 24707–24737. DOI: 10.1007/s11042-019-7283-3

Conway, S. (2016). Teleradiology and telemedicine: They are not equal. *Applied Radiology*, *45*(8), 28–29. https://appliedradiology.com/articles/teleradiology-and-telemedicine-they-are-not-equal. DOI: 10.37549/AR2289

Doğramacı, Y. G. (2020). Telemedicine, health tourism and remote health services: Distance contracts. *İstanbul Hukuk Mecmuası, 78*(2), 657–710. DOI: 10.26650/ihm.2020.78.2.0008

Dorsey, E. R., & Topol, E. J. (2020). State of telehealth. *The New England Journal of Medicine*, *382*(18), 1670–1671. DOI: 10.1056/NEJMp2003107

Ekinci, B. (2022). Remote health service delivery (telemedicine) project. *Turkey Health Literacy Journal*, *3*(2), 122–124.

Free, C., Phillips, G., Watson, L., Galli, L., Felix, L., Edwards, P., Patel, V., & Haines, A. (2013). The effectiveness of mobile-health technologies to improve health care service delivery processes: A systematic review and meta-analysis. *PLoS Medicine*, *10*(1), e1001363. DOI: 10.1371/journal.pmed.1001363 PMID: 23458994

Ganapathy, K. (2020). Space medicine: The ultimate in remote health care. *Telehealth and Medicine Today*, *5*(2), 1–4. DOI: 10.30953/tmt.v5.178

Garzotto, F., Comoretto, R. I., Ostermann, M., Nalesso, F., Gregori, D., Bonavina, M. G., Zanardo, G., & Meneghesso, G. (2021). Preventing infectious diseases in intensive care unit by medical devices remote control: Lessons from COVID-19. *Journal of Critical Care*, *61*, 119–124. DOI: 10.1016/j.jcrc.2020.10.014 PMID: 33157307

Gaydos, J. (2019). *Audio visual connection: Brief history of telemedicine*. HMP Global Learning Network. https://www.hmpgloballearningnetwork.com/site/twc/articles/audio-visual-connection-brief-history-telemedicine

Göde, A. (2023). Uzaktan sağlık hizmetlerinin yeri ve geleceği. [The place and future of remote health services] In Söyler, S., & Çavmak, D. (Eds.), *Modern sağlık yönetiminde temel konular* (pp. 183–201). Eğitim Publishing House.

Grand View Research. (2025). *Remote healthcare market size, share & trends analysis report*. https://www.grandviewresearch.com/industry-analysis/remote-healthcare-market

Gu, D., Humbatova, G., Xie, Y., Yang, X., Zolotarev, O., & Zhang, G. (2021). Different roles of telehealth and telemedicine on medical tourism: An empirical study from Azerbaijan. *Health Care*, *9*(8), 1073. DOI: 10.3390/healthcare9081073 PMID: 34442210

Haselkorn, A., Coye, M. J., & Doarn, C. R. (2007). The future of remote health services: Summary of an expert panel discussion. *Telemedicine Journal and e-Health*, *13*(3), 341–347. DOI: 10.1089/tmj.2006.0078 PMID: 17603837

Health Resources & Services Administration. (2022). *What is telehealth?* https://www.hrsa.gov/telehealth/what-is-telehealth

HealthSnap. (2024). *The evolution of remote care management*. https://healthsnap.io/the-evolution-of-remote-care-management/

Hussain, A., Wenbi, R., da Silva, A. L., Nadher, M., & Mudhish, M. (2015). Health and emergency-care platform for the elderly and disabled people in the Smart City. *Journal of Systems and Software*, *110*, 253–263. DOI: 10.1016/j.jss.2015.08.041

Hwei, L. R. Y., & Octavius, G. S. (2021). Potential advantages and disadvantages of telemedicine: A literature review from the perspectives of patients, medical personnel, and hospitals. *Journal of Community Empowerment for Health*, *4*(3), 180–186. DOI: 10.22146/jcoemph.64247

Institute of Medicine. (1996). *Telemedicine: A guide to assessing telecommunications in health care*. National Academies Press., DOI: 10.17226/5296

Islam, S. M. R., Kwak, D., Kabir, M. H., Hossain, M., & Kwak, K.-S. (2015). The Internet of Things for health care: A comprehensive survey. *IEEE Access : Practical Innovations, Open Solutions*, *3*, 678–708. DOI: 10.1109/ACCESS.2015.2437951

Iyawa, G. E., Herselman, M., & Botha, A. (2016). Digital health innovation ecosystems: From systematic literature review to conceptual framework. *Procedia Computer Science*, *100*, 244–252. DOI: 10.1016/j.procs.2016.09.149

Javed, I. T., Alharbi, F., Bellaj, B., Margaria, T., Crespi, N., & Qureshi, K. N. (2021). Health-ID: A blockchain-based decentralized identity management for remote healthcare. *Health Care*, *9*(6), 712. DOI: 10.3390/healthcare9060712 PMID: 34200778

Jiang, F., Jiang, Y., Zhi, H., Dong, Y., Li, H., Ma, S., Wang, Y., Dong, Q., Shen, H., & Wang, Y. (2017). Artificial intelligence in healthcare: Past, present and future. *Stroke and Vascular Neurology*, *2*(4), 230–243. DOI: 10.1136/svn-2017-000101 PMID: 29507784

Jordanova, M., & Lievens, F. (2011). Global telemedicine and eHealth: A synopsis. In *2011 E-Health and Bioengineering Conference (EHB)* (pp. 1–6). IEEE. DOI: 10.1109/EHB.2011.6107668

Keesara, S., Jonas, A., & Schulman, K. (2020). Covid-19 and health care's digital revolution. *The New England Journal of Medicine*, *382*(23), e82. DOI: 10.1056/NEJMp2005835 PMID: 32240581

Krupinski, E. A., & Bernard, J. (2014). Standards and guidelines in telemedicine and telehealth. *Health Care*, *2*(1), 74–93. DOI: 10.3390/healthcare2010074 PMID: 27429261

Kruse, C. S., Soma, M., Pulluri, D., Nemali, N. T., & Brooks, M. (2017). The effectiveness of telemedicine in the management of chronic heart disease—A systematic review. *JRSM Open*, *8*(3), 2054270416681747. DOI: 10.1177/2054270416681747 PMID: 28321319

Madsen, C., Poropatich, R., & Koehlmoos, T. P. (2023). Telehealth in the Military Health System: Impact, obstacles, and opportunities. *Military Medicine*, *188*(Supplement_1), 15–23. DOI: 10.1093/milmed/usac207 PMID: 36882030

Mangone, E. R., Agarwal, S., L'Engle, K., Lasway, C., Zan, T., van Beijma, H., Orkis, J., & Karam, R. (2016). Sustainable cost models for mHealth at scale: Modeling program data from m4RH Tanzania. *PLoS One*, *11*(1), e0148011. DOI: 10.1371/journal.pone.0148011 PMID: 26824747

Marescaux, J., Leroy, J., Gagner, M., Rubino, F., Mutter, D., Vix, M., Butner, S. E., & Smith, M. K. (2001). Transatlantic robot-assisted telesurgery. *Nature*, *413*(6854), 379–380. DOI: 10.1038/35096636 PMID: 11574874

Mathews, D., Abernethy, A., Butte, A. J., Glicksberg, B. S., & Kulikowski, C. (2023). *Telehealth and mobile health case study for understanding and anticipating emerging science and technology* (NAM Perspectives). National Academy of Medicine. DOI: 10.31478/202311e

Menachemi, N., & Collum, T. H. (2011). Benefits and drawbacks of electronic health record systems. *Risk Management and Healthcare Policy*, *4*, 47–55. DOI: 10.2147/RMHP.S12985 PMID: 22312227

Morley, J., Machado, C. C. V., Burr, C., Cowls, J., Joshi, I., Taddeo, M., & Floridi, L. (2020). The ethics of AI in health care: A mapping review. *Social Science & Medicine*, *260*, 113172. DOI: 10.1016/j.socscimed.2020.113172 PMID: 32702587

Mosa, A. S. M., Yoo, I., & Sheets, L. (2012). A systematic review of healthcare applications for smartphones. *BMC Medical Informatics and Decision Making*, *12*(1), 67. DOI: 10.1186/1472-6947-12-67 PMID: 22781312

Munnecke, T. H., & Kuhn, I. M. (1989). Large-scale portability of hospital information system software within the Veterans Administration. In *Proceedings of the Annual Symposium on Computer Application in Medical Care* (pp. 133–137). American Medical Informatics Association., https://www.ncbi.nlm.nih.gov/pmc/articles/PMC2244995/ DOI: 10.1007/978-1-4612-3488-3_8

National Consortium of Telehealth Resource Centers. (2021). *History of telehealth.* https://telehealthresourcecenter.org/wp-content/uploads/2021/11/History_of_Telehealth.pdf

NEJM Catalyst. (2018). What is telehealth? *NEJM Catalyst Innovations in Care Delivery*, *4*(2). DOI: 10.1056/CAT.18.0268

Nesbitt, T. S. (2012). The evolution of telehealth: Where have we been and where are we going? In Lustig, T. A. (Ed.), *The role of telehealth in an evolving health care environment* (pp. 11–16). National Academies Press.

Norman, C. D., & Skinner, H. A. (2006). eHealth literacy: Essential skills for consumer health in a networked world. *Journal of Medical Internet Research*, *8*(2), e9. DOI: 10.2196/jmir.8.2.e9 PMID: 16867972

Nouri, S., Khoong, E. C., Lyles, C. R., & Karliner, L. (2020). Addressing equity in telemedicine for chronic disease management during the Covid-19 pandemic. *NEJM Catalyst Innovations in Care Delivery*, *1*(3). DOI: 10.1056/CAT.20.0123

Obermeyer, Z., Powers, B., Vogeli, C., & Mullainathan, S. (2019). Dissecting racial bias in an algorithm used to manage the health of populations. *Science*, *366*(6464), 447–453. DOI: 10.1126/science.aax2342 PMID: 31649194

Pallotta, G. (2021). *Analysis and development of a tele-health system to support remote areas* [Doctoral dissertation, University of Camerino]. UniCam Eprints. https://pubblicazioni.unicam.it/retrieve/0bdcc121-fde0-4c54-bfbf-4a3927e33f7d/PALLOTTA%20GRAZIANO%20PHD%20THESIS%2023.06.pdf

Patel, S. Y., Mehrotra, A., Huskamp, H. A., Uscher-Pines, L., Ganguli, I., & Barnett, M. L. (2021). Variation in telemedicine use and outpatient care during the COVID-19 pandemic in the United States. *Health Affairs*, *40*(2), 349–358. DOI: 10.1377/hlthaff.2020.01786 PMID: 33523745

Peng, I. (2022). *A history of telemedicine in America*. RexMD. https://rexmd.com/learn/a-history-of-telemedicine-in-america

Picozzi, P., Nocco, U., Puleo, G., Labate, C., & Cimolin, V. (2023). Telemedicine and robotic surgery: A narrative review to analyze advantages, limitations and future developments. *Electronics (Basel)*, *13*(1), 124. DOI: 10.3390/electronics13010124

Pramanik, P. K. D., Pareek, G., & Nayyar, A. (2019). Security and privacy in remote healthcare: Issues, solutions, and standards. In Tripathy, B. K., & Acharjya, D. P. (Eds.), *Telemedicine technologies* (pp. 201–225). Academic Press., DOI: 10.1016/B978-0-12-816948-3.00014-3

Puri, V. (2021). Telemedicine history and its advantages. *General Medicine: Open Access*, *9*(10), 1–2. DOI: 10.35248/2327-5146.21.9.351

Rinde, E., & Balteskard, L. (2002). Is there a future for telemedicine? *Lancet*, *359*(9322), 1957–1958. DOI: 10.1016/S0140-6736(02)08845-1 PMID: 12076546

Rouidi, M., Hamdoune, A., Choujtani, K., & Chati, A. (2022). TAM-UTAUT and the acceptance of remote healthcare technologies by healthcare professionals: A systematic review. *Informatics in Medicine Unlocked*, *32*, 101008. DOI: 10.1016/j.imu.2022.101008

Roy, J., Levy, D. R., & Senathirajah, Y. (2022). Defining telehealth for research, implementation, and equity. *Journal of Medical Internet Research*, *24*(4), e35037. DOI: 10.2196/35037 PMID: 35416778

Rural Telehealth Evaluation Center. (2022). *Telehealth: Current definitions and future trends*. University of Arkansas for Medical Sciences. https://idhi.uams.edu/rtec/wp-content/uploads/sites/4/2022/05/Telehealth-Definitions-Paper-06MAY2022-1.pdf

Ryu, S. (2010). History of telemedicine: Evolution, context, and transformation. *Healthcare Informatics Research*, *16*(1), 65–66. DOI: 10.4258/hir.2010.16.1.65 PMID: 22509475

Saeed, S. A., & Masters, R. M. (2021). Disparities in health care and the digital divide. *Current Psychiatry Reports*, *23*(9), 61. DOI: 10.1007/s11920-021-01274-4 PMID: 34297202

Shachar, C., Engel, J., & Elwyn, G. (2020). Implications for telehealth in a post-pandemic future: Regulatory and privacy issues. *Journal of the American Medical Association*, *323*(23), 2375–2376. DOI: 10.1001/jama.2020.7943 PMID: 32421170

Shiferaw, F., & Zolfo, M. (2012). The role of information communication technology (ICT) towards universal health coverage: The first steps of a telemedicine project in Ethiopia. *Global Health Action*, *5*(1), 15638. DOI: 10.3402/gha.v5i0.15638 PMID: 22479235

Shigekawa, E., Fix, M., Corbett, G., Roby, D. H., & Coffman, J. (2018). The current state of telehealth evidence: A rapid review. *Health Affairs*, *37*(12), 1975–1982. DOI: 10.1377/hlthaff.2018.05132 PMID: 30633674

Shirzadfar, H., & Lotfi, F. (2017). The evolution and transformation of telemedicine. *International Journal of Biosensors & Bioelectronics*, *3*(4), 303–306. DOI: 10.15406/ijbsbe.2017.03.00070

Smith, J. D., Margolis, S. A., Ayton, J., Ross, V., Chalmers, E., Giddings, P., Baker, L., Kelly, M., & Love, C. (2008). Defining remote medical practice. *The Medical Journal of Australia*, *188*(3), 159–161. DOI: 10.5694/j.1326-5377.2008.tb01561.x PMID: 18241174

Smolić, Š., Blaževski, N., & Fabijančić, M. (2022). Remote healthcare during the COVID-19 pandemic: Findings for older adults in 27 European countries and Israel. *Frontiers in Public Health*, *10*, 927367. DOI: 10.3389/fpubh.2022.921379 PMID: 35910874

Steindal, S. A., Nes, A. A. G., Godskesen, T. E., Holmen, H., Winger, A., Österlind, J., Dihle, A., & Klarare, A. (2023). Advantages and challenges of using telehealth for home-based palliative care: Systematic mixed studies review. *Journal of Medical Internet Research*, *25*, e43684. DOI: 10.2196/43684 PMID: 36912876

Thayer, J., & Dreisbach-Williams, S. (2023). Early innovations in maritime telemedical services: The KDKF Radio Medico Station. *Journal of the Medical Library Association: JMLA*, *111*(1–2), 625–630. DOI: 10.5195/jmla.2023.1567 PMID: 37312806

Topol, E. J. (2019). High-performance medicine: The convergence of human and artificial intelligence. *Nature Medicine*, *25*(1), 44–56. DOI: 10.1038/s41591-018-0300-7 PMID: 30617339

Tornvall, I., Kenny, D., Wubishet, B. L., Russell, A., Menon, A., & Comans, T. (2025). Economic evaluations of mHealth interventions for the management of type 2 diabetes: A scoping review. *Journal of Diabetes Science and Technology*, *19*(1), 179–190. DOI: 10.1177/19322968231183956 PMID: 37395212

Totten, A. M., Womack, D. M., Eden, K. B., McDonagh, M. S., Griffin, J. C., Grusing, S., & Hersh, W. R. (2016). *Telehealth: Mapping the evidence for patient outcomes from systematic reviews* (Technical Brief No. 26). Agency for Healthcare Research and Quality. https://www.ncbi.nlm.nih.gov/books/NBK379320/

Vegesna, A., Tran, M., Angelaccio, M., & Arcona, S. (2017). Remote patient monitoring via non-invasive digital technologies: A systematic review. *Telemedicine Journal and e-Health*, *23*(1), 3–17. DOI: 10.1089/tmj.2016.0051 PMID: 27116181

Wakerman, J. (2004). Defining remote health. *The Australian Journal of Rural Health*, *12*(5), 210–214. DOI: 10.1111/j.1440-1854.2004.00607.x PMID: 15588265

Warshaw, E. M., Lederle, F. A., Grill, J. P., Gravely, A. A., Bangerter, A. K., Fortier, L. A., Bohjanen, K. A., Chen, K., Lee, P. K., Rabinovitz, H. S., Johr, R. H., Kaye, V. N., Bowers, S., Wenner, R., Askari, S. K., Kedrowski, D. A., & Nelson, D. B. (2009). Accuracy of teledermatology for nonpigmented neoplasms. *Journal of the American Academy of Dermatology*, *60*(4), 579–588. DOI: 10.1016/j.jaad.2008.11.892 PMID: 19217689

Wilson, F. A., Rampa, S., Trout, K. E., & Stimpson, J. P. (2017). Reimbursements for telehealth services are likely to be lower than non-telehealth services in the United States. *Journal of Telemedicine and Telecare*, *23*(4), 497–500. DOI: 10.1177/1357633X16652288 PMID: 27260264

Wootton, R., Geissbuhler, A., Jethwani, K., Kovarik, C., Person, D. A., Vladzymyrskyy, A., Zanaboni, P., & Zolfo, M. (2012). Long-running telemedicine networks delivering humanitarian services: Experience, performance and scientific output. *Bulletin of the World Health Organization*, *90*(5), 341–347. DOI: 10.2471/BLT.11.099143 PMID: 22589567

World Health Organization. (2010). *Telemedicine: Opportunities and developments in Member States*. https://www.who.int/goe/publications/goe_telemedicine_2010.pdf

Zundel, K. M. (1996). Telemedicine: History, applications, and impact on librarianship. *Bulletin of the Medical Library Association*, *84*(1), 71–79. https://www.ncbi.nlm.nih.gov/pmc/articles/PMC226126/ PMID: 8938332

Chapter 5
Enhancing Smart Home User Interfaces With Emerging Technologies

Rudra Shekhar Basak
School of Computer Engineering, Kalinga Institute of Industrial Technology (KIIT), Bhubaneswar, India

Hitesh Mohapatra
https://orcid.org/0000-0001-8100-4860
School of Computer Engineering, Kalinga Institute of Industrial Technology (KIIT), Bhubaneswar, India

Bedanta Panigrahy
https://orcid.org/0009-0001-0463-6554
School of Computer Engineering, Kalinga Institute of Industrial Technology (KIIT), Bhubaneswar, India

ABSTRACT

As smart home technology becomes more prevalent, optimizing user interface (UI) design is essential to enhance user experience and unlock the full potential of home automation. This paper explores key factors that influence user interaction and satisfaction by analyzing challenges and opportunities in smart home UI design. Drawing on principles from HCI, cognitive psychology, and design thinking, we propose a framework emphasizing usability, personalization, and flexibility. We review current literature, assess emerging technologies like voice assistants, gesture recognition, and AI algorithms for proactive UI optimization, and provide actionable insights to guide future smart home UI development.

DOI: 10.4018/979-8-3373-3099-0.ch005

1. INTRODUCTION

The rise of smart homes is transforming the way we live by creating intelligent ecosystems that can understand and respond to our needs. However, to truly unlock the potential of these connected devices, we need interfaces that make it easier for people to interact with technology. This paper explores the critical role of Human-Computer Interaction (HCI) in shaping the future of smart home networks (Allifah & Zualkernan, 2022). In recent years, the term smart has become synonymous with technologies that incorporate artificial intelligence to benefit humanity. Key goals have been established, and smart technologies have become a major driving force behind pioneering concepts such as smart home design. Advances in intelligent products and services have led to a significant increase in device and data connectivity across the globe. This trend has had a substantial impact on the rapidly growing global smart home industry. Given the benefits of smart technologies and their market potential, there has been a surge of interest among researchers in smart home technologies (Asare-Bediako et al., 2013).

Rapid advances in automation have led to the emergence of the smart home industry, giving rise to the term "clever home." This industry is experiencing steady growth due to market success and increasing demand. The World Economic Forum (WEF) forecasts that the industry could be worth US$13 billion by 2030, indicating sustained growth and future potential. According to Statista, the smart home market was projected to reach USD 99.41 billion globally by 2021 (Bhalotia et al., 2023). Both forecasts and research focus on further developments in smart home appliances. As the industry expands, expectations are likely to rise as well (Brahman et al., 2015). Initially seen as a mundane feature, the smart home has evolved into a solution for enhancing efficiency, desirability, and security. Studies show that smart homes can reduce overall energy costs, which may have a significant impact. While a single smart home may not reveal the full potential of this technology, the collective effect is substantial (Debnath et al., 2021). Smart homes also have an important role in home security systems, where sensors help maintain a safe environment. Furthermore, they contribute to enriching the home environment, which is their largest market. When effectively implemented, smart home technologies can greatly benefit the disabled, elderly, and ill. Applications such as motion detection and image recognition systems offer assistive technologies for individuals with age- or condition-related limitations. Virtual reality systems are also being utilized in similar contexts (Dehury & Sahoo, 2016).

The smart home has become a highly promising area in home automation and management. The term "clever home" extends beyond human dwellings, encompassing broader technical implications such as intelligent living and lifestyle. Its integration with technologies like smart cities, smart manufacturing, and smart states expands the concept beyond individual residences (Diwakar et al., 2025). The modern Internet of Things (IoT) aims to provide services through intelligent systems that prioritize user convenience and precision. Researchers are conducting numerous studies to develop smart environments, including smart homes, smart grids, and industrial IoT facilities. Typically, IoT-based smart home technologies offer features that surpass those of traditional network systems. Devices within the home connect automatically with one another to enhance everyday life (Erdinc et al., 2015). As smart technology evolves rapidly, smart home companies worldwide are exploring new strategies to engage older adults in adopting their products. These efforts aim to boost revenue streams, drive innovation, and provide seniors with safer, healthier, and more independent living environments (Ewais et al., 2018). This aligns with the United Nations' third and ninth Sustainable Development Goals "Good Health and Well-being" and "Industry, Innovation and Infrastructure" which promote quality of life for all ages, safe construction, inclusive and sustainable employment, and technological advancement. Fig.1 presents the applications of IoT in several sectors.

Figure 1. IoT application is smart city

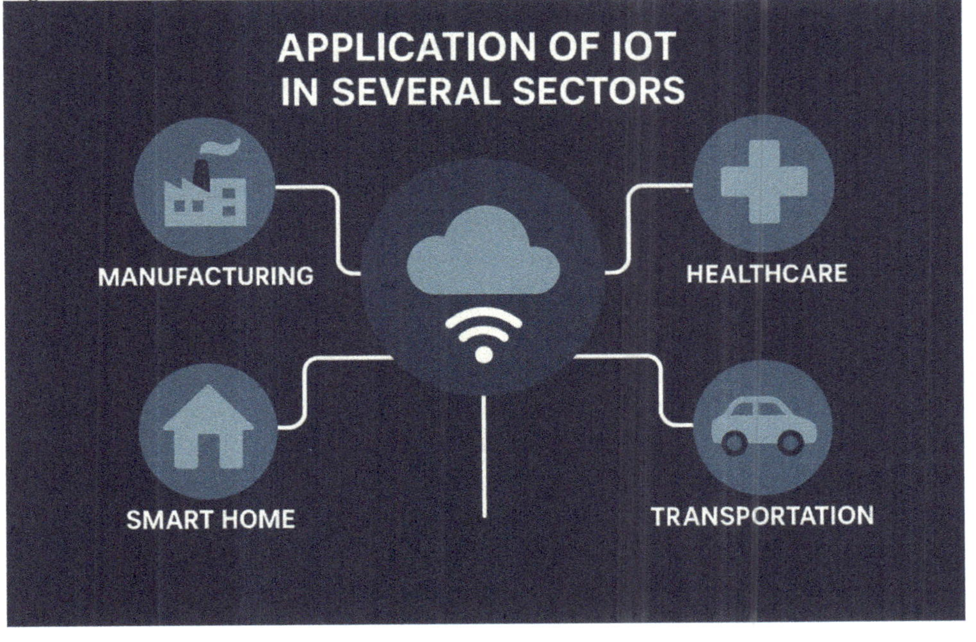

Smart houses provide residents with comfortable, fully managed, and secure living environments. Additionally, smart homes can save energy and money, with potential benefits gained through the use of clean and renewable energy systems. On a broader scale, the possibility of national energy shortages is motivating more governments to support the adoption of smart home technologies (Fthenakis & Kim, 2009). Several countries have already implemented various laws, regulations, and support programs to encourage the integration of smart homes, including incentives for heating system efficiency, energy storage initiatives, and the adoption of smart meters—for example, through the European Standard EN 15232 and the Building Energy Performance Directive 2010/31/EU. In line with the European Commission and the Energy Roadmap 2050, the growing energy demand in residential areas is driving the deployment of smart home technologies (Gao et al., 2020). To monitor and adapt to environmental conditions, smart homes automate the control of specific devices, such as lighting and temperature, based on changes in weather and other external factors.

Modern smart control systems offer numerous advanced features that go well beyond traditional adjustments. They can monitor both the environment and the activities of the home's occupants (Hasan et al., 2018), automatically execute pre-programmed tasks, and operate devices on preset schedules, either independently or based on user preferences. In addition to simplifying daily life, smart homes focus on energy efficiency, reducing peak loads, lowering energy costs, and cutting greenhouse gas emissions. Smart homes can be analyzed from various perspectives, including network design, social implications, thermal behavior, technological advancements, and emerging trends (Hubert & Grijalva, 2012). Moreover, the monitoring and modeling of smart appliances through smart meters are crucial for accurate load forecasting. Recently, energy authorities have revised residential energy pricing structures to encourage homeowners to better manage their demand. Unlike earlier studies, this paper introduces the concept of energy- and cost-efficient smart homes and discusses two different approaches to Smart Home Energy Management Systems (SHEMS): offline load scheduling and real-time control. It also briefly explores the potential impact of specific smart home energy usage patterns on future smart grids (Jidong Wang et al., 2012).

Research on smart refrigerators primarily focuses on technological innovation and the development of intelligent product features. For example, in a study on intelligent refrigeration systems using Internet of Things (IoT) technology, Gupta Sharma et al. proposed using IoT to create smart refrigerators capable of managing the contents within them. The study describes how a smart refrigerator can operate by determining when to restock food and identifying the type and quantity of items stored (Jo et al., 2013). This research approach differs from that of Wu et al. and Dekoninck et al., who focus on the overall design of an affordable smart refrigerator incorporating IoT technology. However, there is still limited research dedicated to optimizing the user experience of smart refrigerators specifically for older consumers in the current technological landscape.

1.1. Role of Advanced Technologies in Smart Home Interface (SHI)

The role of advanced technologies in smart home interfaces has expanded rapidly, revolutionizing how users interact with their living spaces. Central to this transformation is the integration of intelligent systems that provide seamless, context-aware, and anticipatory user experiences. Artificial Intelligence (AI) plays a crucial role by enabling virtual assistants and voice-based interactions capable of understanding natural language, recognizing user intent, and learning behavioral patterns to deliver personalized responses. This adaptability improves usability and reduces cognitive effort, making the smart home interface intuitive rather than reliant on explicit commands or manual control. Machine learning algorithms embedded in these systems continuously process data from sensors, appliances, and user behaviors to identify patterns and anomalies (Maelen et al., 2021). This enables a shift from reactive to proactive interfaces, where actions are suggested or automated based on user preferences. For instance, lighting and temperature can be automatically adjusted according to the time of day, occupancy, and individual comfort levels. These intelligent predictions not only enhance user satisfaction but also promote energy efficiency and sustainability, aligning smart home technologies with broader environmental objectives (Naik et al., 2023). Fig.2 illustrates the role of technologies in SHI.

Figure 2. Role of advanced technologies in smart home interface

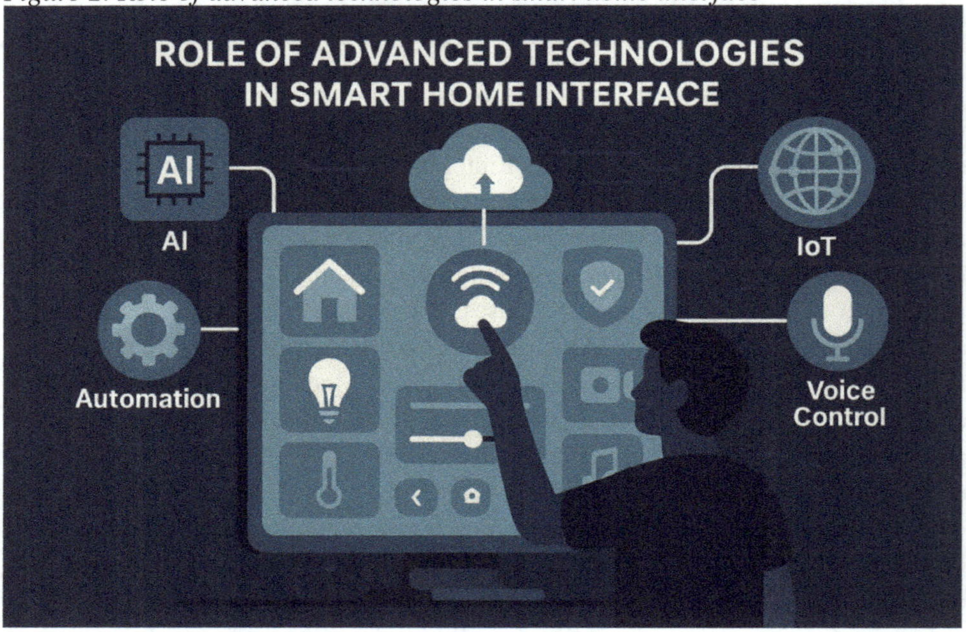

Computer vision significantly enhances the smart home interface experience by enabling gesture recognition, facial authentication, and spatial awareness. AI-integrated cameras can identify users and tailor the interface to their individual profiles, offering personalized settings and increased security. Gesture-based controls provide a touchless mode of interaction, which is particularly beneficial in situations such as cooking or for users with accessibility needs (Gao & Patras, 2024). Augmented Reality (AR) is also emerging as a powerful interface layer, offering immersive visualizations for controlling home systems, virtually placing furniture, and providing interactive overlays that assist users with troubleshooting or maintenance tasks. The Internet of Things (IoT) continues to serve as the foundational element that connects all devices within the smart home ecosystem. Challenges related to interoperability—common in earlier systems—are now being addressed through edge computing and the adoption of standardized communication protocols. These advancements support real-time data processing and secure, device-to-device communication, enabling low-latency, distributed intelligence that ensures faster, more reliable user interactions without the constant need for cloud connectivity (Abdaoui et al., 2023).

Voice interfaces, enhanced by advances in natural language processing, have evolved from basic command-driven tools into conversational systems capable of managing multi-turn dialogues, interpreting contextual cues, and executing complex task sequences. When integrated with ambient computing systems, these interfaces create seamless, screen-free interactions that allow users to engage naturally with their environment. Biometric technologies such as fingerprint scanning, retina recognition, and voiceprint identification are increasingly being incorporated into smart home interfaces, offering improved security while streamlining authentication processes (Mishra & Garg, 2024). These biometric methods not only reinforce access control but also personalize the user experience by adapting the interface based on the recognized individual. This convergence of security and personalization highlights the growing demand for smart homes that are not only secure but also intelligently responsive to the unique needs of their occupants.

Furthermore, the emergence of emotion recognition and affective computing adds a layer of emotional intelligence to smart home systems. By analyzing vocal tone, facial expressions, or physiological signals, these interfaces can adapt their responses to the user's emotional state, enabling empathetic interactions and enhancing overall comfort. For instance, emotionally aware systems might play calming music when stress is detected or adjust lighting to create a more soothing atmosphere (Verma, 2023). In essence, the integration of advanced technologies into smart home interfaces is transforming human-machine interaction from a purely transactional process into a more holistic, human-centered experience. These technologies enable interfaces to evolve beyond mere control panels into intelligent companions that understand, anticipate, and respond with sensitivity and insight. As these innovations continue to develop and merge, the smart home interface of the future will likely become an invisible yet ever-present presence, seamlessly aligning technology with the rhythms and subtleties of everyday life.

1.2. Design Principles for Intuitive and Adaptive Smart Home Interfaces

Designing intuitive and adaptive smart home interfaces demands a deep understanding of human behavior alongside the technological capabilities that can effectively respond to it. Usability is central to a successful interface systems must be simple, coherent, and contextually relevant, minimizing the learning curve and enabling users of all ages and technical backgrounds to interact effortlessly. This requires a user-centered design approach, where the interface is shaped around users' needs, habits, and expectations rather than the constraints of the underlying technology. The ultimate goal is to make complex systems feel invisible, allowing users to engage with their environment naturally and without friction (Zhang & Li, 2019). Consistency is a key design principle, ensuring uniformity in visual layout, interaction patterns, and response behaviors across various devices and input methods. Whether users interact via voice assistant, mobile app, wall panel, or gesture control, the experience should remain seamless and predictable, fostering trust and encouraging long-term use. Additionally, interfaces must be context-aware and capable of adapting dynamically to factors such as location, time of day, user presence, and individual preferences. For example, a lighting control interface could prioritize different settings at night compared to daytime, or automatically align with a user's evening routine, eliminating the need for manual adjustments.

Adaptivity in smart home interfaces goes beyond basic responsiveness by learning from user behavior and evolving to anticipate individual needs. Interfaces should personalize layouts and recommendations based on usage patterns while upholding user control, privacy, and transparency. Instead of making opaque decisions, systems must present clear options and explanations, empower users and foster a sense of ownership. Accessibility is equally vital interfaces should support a wide range of physical abilities through features like voice commands, gesture controls, and customizable visual displays (Herzfeld, 2016). Inclusive design principles also ensure usability across different languages and abilities, enriching the experience for all users. Equally important is providing consistent feedback and maintaining system transparency; users should receive clear, timely confirmations of their actions and be able to understand how automations function. This visibility into system behavior reduces confusion, builds trust, and contributes to a more dependable and user-friendly smart home environment (Smirek et al., 2016).

Seamless integration with the physical environment is essential for smart home interfaces to feel intuitive and non-intrusive. Design elements such as wall-mounted touchscreens, ambient lighting, and embedded sensors should harmonize with home aesthetics and remain discreet, appearing only when they provide meaningful value. Equally important are security and ethical design principles. Interfaces must safeguard user data through encryption, secure authentication, and transparent, revocable consent, while incorporating strong protections against misuse. Ethical design also demands that systems respect user intent and avoid manipulative behaviors. Ultimately, effective smart home interfaces achieve a balance between simplicity and intelligence, automation and user control, and innovation and empathy enhancing everyday life while making technology feel like a natural, trustworthy part of the home (Muck & Frohlich, 2013).

1.3. Multimodal Interaction and Context-Awareness in Smart Home Systems

Multimodal interaction and context-awareness have become foundational pillars in the advancement of smart home systems, significantly enhancing the richness, adaptability, and intuitiveness of user experiences. As homes grow more intelligent and interconnected, relying on a single mode of interaction such as touch, voice, or visual control falls short in addressing the varying needs and dynamic contexts of everyday life. Multimodal interaction solves this by enabling users to engage with their smart environments through a combination of input methods, including voice commands, touchscreen controls, gestures, facial expressions, haptic feedback, and gaze tracking. This variety not only boosts accessibility but also mirrors the natural ways humans communicate, providing more fluid and intuitive control (Lin et al., 2023). The core strength of effective multimodal systems lies in their ability to seamlessly interpret and integrate inputs from multiple channels. For example, a user may issue a voice command to dim the lights while pointing to a specific fixture, allowing the system to interpret intent through contextual and combined cues. Achieving this level of interaction requires advanced sensor fusion, natural language processing, and real-time machine learning capable of interpreting complex multimodal inputs. The result is a more human-centric interface that reduces friction and cognitive effort, offering a seamless, responsive, and satisfying smart home experience (Patel & Champaneria, 2016).

Context-awareness enhances smart home interactions by enabling systems to interpret and respond intelligently to situational factors such as location, time of day, environmental conditions, activity history, the presence of others, and even the user's emotional state. Rather than responding uniformly to every input, context-aware systems adapt their behavior for example, understanding that a command like "turn off the lights" can have different implications depending on when and where it is given (Magade & Sharma, 2024). If the system recognizes that the user is watching a movie, it may automatically dim the lights and lower the blinds without needing explicit instructions, using learned behavior and contextual cues. This real-time adaptability not only streamlines user interaction but also supports proactive engagement. Such systems can anticipate needs and perform actions independently, like starting the coffee machine when the user enters the kitchen in the morning or playing calming music when biometric data indicates stress. When designed with transparency and user control, these anticipatory capabilities foster a more natural and emotionally connected relationship between the user and their environment, enhancing both convenience and well-being.

The integration of multimodal interaction and context-awareness significantly enhances the inclusivity, resilience, and personalization of smart home experiences. By offering multiple modes of interaction such as voice, gesture, touch, and gaze these systems ensure that individuals with disabilities or varying abilities are not excluded, as no single modality becomes a barrier to access. In multi-resident households, context-aware systems can differentiate between users, enabling personalized responses while upholding privacy and consistency (Hu et al., 2024). These features also contribute to system robustness; when one interaction mode fails due to noise, connectivity issues, or physical obstructions others can serve as reliable fallbacks, increasing both reliability and user trust. However, realizing such sophisticated capabilities introduces complex design and ethical challenges. Systems must accurately infer user intent without becoming intrusive or making incorrect assumptions, and users must retain control with options to override or adjust automated behaviors. Moreover, the continuous data collection required for context-aware computing raises critical privacy concerns. Transparent data practices, explicit consent mechanisms, and edge computing for localized data processing are essential to protect user privacy and sustain trust. Ultimately, the convergence of multimodal interaction and context-awareness redefines smart home interfaces as dynamic, responsive, and deeply human-centered systems. By interpreting not only commands but also cues, context, and emotions, these technologies transform homes into intelligent environments that adapt and evolve meaningfully with their inhabitants (Hadiprawoto & Ridley, 2023).

1.4. Emotional Intelligence and Empathetic Responses in Smart Home Interfaces

Emotional intelligence in smart home interfaces marks a significant evolution in human-computer interaction, shifting technology from mere functional responsiveness to empathetic engagement. This transformation redefines the smart home as not just a responsive environment, but as a perceptive companion capable of understanding and addressing the emotional needs of its users (Ulutas & Omeroglu, 2012). By integrating advanced sensors, affective computing algorithms, machine learning, and multimodal data interpretation, smart systems can detect emotional cues such as voice inflection, facial expressions, posture, and physiological signals like heart rate and skin conductance. These capabilities allow the home to adapt its behavior in emotionally appropriate ways offering comfort, support, or silence depending on the user's mood. The impact of such interfaces is profoundly human; for instance, a system might detect stress in a user's voice and respond by dimming the lights, lowering ambient noise, and playing soothing music, or recognize signs of sadness through facial analysis and suggest gentle prompts for social interaction, physical activity, or relaxation. By responding to emotional states as well as commands, emotionally intelligent smart homes foster a deeper sense of well-being, empathy, and connection between users and their living environments.

These empathetic responses contribute to creating a sense of psychological safety, making the smart home not only efficient but also emotionally supportive. In households with elderly individuals or those experiencing mental health challenges, such capabilities can be especially vital providing passive monitoring and proactive emotional support in ways that are non-intrusive and non-disruptive. When empathy is embedded into the design of user interfaces, the role of technology shifts from a functional assistant to a compassionate companion, enhancing emotional well-being alongside everyday convenience. Developing these systems requires a nuanced understanding of emotional variability across individuals and cultures (Sesha Bhargavi Velagaleti, 2024). Emotional expression is inherently personal and context-sensitive; what may be perceived as anger in one cultural setting could be interpreted as assertiveness in another. To avoid bias and misinterpretation, emotionally intelligent systems must be trained on diverse, representative datasets and designed to learn and adapt to the specific emotional language of each user. Personalization is essential empathetic responses must feel genuine and supportive rather than artificial or misplaced. Additionally, emotionally intelligent interfaces must strike a careful balance between being proactive and remaining discreet. While a smart home may have the capability to respond to frustration or fatigue with calming interventions, it must do so with subtlety, ensuring it does not intrude or inadvertently heighten emotional distress. The essence of empathetic design lies in its ability to listen without overwhelming, suggest without dictating, and respond without disrupting. Emotional intelligence in smart homes should not aim to mimic human emotion but rather serve as a quiet, adaptive presence an ambient layer of care attuned to the rhythms and nuances of daily emotional life.

Ethical considerations become especially critical in the emotionally aware dimension of smart homes, where systems interpret and respond to users' emotional states. Transparency is essential users must clearly understand how emotional data is captured, analyzed, and stored, and they should retain full control over these features, including the option to disable emotion tracking entirely. Trust is the foundation of emotionally intelligent design; users must feel assured that their emotional vulnerabilities are not being exploited but respected and protected. This means ensuring robust data security, strict privacy protections, and clear communication about the purpose and scope of emotional recognition features. As smart home interfaces become more attuned to the emotional fabric of human life, they shift from being tools of task execution to partners in relational engagement. A home that senses loneliness and suggests a virtual connection with loved ones, or recognizes heightened stress and prompts a restorative break, moves beyond convenience it becomes a quiet ally in well-being. Such systems hold the potential to enhance emotional resilience, provide gentle companionship, and support a more mindful, balanced lifestyle. In this light, the smart home is no longer just a shelter or a web of connected devices; it becomes an emotionally intelligent habitat one that responds not only to what users do, but to how they feel. Moving forward, the design of empathetic smart home interfaces must prioritize compassion, privacy, and personalization, cultivating environments that truly understand and uplift the individuals who inhabit them. The integration of emotional intelligence into everyday living spaces marks a profound shift, transforming the home into a caring, responsive presence that strengthens both quality of life and emotional connection in a world increasingly influenced by digital relationships.

2. LITERATURE REVIEW

The growing popularity of smart homes powered by the Internet of Things (IoT) necessitates a critical examination of user interface (UI) design, as the effectiveness of the user experience (UX) is directly tied to the quality of the UI. This literature review explores current research on smart home UI design, identifying both challenges and opportunities for improvement through user-centered design (UCD) principles. In the context of smart homes, UI design plays a pivotal role in enhancing UX by supporting IoT functionality, accessibility, consistency, responsiveness, and simplicity (Kumar et al., 2024). Usability defined as the ease with which users achieve their goals is essential, and smart home applications benefit from features such as intuitive navigation, clear layout, and efficient task completion. Studies indicate that customized UIs significantly improve user satisfaction and adoption (Lee et al., 2016). As the smart home ecosystem grows to include more devices and user roles, designing scalable interfaces becomes a major challenge. Without proper planning, increased device integration can lead to performance issues, visual clutter, and implementation complexity (Lei et al., 2009). Addressing scalability requires modular UI design, efficient resource management, and flexible architectures that adapt to dynamic changes in system size. Additionally, accessibility is crucial in ensuring smart home interfaces are inclusive for users with diverse abilities. Considerations such as font size, color contrast, and compatibility with assistive technologies like screen readers and voice assistants—are vital to making these systems usable for everyone (Mazen et al., 2013). Ultimately, well-designed UIs empower smart home users by enhancing control, usability, and satisfaction within increasingly complex and connected environments.

- Consistency: A consistent UI design means maintaining consistency across interface types and interfaces within the smart home ecosystem. Consistent design features and communication flows help users anticipate system behavior and move seamlessly between devices and applications. Consistency improves visibility and reduces cognitive load for users (Mohapatra, 2021).
- Feedback: Feedback mechanisms are essential to provide users with real-time feedback on their communication status and system performance. Information provided in smart homes can take various forms, including visual, audible, or tactile signals. Effective feedback makes users aware of the consequences of their actions and helps them make informed decisions.

- Simplicity: Simple UI design seeks to minimize complexity and innovation to create simple and easy-to-understand interfaces. Simple UIs reduce cognitive costs for users and facilitate faster task completion. By focusing on simplicity, smart home UIs are able to increase user satisfaction and acceptance (Nair et al., 2015).
- Methods of Interaction in Smart Homes UI: Smart home UIs use a variety of interaction techniques to accommodate user preferences and interaction scenarios. Common techniques include voice control, gestures recognition, touch and wearing goddesses allowing for intuitive and non-verbal interaction with IoT devices. Gesture-based interfaces offer a novel and immersive way for users to interact with their smart homes.
- Additional Resources: Smartphone, Tablet, and Touch Screens Touch interfaces are common in smartphones, tablets, and touchscreen devices or built into control panels. The touchscreen provides intuitive tactile feedback and interaction, allowing users to work directly with virtual controls and programs. Touch interfaces provide a familiar and easy-to-use interface for smart home environments.
- Wearable Devices: Wearable devices such as smartwatches and fitness trackers, act as simple interfaces for monitoring and managing smart home devices on the go. Wearables can provide notification, alert, and remote-control functionality, enabling seamless integration with smart home ecosystems. Wearable UIs allow users to move around and personalize them (Nimmy et al., 2022).
- Ambient Displays: Ambient displays provide information and feedback in a discreet, non-intrusive manner, integrating into a simple user environment. Ambient displays use technologies such as LED indicators, color-changing lighting, or projection mapping to provide information about device status, weather forecasts, or upcoming events Ambient UIs enhance situational awareness and match home as intelligence is well mixed.
- Technologies to Enhance UI in Smart Homes: Many technologies are used to improve UI design and user interaction in smart homes, including artificial intelligence (AI) and machine learning (ML), augmented reality (AR), virtual reality (VR), sensor technology, and blockchain for security and privacy and there (Pandey et al., 2024).
- Artificial Intelligence and Machine Learning: AI and ML technologies empower smart home systems to understand user preferences, anticipate needs, and optimize interactions. AI-powered virtual assistant search user behavior in smart homes. Sensor data informs UI design decisions, enabling adaptive interfaces that respond to user presence, preferences, and environmental con-

ditions. Sensor-driven UIs enhance automation, energy efficiency, and user comfort in smart home environments (Paputungan et al., 2019).

- Blockchain for Security and Privacy: Blockchain technology offers decentralized and tamper-resistant mechanisms for securing smart home data and transactions. By leveraging blockchain, smart home UIs can enhance privacy, data integrity, and user control over personal information. Blockchain-based UIs enable secure authentication, data sharing, and smart contract execution, fostering trust and transparency in smart home ecosystems.

Challenges and Opportunities:

Despite advances in UI design principles and technologies, many challenges remain in optimizing UIs for smart homes. Privacy concerns, connectivity issues, scalability limitations, energy efficiency considerations, and user acceptance barriers pose significant obstacles to implementing effective smart home interfaces. These challenges highlight the need for a focused approach to designing user-centered, secure, and adaptable systems.

- Privacy Concerns: Personal data collection in smart homes, shared access, unauthorized entry, and negligence raise significant privacy concerns, emphasizing the importance of self-preservation and personal boundaries in UI design. UI designs must incorporate mechanisms that protect user data and respect privacy. Policies, protocols, and procedures must be clearly defined and implemented to ensure user trust and compliance (Paterakis et al., 2015).
- Energy Efficiency: With the rise of battery-powered IoT devices and the need to reduce energy consumption for durability and cost-effectiveness, energy efficiency is a critical consideration in smart home UI design. Poorly optimized UIs—such as those with excessive animations, background processes, or inefficient network interfaces—can drain device batteries and waste energy. Designing energy-efficient UIs requires minimizing computational overhead and optimizing resource usage.
- User Acceptance: User acceptance is essential for the success of smart home UIs, as reluctant or dissatisfied users may resist adopting or continuing to use IoT technologies. Factors influencing acceptance include perceived usefulness, ease of use, trust, and cultural norms. Designing UIs that align with users' preferences, expectations, and cultural contexts can enhance acceptance and adoption. Furthermore, providing adequate education, support, and feedback mechanisms can address user concerns and foster positive attitudes toward smart home technologies (Raj et al., 2025).
- Interoperability: Interoperability refers to the ability of various IoT devices and platforms to communicate and function seamlessly together. The lack

of standardized protocols and compatibility among different devices hinders interoperability within smart home ecosystems. UI design should support integration and collaboration across diverse platforms to ensure a cohesive and user-friendly experience.

- Future Directions: Despite current challenges in smart home UI design, numerous promising avenues for future research and development offer opportunities to enhance user experience and address existing limitations (Rajasekharan & Koivunen, 2014).
- Personalized Interfaces: Personalization holds great potential for improving user satisfaction and engagement in smart home environments. Future UIs should leverage user preferences, behavior patterns, and contextual information to deliver tailored experiences. Personalized interfaces may include adaptive layouts, content recommendations, and proactive assistance features that anticipate user needs and respond dynamically to changing circumstances.
- Context-Awareness: Context-aware UIs can sense and respond to environmental conditions, user activities, and contextual cues in real time. Integrating context-awareness into smart home interfaces enables adaptive and proactive interactions that anticipate user intentions. These systems may utilize sensor data, location information, and machine learning algorithms to infer user preferences, automate tasks, and provide contextually relevant information and services (Shahriyar et al., 2021).
- Multimodal Interaction: Multimodal interaction combines input methods such as voice, gesture, touch, and gaze, enabling more natural and intuitive interactions with smart home devices. Future UIs should incorporate multimodal strategies to accommodate different user preferences and contexts, allowing users to choose the most suitable interaction method. Such interfaces can also enhance accessibility and usability for users with varying abilities and needs.
- Emotional Intelligence in UI: Emotional intelligence in UI design involves understanding and responding to users' emotional states and needs. Future smart home UIs should integrate emotional intelligence capabilities to recognize and adapt to users' moods and emotional cues. These interfaces may use affective computing techniques, such as sentiment analysis and emotion recognition, to personalize interactions, provide empathetic responses, and improve user satisfaction and well-being (Tachibana et al., 2016).
- Integration with Smart Cities: Integration with smart cities represents an emerging trend in UI design, where smart home ecosystems connect seamlessly with urban infrastructure and services. Future UIs could enable interaction between smart homes and city systems, allowing residents to access city-wide resources, services, and data through their home interfaces. Such

integration could support applications in energy management, transportation, healthcare, and public safety, fostering collaboration between households and the broader urban environment.

This segment outlines recent work in the fields of human behavior research—namely, assistive technology, the Internet of Things (IoT), human–computer interaction, and related disciplines—aimed at developing assisted living experiences in technology-enhanced environments such as smart homes and smart cities (Tao et al., 2017). A wireless sensor system designed to monitor and interpret human movement data for activity recognition was proposed by Azkune et al. The system employed a method of activity clustering developed using knowledge engineering principles. Based on these clusters, the system identified patterns of human movement associated with specific activities. The framework incorporated a Convolutional Neural Network (ConvNet) architecture adapted for regression tasks, along with a Support Vector Machine (SVM) classifier for activity detection (Wan et al., 2015). The authors evaluated the performance of their framework by testing it on activity recognition datasets. Additionally, a hidden Markov model-based architecture was proposed to analyze the multimodal characteristics of sensor data for more accurate activity recognition.

The authors utilized a recorded dataset and enhanced its annotation using an off-the-shelf sensor, the Jabra BT250v. This device was employed to enrich activity annotations throughout daily routines, which were then used to train the hidden Markov model-based architecture for activity recognition. A separate framework was developed that incorporated principles from computer vision, image processing, and video data analysis to monitor and detect activities for both individual and multiple users within a designated IoT-enabled environment. This approach combined motion feature data, user appearance information, and the spatiotemporal characteristics of user behavior to train multiple learning models. The authors evaluated their method by testing it on a dataset of activities. Additionally, an artificial neural network-based architecture was developed to track human movement during various activities, with a specific focus on detecting entry and exit events such as entering or exiting a room—within a spatial environment (Zenginis et al., 2022). The system employed IoT-based sensors with distinct functionalities: one sensor was used to detect the presence or absence of the user, while another determined whether the door was open or closed. The authors used a dataset of different activities to evaluate and discuss the performance characteristics of their proposed approach.

3. PROPOSED STUDY

A holistic user interface (UI) design approach for smart homes begins with a user-centered design (UCD) process that actively involves users throughout the entire design lifecycle. This includes conducting ethnographic studies, interviews, and usability testing to deeply understand user needs, preferences, and pain points. Iterative design improvements based on user feedback help ensure both usability and user satisfaction. Task analysis and scenario modeling are essential to identify users' goals and activities within the smart home context. By developing scenario models that illustrate user interaction with smart devices in various situations, designers can create interfaces that support seamless task completion and enhance user productivity. Consistency and intuitiveness are also critical elements of effective UI design. Maintaining uniform design elements, layouts, and interaction patterns across different devices and applications within the smart home ecosystem fosters familiarity and reduces cognitive load. Using familiar metaphors and conventions helps users quickly grasp functionality, while intuitive interfaces minimize the learning curve and effort required for effective use.

Integration of Emerging Technologies:

- Artificial Intelligence (AI) and Machine Learning (ML): Integrate AI-powered virtual assistants that can understand natural language commands, learn user preferences over time, and offer personalized suggestions and automation. Utilize ML algorithms for predictive analytics, anomaly detection, and proactive maintenance of smart home systems.
- Augmented Reality (AR) and Virtual Reality (VR): Develop AR applications that overlay contextual information, device controls, and maintenance instructions onto the physical environment. Create VR simulations for designing and configuring smart home layouts, experimenting with IoT devices, and troubleshooting issues in virtual environments.
- Sensor Networks: Deploy sensor networks throughout the smart home to collect real-time data on environmental conditions, user behavior, and device status. Use sensor data to dynamically adapt UIs, trigger automation rules, and provide contextual feedback to users. Leverage sensor fusion techniques to combine data from multiple sensors for more accurate and reliable insights.

Privacy-Enhancing Technologies:

- Blockchain for Data Security: Implement blockchain-based solutions to secure sensitive information, manage access control, and ensure data integrity in smart home environments. Use blockchain to create tamper-resistant audit logs, cryptographic key management systems, and decentralized identity frameworks that protect user privacy and prevent unauthorized access.

- End-to-End Encryption: Encrypt data transmissions between smart home devices, gateways, and cloud services using robust cryptographic protocols and encryption algorithms. Employ secure key management practices to protect encryption keys and prevent unauthorized interception or tampering. Ensure that personal data remains private and safeguarded from external threats.

Scalable and Energy-Efficient Design:

- Modular Architecture: Design UIs with a modular architecture that supports easy scalability and extensibility as the smart home ecosystem expands. Separate UI components into reusable modules that can be dynamically loaded and unloaded based on user preferences and system requirements. Utilize a microservices architecture to decouple UI functionalities, enhancing scalability, maintainability, and flexibility.
- Energy-Aware UI Optimization: Optimize UI elements and interactions for energy efficiency to minimize power consumption on battery-operated devices and reduce environmental impact. Implement techniques such as dynamic voltage and frequency scaling, adaptive screen brightness, and background task throttling to conserve energy without compromising user experience. Leverage platform-specific power profiling tools to identify energy-intensive UI components and optimize them accordingly.
- User-Centric Innovation: Co-Creation with Users: Encourage collaboration and co-creation with users by involving them in the UI design process through idea sharing, feedback, and feature requests. Organize workshops, focus groups, and design sprints to engage users in ideation, prototyping, and evaluation activities. Integrate user-generated content and customization options into UI designs to empower users and enhance personalization.
- Continuous Improvement: Establish mechanisms for ongoing development and refinement based on user feedback and performance metrics. Monitor user interactions, usability data, and satisfaction scores to identify areas for improvement and iteratively enhance UI designs. Adopt agile development methodologies and release regular updates to meet user needs and adapt to evolving technological trends.

User-Centered Design Approach:

User research forms the cornerstone of designing effective and meaningful smart home interfaces. Through in-depth studies such as interviews, surveys, and direct observations, designers can gather rich qualitative and quantitative insights into user behaviors, preferences, expectations, and the challenges faced when interacting with smart home technologies. These investigations go beyond surface-level analytics to reveal latent needs and motivations that are often overlooked. Understanding what influences user decision-making, which features are most valued or problematic, and how smart technologies are integrated into daily routines provides essential input for informed design and strategic direction. Building on these insights, persona development becomes a vital component of human-centered design. Personas are fictional yet data-driven representations of distinct user types who interact with smart home systems in diverse ways. They reflect specific goals, frustrations, motivations, and behavioral patterns, allowing designers to maintain a clear and empathetic focus on user needs throughout the design process. Whether representing a tech-savvy millennial in a small apartment or an elderly individual seeking accessible automation support, these archetypes ensure that final designs are grounded in real-world user experiences, rather than abstract assumptions.

User journey mapping adds a temporal and emotional dimension to the design process by charting the end-to-end experience of users as they interact with smart home systems. This exercise allows designers to visualize every touchpoint and transition—starting from discovering a device, setting it up, daily usage, to dealing with issues or system failures. By identifying where users feel delight, confusion, or frustration, journey maps help pinpoint critical pain points and moments of opportunity for improvement. This holistic perspective supports the development of features and interactions that are not only functional but also emotionally satisfying. Usability testing is an essential iterative process used to validate design choices and uncover friction in the user interface. Through structured sessions where participants are observed interacting with prototypes or real systems, designers can measure how easily users' complete tasks, where they encounter difficulties, and how they perceive the overall experience. These insights drive informed revisions, ensuring that the interface becomes more intuitive, efficient, and aligned with user expectations with each iteration. Continuous usability testing throughout the development lifecycle helps eliminate assumptions and leads to a polished, user-approved final product.

The framework for smart home services must begin with strategic service design that aligns closely with real user needs and everyday routines. Smart home systems should deliver a diverse range of services such as security monitoring, energy management, health and wellness tracking, and entertainment controls each thoughtfully designed with the end-user in mind. These services should aim to solve meaningful problems and integrate seamlessly into the user's lifestyle. Service design must be both modular and cohesive, allowing users to adopt features incrementally and extend functionality over time without disruption. Assessing the practicality of each service from the user's perspective is critical to ensure it provides real value without introducing complexity or cognitive overload. This practicality assessment centers on the intuitiveness, usability, and daily relevance of each offering. Even the most technically sophisticated features must feel effortless to use and genuinely useful. To validate this, designers often rely on simulated environments, guided user walkthroughs, and long-term field testing to determine whether a feature is both usable and beneficial in realistic, day-to-day contexts.

A seamless integration of services across various devices and platforms is essential for delivering a coherent and satisfying user experience in smart homes. Fragmented ecosystems often result in user frustration, duplicated efforts, and diminished trust in the technology. To prevent this, integration must ensure that devices such as smart thermostats, lighting systems, voice assistants, and security equipment operate harmoniously, sharing data and commands transparently. This unified operation simplifies user interaction, enhances automation capabilities, and strengthens the perception of an intelligent environment that responds consistently, regardless of the interface used. One powerful enhancement to such integration is the use of RSSI (Received Signal Strength Indicator)-based proximity detection, which adds an intelligent layer of contextual awareness. By utilizing Bluetooth or Wi-Fi signals to sense a user's physical presence, smart home systems can dynamically adjust their behavior reducing the need for manual input and enabling personalized, responsive automation. For example, lights can automatically switch on when a person enters a room, or entertainment systems can pause when the user moves away, creating a more natural and intuitive living environment shaped by real-time presence and movement patterns.

Automation based on proximity detection significantly enhances both convenience and personalization in smart home environments. Device settings can be dynamically adjusted according to a user's physical presence, ensuring that the environment consistently reflects individual preferences without the need for manual intervention. This type of automation introduces a layer of ambient intelligence, enabling the home to intuitively adapt to users' routines and behaviors thereby improving comfort, energy efficiency, and operational fluidity. However, the implementation of proximity detection also raises important privacy concerns that must be addressed with care and responsibility. To preserve user trust, systems should be designed using secure, anonymized methods that detect presence without collecting or exposing sensitive personal data. Techniques such as local signal processing, minimal data retention, and user-configurable activation settings help maintain transparency and ensure privacy. Adopting a privacy-by-design approach reassures users that increased convenience does not come at the expense of security. Additionally, offering customization options is vital to accommodate diverse user preferences, habits, and lifestyles. Providing flexibility in automation routines, device behaviors, notification methods, and control interfaces empowers users to shape their environment according to their unique needs. Whether setting a personalized morning routine, selecting preferred notification channels, or adjusting climate controls, customization reinforces a sense of autonomy and satisfaction within the smart home ecosystem.

Voice control integration plays a transformative role in enhancing both accessibility and convenience within smart home environments. Hands-free interaction via voice commands is particularly valuable for users with mobility challenges, enabling effortless control of lighting, climate, entertainment, and security systems. As natural language processing technology continues to advance, voice assistants are becoming more conversational and context-aware, supporting richer, more intuitive dialogues between users and their homes. In parallel, remote access stands out as another critical feature, granting users the flexibility to monitor and manage their homes from virtually anywhere through mobile apps or web interfaces. Whether adjusting the thermostat while commuting, viewing security camera feeds while on vacation, or remotely granting access to a visitor, remote access significantly increases convenience, control, and peace of mind ensuring users stay connected to their living space regardless of their location. From a performance and security perspective, integrating blockchain technology into smart home control services represents a cutting-edge advancement. Blockchain-based security management ensures data integrity, immutability, and resilience against cyber threats. By decentralizing control and maintaining transparent, tamper-resistant records, blockchain protects sensitive user data and provides a verifiable history of device interactions. This is particularly beneficial in scenarios involving access control, audit trails, and multi-user environments, reinforcing both trust and accountability in smart home ecosystems. Leveraging Hyperledger Fabric further optimizes the performance of smart home ecosystems by enabling efficient transaction processing, secure data exchange, and scalable management of services. As a permissioned blockchain framework, Hyperledger Fabric offers robust access controls and privacy features, making it an ideal backbone for secure smart home operations. It supports modular architectures and fine-grained policies, aligning well with the needs of evolving smart environments. Finally, scalability planning is essential for future-proofing smart home systems. As the number of connected devices and users grows, the underlying architecture must be capable of handling increased data volumes, more complex automation, and diverse interaction patterns. Scalability involves optimizing data pipelines, ensuring network stability, and supporting modular service expansion without degrading performance. A scalable system accommodates future innovation while maintaining a consistent, high-quality experience for every user.

- Conduct Consumer Research: Conduct user research to understand the daily needs and preferences of consumers, particularly the elderly and individuals across different age groups. This research should include interviews, surveys, and observations to gather insights into user behavior, preferences, and challenges when interacting with smart home technologies.

- Develop a Framework of Smart Home Services: Create a comprehensive framework of smart home services that emphasizes the practicality of each feature from the user's perspective. This framework should include services related to security, energy management, entertainment, and other essential areas, ensuring they are relevant and valuable to users.
- Implement RSSI-Based Proximity Detection: Introduce RSSI-based proximity detection to improve user comfort and enhance the overall performance of smart home systems. This system would detect users' presence and automatically adjust device settings, thereby optimizing convenience and operational efficiency.
- Control and Adapt Technology to Meet Daily Needs: Adapt smart technologies to fulfill users' daily requirements, which are key drivers of smart home adoption. This involves designing a user-friendly interface that is intuitive, comfortable, and easily customizable to individual needs and preferences.
- Performance Optimization: Enhance the performance of the smart home system by addressing key factors such as security, reliability, and scalability. This could include developing a smart home security management service using blockchain technology and applying performance optimization techniques to platforms like Hyperledger Fabric.

4. CONCLUSION

A promising future direction lies in modeling the behavior of aggregated smart homes and smart cities under various operating conditions to support energy grid stability and performance. The proposed approach addresses key challenges and opportunities in smart home development, emphasizing user needs, technology integration, and performance optimization. By applying these strategies, smart homes can become more accessible, intuitive, and efficient leading to greater user satisfaction and adoption. Imagine a world where your home is truly intelligent aware of your preferences, anticipating your needs, and adapting to your lifestyle. A home that responds to a simple voice command, adjusts lighting, temperature, and music based on your presence, and remains secure, energy-efficient, and connected to its surroundings. This is the promise of smart homes, and it is within reach. Prioritizing user experience and designing systems with end users in mind allows us to unlock the full potential of smart living creating spaces that are not only connected but truly responsive and user-centric. This study also proposes an IoT-based smart home system that intelligently manages devices using categorized and filtered sensor data. By leveraging insights from human-computer interaction (HCI) and emerging technologies, we can enhance user experience, efficiency, and satisfaction in smart environments. Our findings highlight the importance of usability, accessibility, personalization, and adaptability in UI design to meet diverse user needs. Furthermore, integrating advanced technologies such as voice assistants, gesture recognition, and AI-driven personalization holds immense potential for transforming interaction paradigms and embedding technology seamlessly into daily life. As smart home technology evolves, it is crucial for designers, developers, and researchers to focus on creating intuitive, responsive, and intelligent interfaces that empower users and enhance their quality of life.

REFERENCES

Abdaoui, N., Khalifa, I., & Faiz, S. (2023). Creating a personalized recommendation framework in smart shopping by using IoT devices. In *Proceedings of the 8th International Conference on Internet of Things, Big Data and Security* (pp. 200–207). SCITEPRESS. DOI: 10.5220/0011969400003482

Allifah, N. M., & Zualkernan, I. A. (2022). Ranking security of IoT-based smart home consumer devices. *IEEE Access : Practical Innovations, Open Solutions*, *10*, 18352–18369. DOI: 10.1109/ACCESS.2022.3148140

Asare-Bediako, B., Kling, W. L., & Ribeiro, P. F. (2013). Integrated agent-based home energy management system for smart grids applications. In *2013 IEEE PES Innovative Smart Grid Technologies Conference (ISGT)* (pp. 1–5). IEEE. DOI: 10.1109/ISGTEurope.2013.6695332

Bhalotia, N., Kumar, M., Alameen, A., Mohapatra, H., & Kolhar, M. (2023). A helping hand to the elderly: Securing their freedom through the HAIE framework. *Applied Sciences (Basel, Switzerland)*, *13*(11), 6797. DOI: 10.3390/app13116797

Brahman, F., Honarmand, M., & Jadid, S. (2015). Optimal electrical and thermal energy management of a residential energy hub, integrating demand response and energy storage system. *Energy and Building*, *90*, 65–75. DOI: 10.1016/j.enbuild.2014.12.039

Debnath, D., Siddique, A. H., Hasan, M., Faisal, F., Karim, A., Azam, S., & De Boer, F. (2021). Smart electrification of rural Bangladesh through smart grids. In *Lecture notes on data engineering and communications technologies* (Vol. 62, pp. 41–55). Springer., DOI: 10.1007/978-981-15-8677-4_4

Dehury, C. K., & Sahoo, P. K. (2016). Design and implementation of a novel service management framework for IoT devices in cloud. *Journal of Systems and Software*, *119*, 149–161. DOI: 10.1016/j.jss.2016.06.059

Diwakar, R., Sharma, R., Nayak, D., & Mohapatra, H. (2025). Optimizing load distribution in big data ecosystems. In *AI and the revival of big data* (pp. 177–200). IGI Global., DOI: 10.4018/979-8-3693-8472-5.ch008

Erdinc, O., Paterakis, N. G., Pappi, I. N., Bakirtzis, A. G., & Catalão, J. P. S. (2015). Optimal household appliances scheduling under day-ahead pricing and load-shaping demand response strategies. In *2015 48th Hawaii International Conference on System Sciences* (pp. 1462–1471). IEEE. DOI: 10.1109/HICSS.2015.178

Ewais, A. M., El-Azab, R., & Adma, M. A. R. (2018). Stand-alone microgrid energy storage schemes: Comparative study. In *2018 Twentieth International Middle East Power Systems Conference (MEPCON)* (pp. 564–569). IEEE. DOI: 10.1109/MEPCON.2018.8635266

Fthenakis, V., & Kim, H. C. (2009). Land use and electricity generation: A life-cycle analysis. *Renewable & Sustainable Energy Reviews*, *13*(6–7), 1465–1474. DOI: 10.1016/j.rser.2008.09.017

Gao, H., Xu, Y., Yin, Y., Zhang, W., Li, R., & Wang, X. (2020). Context-aware QoS prediction with neural collaborative filtering for Internet-of-Things services. *IEEE Internet of Things Journal*, *7*(5), 4532–4542. DOI: 10.1109/JIOT.2019.2956827

Gao, Z., & Patras, I. (2024). Self-supervised facial representation learning with facial region awareness. In *2024 IEEE/CVF Conference on Computer Vision and Pattern Recognition (CVPR)* (pp. 2081–2092). IEEE. DOI: 10.1109/CVPR52733.2024.00203

Hadiprawoto, T. R., & Ridley, A. L. (2023). Transparent dashboards: Open data practices for promoting competition-as-motivation in business dashboards. In *2023 IEEE 16th Pacific Visualization Symposium (PacificVis)* (pp. 142–146). IEEE. DOI: 10.1109/PacificVis56936.2023.00023

Hasan, M., Anik, M. H., & Islam, S. (2018). Microgrid energy management system for residential microgrid. In *2018 Fifth HCT Information Technology Trends (ITT)* (pp. 364–367). IEEE. DOI: 10.1109/CTIT.2018.8649518

Herzfeld, N. (2016). Human and artificial intelligence: A theological response. In *Human identity at the intersection of science, technology and religion* (pp. 117–130). Routledge., DOI: 10.4324/9781315587431-7

Hu, Y., Hu, W., & Quigley, A. (2024). Towards enhanced context awareness with vision-based multimodal interfaces. In *MobileHCI '24: Proceedings of the 26th International Conference on Mobile Human-Computer Interaction* (Article 24, pp. 1–3). ACM. DOI: 10.1145/3640471.3686646

Jo, H., Kim, S., & Joo, S. (2013). Smart heating and air conditioning scheduling method incorporating customer convenience for home energy management system. *IEEE Transactions on Consumer Electronics*, *59*(2), 316–322. DOI: 10.1109/TCE.2013.6531112

Kumar, S., Mohapatra, H., & Dalai, A. K. (2024). Enhancing energy efficiency in wireless sensor networks via clustering approach. In *2024 4th International Conference on Artificial Intelligence and Signal Processing (AISP)* (pp. 1–6). IEEE. DOI: 10.1109/AISP61711.2024.10870799

Lee, W., Cho, S., Chu, P., Vu, H., Helal, S., Song, W., Jeong, Y., & Cho, K. (2016). Automatic agent generation for IoT-based smart house simulator. *Neurocomputing*, *209*, 14–24. DOI: 10.1016/j.neucom.2015.04.130

Lei, M., Shiyan, L., Chuanwen, J., Hongling, L., & Yan, Z. (2009). A review on the forecasting of wind speed and generated power. *Renewable & Sustainable Energy Reviews*, *13*(4), 915–920. DOI: 10.1016/j.rser.2008.02.002

Lin, G., Li, J. Y., Fazly, A., Pavlovic, V., & Truong, K. (2023). Identifying multimodal context awareness requirements for supporting user interaction with procedural videos. In *CHI '23: Proceedings of the 2023 CHI Conference on Human Factors in Computing Systems* (Article 186, pp. 1–17). ACM. DOI: 10.1145/3544548.3581006

Maelen, C. V., Lievens, E., Vermeulen, J., & Milkaite, I. (2021). AI and data protection: The case of smart home assistants. In *Artificial intelligence and the law* (pp. 173–206). Intersentia., DOI: 10.1017/9781839701047.009

Magade, K., & Sharma, A. (2024). Significant role of IoT in cyber-physical systems, context awareness, and ambient intelligence. In *The next generation innovation in IoT and cloud computing with applications* (pp. 16–34). CRC Press., DOI: 10.1201/9781003406723-2

Mazen, R., Radwan, M., & Abdel-Samiea, M. (2013). Utilization of biomass energy in high-rise buildings. In *2013 4th International Youth Conference on Energy (IYCE)* (pp. 1–3). IEEE. DOI: 10.1109/IYCE.2013.6604200

Mishra, A. R., & Garg, P. (2024). Recent advancements in text summarization with natural language processing. In *A handbook of computational linguistics: Artificial intelligence in natural language processing* (pp. 15–37). Bentham Science Publishers., DOI: 10.2174/9789815238488124020004

Mohapatra, H. (2021). Socio-technical challenges in the implementation of smart city. In *2021 International Conference on Innovation and Intelligence for Informatics, Computing, and Technologies (3ICT)* (pp. 57–62). IEEE. DOI: 10.1109/3ICT53449.2021.9581905

Muck, T. R., & Frohlich, A. A. (2013). Seamless integration of HW/SW components in a HLS-based SoC design environment. In *2013 International Symposium on Rapid System Prototyping (RSP)* (pp. 109–115). IEEE. DOI: 10.1109/RSP.2013.6683966

Naik, D. B., Sri, S. N., Priya, G. M., & Priya, P. S. (2023). Machine learning boosting algorithms to detect the fake user profiles on Instagram. In *2023 International Conference on Quantum Technologies, Communications, Computing, Hardware and Embedded Systems Security (iQ-CCHESS)* (pp. 1–7). IEEE. DOI: 10.1109/iQ-CCHESS56596.2023.10391800

Nair, K., Kulkarni, J., Warde, M., Dave, Z., Rawalgaonkar, V., Gore, G., & Joshi, J. (2015). Optimizing power consumption in IoT based wireless sensor networks using Bluetooth Low Energy. In *2015 International Conference on Green Computing and Internet of Things (ICGCIoT)* (pp. 589–593). IEEE. DOI: 10.1109/ICGCIoT.2015.7380533

Nimmy, K., Sankaran, S., Achuthan, K., & Calyam, P. (2022). Lightweight and privacy-preserving remote user authentication for smart homes. *IEEE Access : Practical Innovations, Open Solutions*, *10*, 176–190. DOI: 10.1109/ACCESS.2021.3137175

Pandey, R., Rajput, I. S., Tyagi, S., Koranga, M., & Sharma, P. K. (2024). Enhancing smart city resilience. In *Advances in computational intelligence and robotics* (pp. 77–90). IGI Global. DOI: 10.4018/979-8-3693-2373-1.ch005

Paputungan, I. V., Al Fitri, M. R., & Oktiawati, U. Y. (2019). Motion and movement detection for DIY home security system. In *2019 IEEE Conference on Sustainable Utilization and Development in Engineering and Technologies (CSUDET)* (pp. 122–125). IEEE. DOI: 10.1109/CSUDET47057.2019.9214684

Patel, A., & Champaneria, T. A. (2016). Fuzzy logic-based algorithm for context awareness in IoT for smart home environment. In *2016 IEEE Region 10 Conference (TENCON)* (pp. 1057–1060). IEEE. DOI: 10.1109/TENCON.2016.7848168

Paterakis, N. G., Erdinç, O., Bakirtzis, A. G., & Catalão, J. P. S. (2015). Optimal household appliances scheduling under day-ahead pricing and load-shaping demand response strategies. *IEEE Transactions on Industrial Informatics*, *11*(6), 1509–1519. DOI: 10.1109/TII.2015.2438534

Raj, S., Sheel, S., Singh, R., Ashar, S., & Mohapatra, H. (2025). Securing smart cities. In *New horizons in leadership* (pp. 487–512). IGI Global., DOI: 10.4018/979-8-3693-6437-6.ch021

Rajasekharan, J., & Koivunen, V. (2014). Optimal energy consumption model for smart grid households with energy storage. *IEEE Journal of Selected Topics in Signal Processing*, *8*(6), 1154–1166. DOI: 10.1109/JSTSP.2014.2361315

Sesha Bhargavi, V.Sesha Bhargavi Velagaleti. (2024). Empathetic algorithms: The role of AI in understanding and enhancing human emotional intelligence. *Journal of Electrical Systems*, *20*(3s), 2051–2060. DOI: 10.52783/jes.1806

Shahriyar, F., Islam, M., Chakraborty, A., Hasan, M., Zaman, H. U., & Siddique, A. H. (2021). Fault and system analysis model of voltage source control based HVDC transmission system. In *2021 12th International Conference on Computing Communication and Networking Technologies (ICCCNT)* (pp. 1–6). IEEE. DOI: 10.1109/ICCCNT51525.2021.9579990

Smirek, L., Zimmermann, G., & Beigl, M. (2016). Just a smart home or your smart home – A framework for personalized user interfaces based on Eclipse Smart Home and Universal Remote Console. *Procedia Computer Science*, *98*, 107–116. DOI: 10.1016/j.procs.2016.09.018

Tachibana, T., Furuichi, T., & Mineno, H. (2016). Implementing and evaluating priority control mechanism for heterogeneous remote monitoring IoT system. In *MobiQuitous '16: Adjunct proceedings of the 13th International Conference on Mobile and Ubiquitous Systems: Computing, Networking and Services* (pp. 239–244). ACM. DOI: 10.1145/3004010.3004040

Tao, M., Ota, K., & Dong, M. (2017). Ontology-based data semantic management and application in IoT- and cloud-enabled smart homes. *Future Generation Computer Systems*, *76*, 528–539. DOI: 10.1016/j.future.2016.11.012

Ulutas, I., & Omeroglu, E. (2012). Maternal attitudes, emotional intelligence and home environment and their relations with emotional intelligence of sixth years old children. In *Emotional intelligence: New perspectives and applications* (pp. 117–132). IntechOpen., DOI: 10.5772/32926

Verma, G. K. (2023). Multimodal fusion framework: Emotion recognition from physiological signals. In *Multimodal affective computing: Affective information representation, modelling, and analysis* (pp. 115–127). Bentham Science Publishers., DOI: 10.2174/9789815124453123010012

Wan, C., Zhao, J., Song, Y., Xu, Z., Lin, J., & Hu, Z. (2015). Photovoltaic and solar power forecasting for smart grid energy management. *CSEE Journal of Power and Energy Systems*, *1*(4), 38–46. DOI: 10.17775/CSEEJPES.2015.00046

Wang, J., Sun, Z., Zhou, Y., & Dai, J. (2012). Optimal dispatching model of smart home energy management system. In *2012 IEEE Innovative Smart Grid Technologies - Asia (ISGT Asia)* (pp. 1–5). IEEE. DOI: 10.1109/ISGT-Asia.2012.6303266

Zenginis, I., Vardakas, J. S., Koltsaklis, N. E., & Verikoukis, C. (2022). Smart home's energy management through a clustering-based reinforcement learning approach. *IEEE Internet of Things Journal*, *9*(17), 16363–16371. DOI: 10.1109/JIOT.2022.3152586

Zhang, W., & Li, W. (2019). A deep reinforcement learning based human behavior prediction approach in smart home environments. In *2019 International Conference on Robots & Intelligent System (ICRIS)* (pp. 59–62). IEEE. DOI: 10.1109/ICRIS.2019.00024

Chapter 6
The Role of Tele-Health Approaches in Home Nutrition Support

Mehmet Özyurt
https://orcid.org/0000-0001-8115-3460
Mardin Artuklu University, Turkey

Çağlar Akçalı
https://orcid.org/0000-0001-8226-9879
Mardin Artuklu University, Turkey

ABSTRACT

The integration of digital technologies into healthcare has transformed home-based nutrition support. Tele-health, especially tele-nutrition, has become essential for delivering personalised dietary counselling and monitoring by overcoming geographical and logistical barriers. This chapter examines the development and implementation of tele-nutrition, particularly in home enteral nutrition (HEN) and chronic disease contexts. Drawing on current evidence, it discusses how mobile applications, wearable technologies, AI-based systems, and hybrid care models improve clinical outcomes, patient engagement, and continuity of care. The chapter also addresses barriers such as limited digital literacy, regulatory inconsistencies, and social inequalities, alongside ethical concerns like informed consent and algorithmic transparency. Policy implications are analysed in relation to reimbursement systems, licensure frameworks, and the legal responsibilities of clinicians. The chapter concludes with strategic recommendations for integrating tele-nutrition into public health infrastructures and outlines research priorities focused on long-term effectiveness, patient-reported outcomes, and inclusive design. By synthesizing multidisciplinary

DOI: 10.4018/979-8-3373-3099-0.ch006

evidence, this chapter provides a comprehensive roadmap for the sustainable integration of tele-health in home-based nutrition support, reinforcing its relevance in achieving equitable, person-centred, and technology-enabled dietary care.

1. INTRODUCTION

The digital health transformation has created a significant change in the delivery of healthcare services in recent years, and this transformation has required the integration of telehealth applications in specific areas such as nutritional support. Telehealth is a method of delivering healthcare services remotely, which has been critical, for example, in pandemics such as COVID-19 or similar situations (Mundi et al., 2021; Mulherin et al., 2020). Telehealth applications can reach more individuals and improve health outcomes by overcoming access barriers (Nelson et al., 2017).

Telehealth applications provide many advantages for individuals who need to receive nutritional support. In particular, patients who need home nutrition support (home enteral nutrition-HEN) can overcome the difficulties they face in traditional face-to-face examinations through telehealth applications. Ma et al. (2025) found that patients receiving enteral nutrition support at home have a high level of acceptance of telehealth applications. In addition, mobile telehealth applications have emerged as an important tool to increase health literacy during nutrition counselling (Bahshur et al., 2020).

Telehealth tools provide great benefits, especially for individuals suffering from chronic diseases. Nelson et al. (2017) present supporting data; research shows that telehealth applications can reach many patients at the same time and provide access to healthcare services. For example, during COVID-19, many people had difficulty accessing healthcare services due to social distancing; however, telehealth minimised these difficulties and enabled patients to receive the nutritional support they needed (Ma et al., 2025).

Customised nutritional support provided by telehealth applications helps individuals to feel better as it adopts a patient-oriented approach. In the study by Nelson et al. (2017), it is associated with the results that individuals receiving home parenteral nutrition (HPN) have high levels of satisfaction with the support provided through telehealth and feel better emotionally. Such support not only provides information about nutrition, but also strengthens the emotional connection between patients and caregivers (Mulherin et al., 2020).

Social support provided by telehealth applications is important in the care of individuals with chronic diseases. The applications allow patients to reduce the stress in their daily lives and receive emotional support (Persoon et al., 2005). This is especially critical for patients who follow dietary methods such as HPN, as these patients often experience a sense of social isolation (Ma et al., 2025). Telehealth support reduces this sense of isolation and creates a positive support network.

In terms of nutritional support, the diversity of resources is also important. Baker et al. (2011) emphasise that integrated telehealth and care management programmes in individuals with chronic diseases are both important in terms of cost-effectiveness and have a critical potential in providing quality and effective care. In addition to nutritional support, these programmes offer important gains in better management of one's health (Mundi et al., 2021).

There are also some challenges in digital health transformation. Mundi et al. (2021) state that financial constraints and structural complexity in healthcare delivery are among the main challenges faced. It has been found that low-income individuals have difficulties in accessing telehealth services and this affects their potential to receive nutritional support (Nelson et al., 2017). Therefore, reforms to overcome financial barriers are vital for effective nutrition support and general health services.

Another advantage of telehealth is the ability to remotely monitor individuals' nutritional status and physical health. Such monitoring enables continuous assessment of patient status and rapid interventions when necessary (Ma et al., 2025). Nelson et al. (2017) show that health data recorded by remote monitoring has positive effects on patient care and enables healthcare professionals to take faster action when needed. Furthermore, the impact of the pandemic on nutritional behaviours should also be addressed. Aalaei et al. (2025) state that their research during COVID-19 emphasises the role of mobile applications in increasing individuals' access to information on healthy lifestyles during this period. In this context, telehealth systems increase the knowledge level of individuals by providing information flow about nutrition and preventing misinformation (Zheng et al., 2016).

Building upon these findings, the use of smart devices and digital platforms not only enables individuals to access health information quickly, but also plays an active role in managing their own health. In the study conducted by Ma et al. (2025), it was observed that the overall satisfaction levels of patients increased with digital platforms used in home enteral nutrition applications. Such applications are considered as an approach that makes individuals feel better and offers significant benefits in their daily lives.

As the integration of mobile and digital tools becomes more common in clinical settings, it is also important to consider how such trends align with broader telehealth advancements in related disciplines. The shift toward telehealth-based service delivery in nutrition has paralleled broader trends observed in other specialties, such as gastroenterology. Telehealth not only enhances patient accessibility but also promotes care continuity and multidisciplinary coordination—especially valuable in managing chronic gastrointestinal and metabolic disorders that require sustained dietary regulation (Kim et al., 2024). Moreover, implementation of hybrid models—combining in-person and virtual visits—has been shown to improve both patient outcomes and satisfaction by allowing greater flexibility and personalization. These findings underscore the potential for tele-nutrition systems to benefit from cross-disciplinary practices that emphasize shared digital workflows and patient-centered engagement.

In the future perspective, digital health transformation will play an even greater role in nutrition support. Developing technologies are evolving in a way that will enable health systems to operate more efficiently and patients to have easier access to the nutritional support they need. In this respect, it is emphasised that health policies should be reshaped to support this transformation (Mundi et al., 2017).

In conclusion, digital health transformation increases the efficiency of the health-care system with various advantages it offers in the field of nutritional support. Telehealth applications facilitate patients' access to healthcare services, provide social support and improve health outcomes. In the coming period, this trend is expected to continue and digital health innovations will radically change the way individuals are reached. Innovative redesign of healthcare services will enable this transformation to continue in a healthy and sustainable manner. To adapt to the rapidly evolving landscape, Kelly (2020) calls for urgent reform in dietetics education and professional development. Digital literacy, data interpretation, and ethical use of AI tools must become core components of training curricula. Without proactive upskilling, dietitians risk becoming passive users of technologies designed by others, which could further marginalize their role in integrated digital health ecosystems. Building interdisciplinary partnerships with technology developers, policy makers, and patients will be essential in co-designing systems that reflect the values and competencies of the profession.

As tele-health platforms become increasingly sophisticated, it is crucial that these technologies accommodate the personal preferences and psychosocial needs of patients receiving HEN. Recent studies show a growing interest in blended food-based tube feedings (BTFs), which not only support nutritional adequacy but also contribute to a sense of normalcy and empowerment among patients and caregivers (Pentiuk, 2011; Martin & Gardner, 2017). The ability to customise enteral feeds with natural ingredients has been associated with improved tolerance, reduced gastrointestinal symptoms, and enhanced quality of life—benefits that tele-health platforms could amplify by offering virtual dietitian consultations and educational content for safe BTF preparation (Pentiuk, 2011; Gibson & Roberfroid, 1995). Thus, integrating these evolving feeding preferences into tele-health infrastructure aligns digital innovation with patient-centred care.

The proliferation of mobile applications and smart devices has significantly reshaped how patients engage with their nutritional care. Mobile health apps now enable real-time tracking of food intake, macronutrient distribution, and lifestyle habits, providing a robust platform for continuous patient engagement and self-management (Limketkai et al., 2021). These apps not only enhance adherence through feedback loops but also offer providers the opportunity to monitor trends and provide timely interventions. For example, apps that integrate dietary recall with visual tracking reduce the risk of underreporting and recall bias—common limitations in traditional dietary assessments (Ventura et al., 2006). This synergy between self-monitoring and professional oversight demonstrates the potential for tele-health platforms to evolve into hybrid models that combine digital autonomy with clinical accountability.

2. TELE-NUTRITION AND AVAILABILITY

In these days, the transformation of health services, combined with technology, has led to the emergence of new and effective methods in the provision of nutrition services. Tele-nutrition is a model that aims to provide nutrition counselling to individuals integrated with distance health services. This model attracts attention with its effects on both physical and mental health. Tele-nutrition systems are implemented using various digital platforms to monitor the health status of patients, correct dietary habits and improve overall health (Kelly et al., 2023; Kelly et al., 2022; Nguyen et al., 2024).

The feasibility of tele-nutrition systems is possible by integrating these systems into home care services and providing individuals with easy access to health services. Remote nutrition counselling offers a great advantage, especially for patients living in rural and marginal areas (Nguyen et al., 2024). Especially for elderly individuals, difficulties in technical knowledge and device use should be taken into consideration. Research shows that functional requirements designed for older people have positive effects on their nutritional status. In this context, visual elements such as clear graphics and alert systems increase the effectiveness of home health systems (Shamsabadi et al., 2023).

Tele-nutrition platforms must not only provide educational support but also address logistical and systemic challenges frequently experienced in home care settings. One of the most significant barriers reported in the literature is the fragmented nature of care transitions from hospital to home, which often leads to inadequate instruction, mismanagement of enteral supplies, and increased risk of readmission (Schneider et al., 2001; Hall et al., 2014). These issues can be mitigated through digitally supported coordination models that involve registered dietitians, home care teams, and supply chain operators in a unified system. Evidence suggests that interventions incorporating care continuity protocols and telehealth-assisted monitoring significantly reduce malnutrition rates and hospitalisations in HEN patients (Hall et al., 2014).

Another important component of tele-nutrition systems is remote monitoring and information sharing. These systems allow patients to monitor their daily calorie intake, food consumption and health status. Remote nutrition counselling also provides real-time feedback and support to improve patient motivation. For example, in tele-nutrition counselling studies applied in individuals with spinal cord injury, it is important to identify strategies that support individuals to achieve their goals (Wood et al., 2021). Tele-nutrition has attracted more attention during the COVID-19 pandemic and has been observed to play an important role in ensuring continuity of healthcare services (Tewksbury et al., 2021).

Recent innovations in wearable technologies, particularly smartwatches and wrist-based sensors, have opened new avenues for passive data collection in nutritional care. These devices can monitor physical activity, heart rate variability, and even detect hand-to-mouth movements—providing proxy markers for dietary intake and functional status (Dong et al., 2014; Limketkai et al., 2021). Their integration into tele-nutrition platforms allows for remote, objective assessments that supplement or even replace self-reported measures. Importantly, clinicians report that patient-generated health data from wearables can be useful in initiating care discussions and tailoring nutritional interventions, particularly in populations with chronic illnesses or mobility limitations (Alpert et al., 2020).

It is stated that various social, cultural and technological barriers must be overcome in order for an effective tele-nutrition application to be successful. It is important to provide user trainings and support systems to increase the effectiveness of tele-nutrition applications. Previous studies have shown that remote delivery of nutrition counselling services helps to significantly improve nutritional quality compared with face-to-face services (Norouzi et al., 2024). However, it is also emphasised that methods such as video calls and telephone counselling have some limitations. The inability to meet the need for physical examination may pose a challenge for older individuals and social groups that are not familiar with technology (Prat et al., 2024).

Building on the recognition of these challenges, a successful tele-nutrition model must also integrate individual-level determinants that affect service uptake and effectiveness. It is of great importance to consider individual differences and needs in the development of the implementation model of tele-nutrition systems. In this framework, individuals' health status, lifestyles, socio-economic status and technological competences should be taken into account. In addition, it is stated that the education of health professionals should also be emphasised. Research in the field of nutrition shows that tele-nutrition has positive effects on patient satisfaction and health outcomes (Bergerot et al., 2024; Assaad et al., 2024).

As digital health technologies increasingly integrate into healthcare systems, the role of dietitians is undergoing substantial transformation. Kelly (2020) argues that the profession of dietetics must confront a digital disruption that challenges traditional models of care, communication, and professional identity. From algorithm-based dietary planning tools to AI-driven nutrition chatbots, many functions previously seen as core to the profession are now being shared with—or replaced by—digital systems. While these innovations offer opportunities to expand reach and standardize care, they also raise questions about the future competencies required of nutrition professionals in telehealth environments.

Despite its advantages, telehealth systems must be adapted to address disparities in access caused by digital illiteracy, limited broadband connectivity, or low socioeconomic status. Kim et al. (2024) emphasize that patients from underserved communities, including racial and ethnic minorities, face greater barriers to utilizing digital platforms for healthcare. These barriers can limit the effectiveness of remote nutrition services, particularly in populations with pre-existing dietary vulnerabilities. Thus, tele-nutrition programs must incorporate culturally and linguistically tailored education materials and low-bandwidth compatible platforms to promote inclusive engagement.

3. HISTORICAL DEVELOPMENT OF TELEHEALTH IN NUTRITION SUPPORT

The historical development of telehealth in nutrition support has evolved significantly, particularly in recent years due to technological advancements and the exigencies of the COVID-19 pandemic. Telehealth modalities, often classified under the umbrella of "telenutrition," utilize telecommunications technology to deliver nutritional counseling and interventions remotely (Eid et al., 2024; Mundi et al., 2021). This evolution can be traced through various stages, from early telephonic consultations to the current use of sophisticated telehealth platforms that incorporate video conferencing, mobile applications, and real-time monitoring of patient progress.

Initially, the concept of delivering healthcare remotely emerged in the late 19th century, primarily relying on telephone communications to address patient needs (Mundi et al., 2021). However, the true expansion of telehealth services, particularly in the context of nutrition support, did not take root until the integration of digital technologies became commonplace. Telenutrition services rapidly expanded during the COVID-19 pandemic, as lockdowns and social distancing measures necessitated a shift from traditional in-person consultations to remote interactions (Bas et al., 2023; Mehta et al., 2020). Studies have shown that telehealth not only provided continuity in care but also increased access for patients, particularly those in rural or underserved areas where traditional healthcare services may have been limited (Pfeil and Shellhaas, 2023; Nguyen et al., 2024).

The early adoption of telehealth in nutrition support consisted mostly of one-on-one nutritional assessments and counseling via phone calls. However, as technology advanced, this modality transformed into comprehensive telehealth systems capable of providing a range of services, including nutritional assessments, personalized meal plans, and ongoing support through various digital platforms (Mundi et al., 2021; Kelly et al., 2023). In this regard, a systematic review by Kelly et al. (2023) delineates the effectiveness of telehealth interventions in achieving improved nutritional outcomes compared to traditional in-person consultations.

Telehealth's integration into nutrition support practices highlighted the flexibility and accessibility of such services, allowing healthcare professionals to better tailor their approaches to individual patient needs. The correlation between dietitian engagement and patient outcomes facilitates the development of personalized interventions supported by continuous monitoring (Eid et al., 2024; Kelly et al., 2023). Moreover, this evolution paved the way for the emergence of evidence-based practices that inform virtual nutrition counseling (Shah et al., 2021).

The pandemic catalyzed an unprecedented surge in the adoption of telehealth services. A study by Raz et al. (2024) emphasized how practitioners adapted their nutritional counseling practices to online formats, providing insights into new methodologies that emerged from necessity. This includes virtual educational workshops, the use of mobile health applications to track dietary intake, and the establishment of support networks for weight management (Pfeil and Shellhaas, 2023; Eid et al., 2024). A well-documented example of this phenomenon is seen in oncology patients, who benefited significantly from telenutrition services during the pandemic as they faced unique challenges related to their care and dietary needs (Hogan et al., 2024; Arem et al., 2022).

Moreover, challenges to the implementation of telehealth in nutrition support cannot go unmentioned. Some research suggests barriers such as patients' preferences for in-person consultations, lack of familiarity with technology, and varying levels of digital literacy among patient populations (Assaad et al., 2024; Arem et al., 2022). Mixed-method studies have revealed that while some patients appreciated the convenience of telehealth, others felt that face-to-face interactions were vital for effective communication and the establishment of therapeutic relationships (Alhuwayfi et al., 2023; Trivedi et al., 2024). The challenge lies not only in adapting to a new mode of service delivery but in ensuring that patients continue to receive high-quality care that meets their psychological and educational needs.

The incorporation of telehealth practices has also led to the development of innovative strategies for engaging patients in their nutrition journeys. Many studies articulated the significance of integrating family support and social interaction into telehealth platforms to bolster patient commitment and adherence to dietary interventions (Bookari et al., 2023; Latif et al., 2024). For instance, nutritional monitoring and coaching that include family participation have been shown to improve compliance among patients undergoing various dietary interventions (Kirk et al., 2022; Eid et al., 2024).

4. POLICY, REGULATORY, AND LEGAL CONSIDERATIONS

As tele-health approaches emerge as increasingly viable alternatives in the provision of home nutrition support, understanding the associated policy, regulatory, and legal considerations becomes imperative. The COVID-19 pandemic served as a catalyst for the rapid adoption of telehealth services, including home nutrition support, highlighting both opportunities and challenges that are directly influenced by existing and evolving regulations.

4.1. Regulatory Frameworks for Tele-Health

The rapid expansion of telehealth was expedited by various states and federal authorities enacting temporary legislative measures that relaxed previously stringent regulations regarding virtual service delivery. This included modifications to licensure requirements, reimbursement policies, and practice standards, allowing healthcare professionals, including registered dietitian nutritionists (RDNs), to deliver services virtually across state lines (Mehta et al., 2020). The Centers for Medicare and Medicaid Services (CMS) notably expanded telehealth coverage, facilitating remote nutrition consultations during the pandemic (Mundi et al., 2021).

However, these temporary measures necessitate a more permanent evaluation. Many experts emphasize the need for ongoing dialogue around how post-pandemic regulations will shape the future landscape of telehealth (Williams et al., 2024). Without lasting policy frameworks, the sustainability of these services may be compromised. For instance, significant discrepancies in telehealth utilization rates persist across state lines, with some states implementing long-term or permanent policies while others have reverted to stricter regulations (Mehta et al., 2020).

4.2. Legal Implications of Tele-Health

Legal considerations related to tele-health are multifaceted, encompassing patient privacy, data security, and liability issues. The Health Insurance Portability and Accountability Act (HIPAA) regulations have been integral in dictating how telehealth services should maintain patient confidentiality. The pandemic prompted some flexibility in HIPAA enforcement in light of the urgent need for care; nevertheless, the transition to telehealth requires providers to ensure they have adequate security measures in place to protect sensitive health information (Shah et al., 2021).

Moreover, legal implications arise concerning malpractice, especially when employing remote modalities for assessment and treatment planning in nutrition care. Providers may encounter broader challenges if telehealth consultations lead to adverse health outcomes due to inadequate interpretations of dietary needs based on limited assessment capabilities compared to in-person evaluations (Mauldin et al., 2021). This scenario raises questions of liability and whether traditional standards of care are applicable in a virtual context (Shah et al., 2021).

With the increasing use of consumer-grade health tracking tools in clinical nutrition, regulatory clarity is becoming essential. Devices such as smartwatches and continuous glucose monitors may eventually influence clinical decision-making, yet many remain outside formal FDA regulation unless they are explicitly used for diagnostic or therapeutic purposes (Foster & Torous, 2019; Limketkai et al., 2021). The FDA's Digital Health Software Precertification Program offers a potential pathway for low-risk wearable devices to gain clearance, but clinicians must remain aware of the limitations in data accuracy, user interpretation, and privacy implications. Ensuring secure data transmission, particularly when integrated with electronic health records (EHR), is crucial to maintaining patient trust and legal compliance.

4.3. Economic and Reimbursement Policies

Reimbursement policies are significant barriers to the consistent implementation of telehealth in nutrition services (Porteny et al., 2025). Different insurance providers have evolved varied coverage mechanisms for telehealth services; however, inconsistencies can deter clinicians from fully adopting these models. Nationally, findings indicate that some insurance plans are reluctant to cover these services unless stringent documentation and justification are provided (Ong et al., 2024).

In the wake of the COVID-19 crisis, some reimbursement policies have adapted more favorably toward telehealth strategies (McBain et al., 2023). However, ongoing advocacy is essential to ensure that these changes are acknowledged and retained, allowing flexibility to support a broader range of tele-nutrition services, particularly for marginalized groups who may struggle to access nutrition support otherwise (Zhai et al., 2023).

4.4. Ethical Considerations

Ethics in telehealth extends beyond patient confidentiality to encompass equity in access to services. The shift to telehealth has the potential to exacerbate existing healthcare disparities if specific population segments are disadvantaged due to technological literacy or resource availability (Arem et al., 2022). Ensuring that telehealth serves not only well-resourced consumers but also those in underserved communities is crucial. Interventions that incorporate methods to enhance digital literacy among patients are paramount (Turner et al., 2022).

Also germane is the ethical consideration surrounding informed consent in a telehealth context. Patients must be adequately informed about the nature of telehealth interactions, associated risks, and the limitations inherent to virtual consultations compared to traditional face-to-face engagements (Gajarawala & Pelkowski, 2021).

The increasing use of automation and data-driven platforms in dietetic care raises new ethical considerations. Kelly (2020) emphasizes that while digital solutions offer scale and efficiency, they can dilute the personalised and empathetic nature of nutrition counselling. Ethical practice in tele-nutrition must therefore balance the benefits of automation with the humanistic elements of care, ensuring that digital tools do not compromise the dignity, preferences, and values of patients. Furthermore, the lack of well-established professional standards for digital dietetic practices makes it more difficult to determine accountability and clearly define professional roles.

Additionaly from an ethical perspective, ensuring equitable access to telehealth remains a major concern. As Kim et al. (2024) point out, digital exclusion not only reinforces existing health disparities but also violates the principle of justice in care delivery. Patients who lack digital competence or equipment may be unintentionally excluded from innovative services. In nutrition care, this can translate into missed education, delayed follow-up, and unaddressed malnutrition. Ethical tele-nutrition design should therefore prioritize user-friendly interfaces, multilingual support, and alternative modalities such as telephone or hybrid follow-up for at-risk groups.

In addition to data protection and consent, Ahmadi (2024) notes that ethical concerns also arise from the opacity of AI systems. Many AI-based recommendations in digital nutrition platforms are generated through complex algorithms that lack explainability. This raises challenges for patient autonomy and trust. To address this, the use of explainable AI (XAI) models that offer transparent, interpretable outputs is recommended to ensure responsible integration of technology in dietetic care.

5. HOME NUTRITION SUPPORT APPLICATIONS OF TELE-HEALTH APPROACHES ON COUNTRY BASIS

The COVID-19 pandemic has led to rapid adoption of telehealth practices on a global scale, supporting continuity of care by reducing the risk of infection for patients receiving nutritional support at home. For example, the rate of telemedicine use in the USA increased from 11% before the pandemic to 46% in 2020

(Ramirez-Vega et al., 2022). Disruptions in routine tests and controls have led to interruptions in home parenteral/enteral nutrition services; however, many centres have rapidly introduced remote monitoring and counselling systems (Mundi et al., 2021). International organisations (The European Society of Parenteral and Enteral Nutrition (ESPEN), The American Society for Parenteral and Enteral Nutrition (ASPEN) have recommended prioritising telehealth applications by reducing face-to-face visits (Lal et al., 2020; Wells Mulherin et al., 2020). In this section, models and disseminable practices developed during the pandemic period are discussed with examples from different countries.

In Turkey, tele-health applications in home nutrition support have expanded notably, particularly through telenutrition services provided by licensed dietitians for chronic disease management and special patient groups. These services employ live video conferencing, mobile applications, social media, SMS, and e-mail to deliver medical nutrition therapy, ensuring continuity of care for individuals with mobility limitations or those living in remote areas. During the COVID-19 pandemic, telehealth became a vital alternative to face-to-face consultations, supporting dietary monitoring, patient education, and treatment adherence in conditions such as obesity, diabetes, phenylketonuria, and inflammatory bowel disease. For example, patients with phenylketonuria were successfully monitored via telecommunication tools, maintaining metabolic control and improving dietary compliance during lockdowns.

Similarly, in inflammatory bowel disease management, telenutrition has provided cost-effective, accessible, and personalised dietary counselling, enabling regular monitoring and symptom management despite limited specialist availability. However, challenges such as lack of standardisation, technological barriers, and insurance reimbursement issues remain. Current literature emphasises the need for national strategies, legal frameworks, and professional training to integrate telenutrition sustainably into Turkey's healthcare system (Güney Coşkun et al., 2023; Muslu, 2022).

The United States has made significant progress in the delivery of home nutritional support services through telehealth during the COVID-19 pandemic, with licensing and reimbursement restrictions temporarily lifted in 2020, allowing these services to be rapidly integrated into the digital environment. In a study led by the Mayo Clinic, a telehealth model including steps such as technology selection, virtual examination protocols and team-patient trainings was successfully implemented (Mundi et al., 2021). In this way, the follow-up of patients in need of chronic nutritional support could be continued uninterruptedly in the home environment; it was demonstrated that tele-nutrition applications can be as effective as face-to-face approaches.

Canada has developed pioneering practices in the field of home nutritional support by overcoming the access difficulties created by its vast geographical structure through telehealth applications. A tele-medicine programme initiated by Toronto General Hospital in Ontario in the early 2000s enabled total parenteral nutrition

(TPN) patients living in rural areas to make video calls with the specialist team at the centre. In the evaluations of 81 teleconferences conducted, it was reported that patient satisfaction was above 85% during the implementation period between 2002 and 2007, and it was determined that remote consultations and follow-ups provided significant cost and time savings. For example, approximately 724 Canadian dollars in travelling and accommodation costs were avoided by telehealth. The catheter sepsis rate of 0.89 per 1000 catheter-days supports the clinical safety of the practice (Saqui et al., 2007). In line with these positive results, it is recommended that telehealth services in Canada should be integrated into home nutrition support on a national scale.

The United Kingdom is among the European countries that stand out with successful practices for the follow-up of patients receiving home parenteral nutrition (HPN) via telehealth. In the UK, at a national intestinal failure unit in Salford, routine 3-6 monthly follow-ups of HPN patients have been carried out via video calls since 2015. This system eliminated the need for patients to physically travel to the health centre, avoiding an average journey of 56.7 miles per patient. In the evaluations conducted, no adverse clinical outcomes were detected in 25 patients monitored by telehealth; 63% of the patients stated that they were satisfied with remote follow-up, and the overall satisfaction level was reported as 85 out of 100. In addition, in this group, the rate of emergency hospitalisation due to nutrition therapy remained at a low level of 8% (Cloutier et al., 2020). These data show that telehealth applications offer a safe and effective follow-up model that can replace face-to-face visits.

Similarly, during the COVID-19 pandemic in the UK and France, patient monitoring via telephone and video calls has become widespread in order to reduce face-to-face visits (Pironi et al., 2016; Sasegbon et al., 2025). Centres such as Paris Beaujon Hospital continued to care for patients by using telehealth technologies effectively in this process. The importance of this approach was emphasised in ESPEN (2020) guidelines and France was among the contributing countries in a multinational study published in 2025. In the study, 96% of the physicians participating in the study stated that video-based HPN interviews met all the needs of the patients; 57% stated that these interviews provided services of equivalent quality to face-to-face examinations. Supporting the practices in France with standardised protocols and training materials resulted in positive feedback from both healthcare professionals and patients (Sasegbon et al., 2025).

Italy has a well-established infrastructure in the field of home enteral and parenteral nutrition services and is among the countries that are rapidly integrating telehealth applications with these services. The Home Artificial Nutrition (HAN) registry system, initiated by the Italian Society for Enteral and Parenteral Nutrition (SINPE) (2014) in 2005, provides coordination of HPN and HEN services throughout the country. The prevalence of patients per million people increased from 195.6 in

2005 to 325.5 in 2012; it was observed that developments in regional health services as well as the spread of telehealth practices played an important role in this 66% increase. During the COVID-19 pandemic, 60-95% of medical assessments were conducted virtually, and patients receiving home nutritional support were monitored through regular telephone and video-based calls (Hincapié et al., 2020; Pironi et al., 2005; Pironi et al., 2017; Ramirez-Vega et al., 2022). This practice shows that by integrating a strong national home care system with telehealth technologies, uninterrupted and safe nutritional treatment can be maintained even in times of crisis.

Switzerland has made a significant contribution to the literature in this field with a multicentre survey study evaluating the attitudes of patients receiving home nutrition support towards digital health solutions. In a study evaluating the views of 35 patients receiving home parenteral nutrition (HPN) on eHealth applications, 86% of the participants reported that they had access to digital devices and 63% actively used health applications between 2020-2021. Features such as data tracking, checklists, educational content and video calls were considered important by patients; 74% stated that they were willing to enter their own health data into the system (Schönenberger et al., 2022). The results obtained show that HPN patients in Switzerland are highly ready and willing to use digital health technologies and provide a strong basis for the applicability of tele-nutrition applications.

Argentina stands out as one of the successful examples in Latin America for telehealth monitoring of patients receiving home parenteral nutrition (HPN) during the COVID-19 pandemic. In line with the recommendations of international organisations such as ESPEN and ASPEN, patient monitoring was conducted via telephone or online platforms, and personal protective equipment protocols were carefully implemented when face-to-face visits were mandatory (Barclay et al., 2021; Lal et al., 2020; Wells Mulherin et al., 2020). In the study conducted by Crivelli et al. (2022), 380 HPN patients were regularly monitored via telehealth by a multidisciplinary team providing a specialised home care service during the period of strict curfew restrictions. During the follow-up period, routine blood tests, individual nutritional planning and catheter care were maintained without interruption; the COVID-19 infection rate was reported as only 3.15%. Most infected patients recovered with mild symptoms; the rate of serious complications remained low. In addition, in the same study, 111 catheter infections were detected in the telemedicine-assisted follow-up model and the rate per 1000 catheter-days was reported to be below the international acceptance limits (Crivelli et al., 2022). Thus, it has been demonstrated that telehealth has the potential not only to reduce the risk of infectious diseases, but also to maintain continuity and quality of care.

China is one of the countries that can effectively scale telehealth applications in home nutritional support, with its large population and predisposition to digital solutions. The Tele-Medicine Supported Home Enteral Nutrition Service (HENST) model developed by a university hospital in Sichuan province has led to a significant increase in the number of patients and frequency of telemedicine follow-up between 2018 and 2022. Within the scope of this model, a total of 3,710 tele-medicine visits were conducted with 1,437 patients as of 2022, and the remote monitoring rate increased to 35.8%. Patients were satisfied with the telehealth model, especially in terms of time and cost savings; 98.7% of the participants reported satisfaction with the service. This model stands out as one of China's effective and applicable telehealth examples in this field by offering an affordable and accessible care approach that can replace face-to-face visits in patient follow-up (Ma et al., 2025).

Australia has been one of the early adopters of telehealth applications due to its large surface area and rural population structure. In this context, dietetic services have started to be provided through telephone and video-based platforms, and successful results have been achieved especially in hard-to-reach areas and special patient groups. In a pilot study conducted at the Royal Brisbane & Women's Hospital in Queensland, swallowing and nutritional rehabilitation after head and neck cancer treatment was provided through telehealth; patients were able to receive guidance from dietitians and speech therapists online without visiting the hospital. Patients reported a high level of satisfaction with the service provided; especially time saving and the elimination of the need for physical transport were cited as the main advantages (Collins et al., 2017). Kelly et al. (2020) emphasised that tele-dietitian services are an effective and cost-effective intervention model and suggested that these practices should be disseminated across health systems. In this context, the elderly, individuals with chronic diseases and those living in rural areas can regularly access nutrition counselling at home. The Australian experience shows that telehealth offers a flexible, accessible and effective model of care for medical nutrition treatments, even in specialised areas.

Mexico has effectively utilised its long-standing telehealth infrastructure to support public health during the COVID-19 pandemic. Locatel, a telephone and internet-based counselling line that has been operating in the capital city of Mexico City for more than 40 years, turned into a platform where requests for information and medical support related to COVID-19 intensified during the pandemic (Ramirez-Vega et al., 2022). Thanks to telehealth, patients' access to basic services without going to the hospital has prevented overload in the health system. Mexican health authorities see ICT as a strategic tool to increase access to health services and emphasise the potential of this approach to reduce social inequalities and support development (Bowles et al., 2021; Zagmutt et al., 2020). In the field of nutrition, tele-dietetic practices called 'telenutrition' came to the agenda with the pandemic; measurements made in face-to-face interviews started to be carried out remotely with methods supported by family participation (Ramirez-Vega et al., 2022). Mexico's vision is to make telenutrition services a permanent component of the health system and to expand digital counselling and education. This approach demonstrates rapid adaptation to pandemic conditions and the potential for digital transformation of nutrition services (Barazzoni et al., 2020; Ramirez-Vega et al., 2022).

6. FUTURE STRATEGIC RECOMMENDATIONS AND RESEARCH DIRECTIONS FOR TELE-HEALTH APPROACHES IN HOME NUTRITION SUPPORT

The landscape of healthcare delivery has fundamentally transformed with the expansion of tele-health services, particularly in the realm of home-based nutrition support. As digital health solutions become increasingly embedded in public health systems, the need for strategic frameworks and evidence-based guidance becomes more urgent. This proposal outlines future directions to strengthen the tele-health ecosystem in nutritional care, focusing on regulation, reimbursement, literacy, multidisciplinary collaboration, research priorities, technological advancement, and equity in access.

One of the foremost challenges in tele-health implementation is the inconsistency in regulatory frameworks across jurisdictions. The rapid expansion of digital health services, accelerated during global health crises, exposed gaps in existing policies. Inconsistent regulations—ranging from licensure and service definitions to quality and privacy standards—can limit the scalability and sustainability of tele-nutrition interventions (Brunton et al., 2021; Jeri et al., 2023). To address this, there is a pressing need to establish national or cross-regional standards that ensure both quality assurance and professional accountability. Policymakers should collaborate with healthcare professionals to create regulatory frameworks that cover licensure, reimbursement modalities, and technology standards specific to nutrition services.

Equally important is the development of equitable reimbursement systems. Disparities in tele-nutrition reimbursement policies remain a barrier to widespread provider adoption. Payment inequities across service modalities can discourage clinicians from offering tele-health services, thereby restricting patient access (Mundi et al., 2021; Khan et al., 2022). Future strategies should advocate for payment parity between virtual and in-person consultations and promote value-based reimbursement models that reward positive health outcomes, particularly in chronic disease management.

Another critical area is digital literacy and technological accessibility. The effectiveness of tele-health relies not only on system readiness but also on users' ability to engage meaningfully with the technology. However, significant disparities persist in patients' digital competence and access to necessary devices or internet connectivity (Butzner & Cuffee, 2021; Herbert et al., 2023). Empowering individuals through structured digital literacy programs—such as mobile tutorials, help desks, or community workshops—can mitigate these disparities and ensure that tele-nutrition platforms are inclusive and user-friendly.

Holistic care models that incorporate multidisciplinary approaches have shown promising results in improving patient outcomes. Integrated tele-health models involving professionals from different disciplines—such as dietitians, mental health experts, and exercise physiologists—are more effective in managing complex conditions (Galvão et al., 2022). Including family members in nutrition consultations has also been linked to improved patient engagement and better adherence to dietary recommendations (Brunton et al., 2021). Developing care pathways that emphasize collaborative planning and shared decision-making is essential for sustaining long-term behavioral change.

Evidence from gastroenterology further supports the integration of tele-nutrition into multidisciplinary care models. Kim et al. (2024) report that remote care platforms that incorporate not only physicians and nurses, but also dietitians and behavioral health professionals, improve clinical outcomes and patient satisfaction. These collaborative systems are particularly valuable for managing complex nutritional conditions—such as those requiring enteral or elimination diets—where psychological adherence and metabolic monitoring are critical. Expanding tele-nutrition to include mental health, pharmacy, and physical therapy input may further strengthen its utility in chronic care frameworks.

Despite growing acceptance, research in tele-nutrition has often focused on short-term outcomes, neglecting longitudinal impacts and behavioral adaptation over time. Existing studies have yet to fully capture the long-term clinical, psychological, and economic implications of digital nutrition interventions (Khan et al., 2022). While digital nutrition services have shown short-term efficacy, there remains a substantial gap in understanding the long-term impact of HEN interventions on patient-reported outcomes. To address this gap, validated tools that assess patient-reported outcomes in home enteral nutrition have gained attention in recent years. The NutriQoL® questionnaire, specifically developed for individuals receiving HEN, enables systematic evaluation of health-related quality of life in clinical and research settings (Hinchliffe et al., 2022). This instrument considers both physical and psychosocial dimensions of patient well-being, including issues of social participation, autonomy, and feeding-related burden. As tele-health systems evolve, integrating digital versions of NutriQoL® into remote monitoring platforms could facilitate real-time tracking of patient satisfaction and psychosocial adaptation, ensuring a more holistic approach to tele-nutrition. Such integration would also allow providers to proactively identify patients at risk of poor quality of life and tailor interventions accordingly. Reddy and Malone (1998) found that although HEN can reduce hospitalisation and improve functional outcomes, many patients report social isolation and emotional distress without appropriate follow-up mechanisms.

Instruments like the NutriQoL®, designed to evaluate the quality of life in patients receiving HEN, still require broader validation and digital integration to be applied effectively in tele-health contexts (Cuerda et al., 2016).

The development of patient-centred, AI-supported tele-nutrition systems capable of real-time feedback, bidirectional communication, and personalised, evidence-based recommendations is pivotal for improving long-term adherence and satisfaction. Such systems, as Ahmadi (2024) notes, can leverage wearable technologies and mobile applications for continuous monitoring of physiological signals, treatment adherence, and lifestyle factors, generating early alerts for deviations in health parameters and providing actionable insights to clinicians and patients. By dynamically adapting dietary recommendations to evolving patient data, these platforms can enhance engagement, outcomes, and informed decision-making, provided they are implemented alongside clinical restructuring, interdisciplinary training, regulatory alignment, ethical safeguards, and ongoing evaluation of their clinical and cost-effectiveness.

Future research can focus on embedding such tools into tele-nutrition dashboards to allow for real-time assessment of psychosocial well-being alongside clinical parameters. Future research also should adopt robust, theory-driven frameworks to evaluate tele-nutrition strategies. For instance, employing behavioral models like the COM-B (Capability, Opportunity, Motivation – Behavior) model may offer insights into how digital tools influence eating behaviors. Moreover, cost-effectiveness analyses are vital for demonstrating the economic value of tele-health services to healthcare systems and insurers (Kelly et al., 2023).

Additionally, reimbursement complexity remains a critical factor influencing both access to and sustainability of home-based nutrition support. Data indicate that Medicare and Medicaid often prioritise synthetic polymeric formulas due to cost considerations, making food-based formulations less accessible without documented allergies or intolerances (Martin & McGinnis, 2016). As digital health platforms evolve, there is a growing opportunity to document intolerance episodes and upload clinical justifications through real-time systems, improving eligibility for reimbursement. Reforming digital documentation standards may thus enhance equity in nutrition access, particularly among vulnerable populations reliant on public insurance systems.

The integration of emerging technologies offers vast potential for transforming home-based nutrition care. Artificial intelligence and machine learning can help personalize dietary advice, detect patterns in dietary behaviors, and predict adherence risks. These technologies also offer opportunities for real-time feedback and decision support, strengthening the clinician-patient relationship. Such innovations could pave the way for more efficient triaging, tailored recommendations, and proactive care management.

Artificial intelligence (AI) applications are rapidly transforming the scope of personalized nutrition care. Early clinical models have demonstrated that machine learning algorithms can outperform traditional dietary prediction methods by incorporating individual-level data such as microbiota composition, lifestyle patterns, and biometric indicators (Zeevi et al., 2015). These approaches offer improved accuracy in diet optimization, particularly in predicting post-prandial glycemic responses and generating tailored meal plans. As these systems become more refined, integrating AI-driven tools into tele-nutrition platforms could provide dynamic feedback loops that adapt to patients' evolving health status and dietary needs in real-time (Limketkai et al., 2021)

While emerging technologies offer remarkable opportunities for personalization and efficiency, equal attention must be paid to ensuring that these advancements are equitably distributed across diverse user groups. Lastly, it is imperative to ensure that tele-health services are adaptable to the diverse needs of populations, particularly underserved or marginalized communities. Access gaps due to geographic, economic, linguistic, or cultural barriers must be actively addressed through inclusive system design and culturally responsive care models (Jeri et al., 2023). This includes offering services in multiple languages, designing mobile-compatible platforms for low-bandwidth environments, and partnering with local organizations to build trust and awareness.

In conclusion, the future of tele-health in home nutrition support holds substantial promise, yet its success hinges on comprehensive and strategic approaches. Strengthening regulatory clarity, aligning reimbursement policies, expanding digital education, fostering interdisciplinary collaboration, investing in long-term research, leveraging innovation, and ensuring equitable access are all essential steps. As digital health continues to evolve, tele-nutrition should not be viewed merely as a temporary solution but as a foundational component of modern nutrition care delivery. Evidence-based policies and inclusive practices can make tele-health a transformative force in advancing public health and nutritional well-being at home.

REFERENCES

Aalaei, S., Firouraghi, N., Aalaei, M., Karbin, K., Bararbakhti, H., Nematy, M., & Rezvani, R. (2025). Feasibility of Mobile Telehealth for Health Literacy Enhancement via Nutritional Counseling during COVID-19. Journal of Nutrition. *Fasting and Health*, *13*(1), 24–34.

Ahmadi, A. (2024). Digital health transformation: Leveraging ai for monitoring and disease management. [IJBLS]. *International Journal of BioLife Sciences*, *3*(1), 10–24.

Alpert, J. M. (2020). Secondary care provider attitudes towards patient-generated health data from smartwatches. npj. *Digital Medicine*, *3*(1), 1–7. PMID: 32140569

Arem, H., Moses, J., Cisneros, C., Blondeau, B., Nekhlyudov, L., Killackey, M., & Pratt-Chapman, M. L. (2022). Cancer provider and survivor experiences with telehealth during the COVID-19 pandemic. *JCO Oncology Practice*, *18*(4), e452–e461. DOI: 10.1200/OP.21.00401 PMID: 34714706

Assaad, M., Chamma, N., Mateev, M., & Rizk, R. (2024). Telehealth during and beyond the covid-19 pandemic: evidence from licensed dietitians in an emerging economy. DOI: 10.1101/2024.09.19.24314030

Baker, L. C., Johnson, S. J., Macaulay, D., & Birnbaum, H. (2011). Integrated telehealth and care management program for Medicare beneficiaries with chronic disease linked to savings. *Health Affairs*, *30*(9), 1689–1697. DOI: 10.1377/hlthaff.2011.0216 PMID: 21900660

Barazzoni, R., Bischoff, S. C., Breda, J., Wickramasinghe, K., Krznaric, Z., Nitzan, D., Pirlich, M., & Singer, P. (2020). ESPEN expert statements and practical guidance for nutritional management of individuals with SARS-CoV-2 infection. *Clinical Nutrition (Edinburgh, Lothian)*, *39*(6), 1631–1638. DOI: 10.1016/j.clnu.2020.03.022 PMID: 32305181

Barazzoni, R., Bischoff, S. C., Breda, J., Wickramasinghe, K., Krznaric, Z., Nitzan, D., Pirlich, M., & Singer, P.The European Society of Parenteral and Enteral Nutrition (ESPEN). (2020). ESPEN expert statements and practical guidance for nutritional management of individuals with SARS-CoV-2 infection. *Clinical Nutrition (Edinburgh, Lothian)*, *39*(6), 1631–1638. DOI: 10.1016/j.clnu.2020.03.022 PMID: 32305181

Barclay, A. R., McGuckin, C., Hill, S., Protheroe, S., & Batra, A. (2021). Exit strategies from the COVID-19 lockdown for children and young people receiving home parenteral nutrition (HPN): Lessons from the BSPGHAN Intestinal Failure Working Group experience. *Frontline Gastroenterology*, *12*(4), 348–353. DOI: 10.1136/flgastro-2020-101598 PMID: 34249323

Bashshur, R. L., Doarn, C. R., Frenk, J., Kvedar, J. C., Shannon, G. W., & Woolliscroft, J. O. (2020). Beyond the covid pandemic, telemedicine, and health care. *Telemedicine Journal and e-Health*, *26*(11), 1310–1313. DOI: 10.1089/tmj.2020.0328 PMID: 32809913

Bergerot, C. D., Bergerot, P. G., Philip, E. J., Ferrari, R., Peixoto, R. M., Crane, T. E., Schmitz, K. H., & Soto-Pérez-de-Celis, E. (2024). Enhancing cancer supportive care: Integrating psychosocial support, nutrition, and physical activity using telehealth solutions. *JCO Global Oncology*, (10), e2400333. DOI: 10.1200/GO-24-00333 PMID: 39509661

Bowles, K. H., McDonald, M., Barron, Y., Kennedy, E., O'Connor, M., & Mikkelsen, M. (2021). Surviving COVID-19 after hospital discharge: Symptom, functional, and adverse outcomes of home health recipients. *Annals of Internal Medicine*, *174*(3), 316–325. DOI: 10.7326/M20-5206 PMID: 33226861

Brunton, C., Arensberg, M., Drawert, S., Badaracco, C., Everett, W., & McCauley, S. (2021). Perspectives of registered dietitian nutritionists on adoption of telehealth for nutrition care during the covid-19 pandemic. *Health Care*, *9*(2), 235. DOI: 10.3390/healthcare9020235 PMID: 33672179

Butzner, M., & Cuffee, Y. (2021). Telehealth interventions and outcomes across rural communities in the United States: Narrative review. *Journal of Medical Internet Research*, *23*(8), e29575. DOI: 10.2196/29575 PMID: 34435965

Cloutier, A., Bond, A., Taylor, M. I., Ablett, J., Teubner, A., Farrer, K., Leahy, G., Abraham, A., & Lal, S. (2020). Successful implementation of remote video consultations for patients receiving home parenteral nutrition in a national UK Centre. *Frontline Gastroenterology*, *11*(4), 280–284. DOI: 10.1136/flgastro-2019-101257 PMID: 32587671

Collins, P. F., Huggins, C. E., Booth, A., & Banks, M. (2017). Telehealth dietetic consultation is effective for patients undergoing head and neck cancer treatment. *Journal of Nutrition and Dietetics*, *74*(1), 7–13. DOI: 10.1111/1747-0080.12345

Coşkun, M. G., Kolay, E., & Basaranoglu, M. (2023). Telenutrition for the management of inflammatory bowel disease: Benefits, limits, and future perspectives. *World Journal of Clinical Cases*, *11*(2), 308.

Crivelli, A., Fabeiro, M., Puga, M., Dieguez, N., Giunta, L., Pochettino, F., Balacco, M., Merlo, G., Garrido, V., Fain, H., Buncuga, M., Martinuzzi, A., Cascarón, M. F., Delgado, N., Capurro, G., Bernardis, V., Ghiglieri, C., Hassam, A., Soria, O., & Fernandez, A. (2022). Care of patients on home parenteral nutrition during the first year of the COVID-19 pandemic: Management of central line-associated bloodstream infections. *Clinical Nutrition ESPEN*, *52*, 250–253. DOI: 10.1016/j.clnesp.2022.11.003 PMID: 36513461

Cuerda, M. C., Apezetxea, A., Carrillo, L., Casanueva, F., Cuesta, F., Irles, J. A., Virgili, M., Layola, M., & Lizan, L. (2016). Development and validation of a specific questionnaire to assess health-related quality of life in patients with home enteral nutrition: NutriQoL®. *Patient Preference and Adherence*, *10*, 2289–2296. DOI: 10.2147/PPA.S110188 PMID: 27853360

Dong, Y., Scisco, J., Wilson, M., Muth, E., & Hoover, A. (2014). Detecting periods of eating during free-living by tracking wrist motion. *IEEE Journal of Biomedical and Health Informatics*, *18*(4), 1253–1260. DOI: 10.1109/JBHI.2013.2282471 PMID: 24058042

Foster, K. R., & Torous, J. (2019). The opportunity and obstacles for smartwatches and wearable sensors. *IEEE Pulse*, *10*(1), 22–25. DOI: 10.1109/MPULS.2018.2885832 PMID: 30872210

Gajarawala, S. N., & Pelkowski, J. N. (2021). Telehealth benefits and barriers. *The Journal for Nurse Practitioners*, *17*(2), 218–221. DOI: 10.1016/j.nurpra.2020.09.013 PMID: 33106751

Galvão, D. A., Taaffe, D. R., Hayne, D., Lopez, P., Lyons-Wall, P., Tang, C. I., Chambers, S. K., Devine, A., Spry, N., Jeffery, E., Kudiarasu, C., Joseph, D., & Newton, R. U. (2022). Weight loss for overweight and obese patients with prostate cancer: A study protocol of a randomised trial comparing clinic-based versus Telehealth delivered exercise and nutrition intervention (the telex trial). *BMJ Open*, *12*(6), e058899. DOI: 10.1136/bmjopen-2021-058899 PMID: 35667725

Gibson, G. R., & Roberfroid, M. B. (1995). Dietary modulation of the human colonic microbiota: Introducing the concept of prebiotics. *The Journal of Nutrition*, *125*(6), 1401–1412. DOI: 10.1093/jn/125.6.1401 PMID: 7782892

Hall, B. T., Englehart, M. S., Blaseg, K., Wessel, K., Stawicki, S. P. A., & Evans, D. C. (2014). Implementation of a dietitian-led enteral nutrition support clinic results in quality improvement, reduced readmissions, and cost savings. *Nutrition in Clinical Practice*, *29*(5), 649–655. DOI: 10.1177/0884533614538285 PMID: 25606646

Herbert, J., Schumacher, T., Brown, L. J., Clarke, E. D., & Collins, C. E. (2023). Delivery of telehealth nutrition and physical activity interventions to adults living in rural areas: A scoping review. *The International Journal of Behavioral Nutrition and Physical Activity*, *20*(1), 110. DOI: 10.1186/s12966-023-01505-2 PMID: 37715234

Hincapié, M. A., Gallego, J. C., Gempeler, A., Piñeros, J. A., Nasner, D., & Escobar, M. F. (2020). Implementation and usefulness of telemedicine during the COVID-19 pandemic: A scoping review. *Journal of Primary Care & Community Health*, *11*, 2150132720980612. DOI: 10.1177/2150132720980612 PMID: 33300414

Hinchliffe, N., Capehorn, M. S., Bewick, M., & Feenie, J. (2022). The potential role of digital health in obesity care. *Advances in Therapy*, *39*(10), 4397–4412. DOI: 10.1007/s12325-022-02265-4 PMID: 35925469

Jeri, A., Lambert, K., Mak, M., & Diamantes, M. (2023). Lessons learnt from rapid implementation of telehealth in a paediatric dietetics' outpatient service: Is there a silver lining beyond the coronavirus pandemic to support patient-centred care? *Dietetics*, *2*(3), 267–277. DOI: 10.3390/dietetics2030019

Kelly, J. T., Allman-Farinelli, M., Chen, J., Partridge, S. R., Collins, C., Rollo, M., Haslam, R., Diversi, T., & Campbell, K. L. (2020). Dietitians Australia position statement on telehealth. *Nutrition & Dietetics: the Journal of the Dietitians Association of Australia*, *77*(4), 406–415. DOI: 10.1111/1747-0080.12619 PMID: 32596950

Kelly, J. T., Collins, P. F., McCamley, J., Ball, L., Roberts, S., & Campbell, K. L. (2021). Digital disruption of dietetics: Are we ready? *Journal of Human Nutrition and Dietetics*, *34*(1), 134–146. DOI: 10.1111/jhn.12827 PMID: 33108029

Kelly, J. T., Law, L., Guzman, K. D., Hickman, I. J., Mayr, H., Campbell, K. L., & Erku, D. A. (2022). Are telehealth-delivered nutrition care interventions cost-effective for managing chronic diseases? a systematic review of all payer perspectives. *Current Developments in Nutrition*, *6*, 842. DOI: 10.1093/cdn/nzac065.026

Kelly, J. T., Law, L., Guzman, K. R. D., Hickman, I. J., Mayr, H. L., Campbell, K. L., & Erku, D. A. (2023). Cost-effectiveness of telehealth-delivered nutrition interventions: A systematic review of randomized controlled trials. *Nutrition Reviews*, *81*(12), 1599–1611. DOI: 10.1093/nutrit/nuad032 PMID: 37016937

Khan, M., Manduchi, B., Rodríguez, V., Fitch, M., Barbon, C., McMillan, H., Hutcheson, K. A., & Martino, R. (2022). Exploring patient experiences with a telehealth approach for the pro-active trial intervention in head and neck cancer patients. *BMC Health Services Research*, *22*(1), 1218. DOI: 10.1186/s12913-022-08554-6 PMID: 36180905

Kim, S., Zhang, Y., Mauldin, K., & Limketkai, B. N. (2024). Advances in Digital Health for Gastrointestinal Nutrition. *Current Treatment Options in Cardiovascular Medicine*, *22*(4), 267–278. DOI: 10.1007/s11938-024-00458-0

Lal, S., Van Gossum, A., Joly, F., Bozzetti, F., Cuerda, C., Lamprecht, G., Mundi, M. S., Staun, M., Szczepanek, K., Wanten, G., Wheatley, C., & Pironi, L. (2020). Considerations for the management of home parenteral nutrition during the SARS-CoV-2 pandemic: A position paper from the Home Artificial Nutrition and Chronic Intestinal Failure Special Interest Group of ESPEN. *Clinical Nutrition (Edinburgh, Lothian)*, *39*(7), 1988–1991. DOI: 10.1016/j.clnu.2020.05.023 PMID: 32487434

Limketkai, B. N., Mauldin, K., Manitius, N., Jalilian, L., & Salonen, B. R. (2021). The age of artificial intelligence: Use of digital technology in clinical nutrition. *Current Surgery Reports*, *9*(7), 20. DOI: 10.1007/s40137-021-00297-3 PMID: 34123579

Ma, Y., Zhang, L., Liu, W., & Chen, X. (2025). Telemedicine-supported home enteral nutrition service (HENST): A five-year regional experience in China. *Asia Pacific Journal of Clinical Nutrition*, *34*(1), 87–95. DOI: 10.1016/j.apjcn.2025.01.010

Martin, K., & Gardner, G. (2017). Home enteral nutrition: Updates, trends, and challenges. *Nutrition in Clinical Practice*, *32*(6), 712–721. DOI: 10.1177/0884533617701401 PMID: 28437132

Martin, K., & McGinnis, C. (2016). Home nutrition support: Ethics and reimbursement. *Nutrition in Clinical Practice*, *31*(3), 325–333. DOI: 10.1177/0884533616639128 PMID: 27072855

Mauldin, K., Gieng, J., Saarony, D., & Hu, C. (2021). Performing nutrition assessment remotely via telehealth. *Nutrition in Clinical Practice*, *36*(4), 751–768. DOI: 10.1002/ncp.10682 PMID: 34101249

McBain, R. K., Cantor, J., Pera, M. F., Breslau, J., Bravata, D. M., & Whaley, C. M. (2023, January). Mental health service utilization rates among commercially insured adults in the US during the first year of the COVID-19 pandemic. [). American Medical Association.]. *JAMA Health Forum*, *4*(1), e224936–e224936. DOI: 10.1001/jamahealthforum.2022.4936 PMID: 36607697

Mehta, P., Stahl, M. G., Germone, M. M., Nagle, S., Guigli, R., Thomas, J., Shull, M., & Liu, E. (2020). Telehealth and nutrition support during the COVID-19 pandemic. *Journal of the Academy of Nutrition and Dietetics*, *120*(12), 1953–1957. DOI: 10.1016/j.jand.2020.07.013 PMID: 32792328

Mulherin, D. W., Walker, R., Holcombe, B., & Guenter, P. (2020). Aspen report on nutrition support practice processes with covid-19: The first response. *Nutrition in Clinical Practice*, *35*(5), 783–791. DOI: 10.1002/ncp.10553 PMID: 32671870

Mundi, M. S., Elfadil, O. M., Bonnes, S. L., Salonen, B. R., & Hurt, R. T. (2021). Use of telehealth in home nutrition support: Challenges and advantages. *Nutrition in Clinical Practice*, *36*(4), 775–784. DOI: 10.1002/ncp.10736 PMID: 34245465

Mundi, M. S., Mohamed Elfadil, O., Bonnes, S. L., Salonen, B. R., & Hurt, R. T. (2021). Use of telehealth in home nutrition support: Challenges and advantages. *Nutrition in Clinical Practice*, *36*(4), 775–784. DOI: 10.1002/ncp.10736 PMID: 34245465

Muslu, M. (2022). Tıbbi Beslenme Tedavisinde Güncel Bir Yaklaşım: Telenütrisyon. *Balıkesir Sağlık Bilimleri Dergisi*, *11*(3), 523–531.

Nelson, E., Yadrich, D. M., Thompson, N., Wright, S., Stone, K. J., Adams, N., Werkowitch, M., & Smith, C. E. (2017). Telemedicine support groups for home parenteral nutrition users. *Nutrition in Clinical Practice*, *32*(6), 789–798. DOI: 10.1177/0884533617735527 PMID: 29016235

Nguyen, G., Furness, K., Croagh, D., Haines, T., & Hanna, L. (2024). Supplemental tube feeding: Qualitative study of patient perspectives in advanced pancreatic cancer. BMJ Supportive &Amp. *Palliative Care*, *14*(e3), e3002–e3010. DOI: 10.1136/spcare-2024-004836 PMID: 38580394

Norouzi, S., Majd, F. A., Rostami, S., Mirzaee, M., Sistani, S., & Ahmadian, L. (2024). Tele-medical nutrition therapy to promote healthy eating and nutrition adherence of chronic patients in the covid-19 pandemic: A pragmatically before-after trial. *Health Science Reports*, *7*(11), e70193. DOI: 10.1002/hsr2.70193 PMID: 39540025

Ong, T., Barrera, J. F., Sunkara, C., Soni, H., Ivanova, J., Cummins, M. R., Schuler, K. R., Wilczewski, H., Welch, B. M., & Bunnell, B. E. (2024). Mental health providers are inexperienced but interested in telehealth-based virtual reality therapy: Survey study. *Frontiers in Virtual Reality*, *5*, 1332874. DOI: 10.3389/frvir.2024.1332874 PMID: 39228388

Pentiuk, S. S., O'Flaherty, T., Santoro, K., Willging, P., & Kaul, A. (2011). Pureed by gastrostomy tube diet improves gagging and retching in children with fundoplication. *JPEN. Journal of Parenteral and Enteral Nutrition*, *35*(3), 375–379. DOI: 10.1177/0148607110377797 PMID: 21527599

Persoon, A., Huisman-de Waal, G., Naber, T. A., Schoonhoven, L., Tas, T., Sauerwein, H., & van Achterberg, T. (2005). Impact of long-term HPN on daily life in adults. *Clinical Nutrition (Edinburgh, Lothian)*, *24*(2), 304–313. DOI: 10.1016/j.clnu.2004.12.009 PMID: 15784493

Pironi, L., Arends, J., Bozzetti, F., Cuerda, C., Gillanders, L., Jeppesen, P. B., Joly, F., Kelly, D., Lal, S., Staun, M., Szczepanek, K., Van Gossum, A., Wanten, G., & Schneider, S. M. (2016). ESPEN guidelines on chronic intestinal failure in adults. *Clinical Nutrition (Edinburgh, Lothian)*, *35*(2), 247–307. DOI: 10.1016/j.clnu.2016.01.020 PMID: 26944585

Porteny, T., Brophy, S. A., & Burroughs, E. (2025). Experiences of telehealth reimbursement policies in federally qualified health centers. *JAMA Network Open*, *8*(2), e2459554–e2459554. DOI: 10.1001/jamanetworkopen.2024.59554 PMID: 39937474

Prat, V. D., Pedrazzoli, P., & Caccialanza, R. (2024). Nutritional care for cancer patients: Are we doing enough? *Frontiers in Nutrition*, *11*, 1361800. DOI: 10.3389/fnut.2024.1361800 PMID: 38721029

Ramirez-Vega, D., Salinas-Cortes, M., Melendez-Coral, M., Cordell, G. A., & Rodriguez-Garcia, A. (2022). The evolution of nutrition intervention during the COVID-19 pandemic. *Ciencia & Saude Coletiva*, *27*(8), 3053–3061. DOI: 10.1590/1413-81232022278.04082021 PMID: 35894318

Reddy, P., & Malone, M. (1998). Cost and outcome analysis of home parenteral and enteral nutrition. *JPEN. Journal of Parenteral and Enteral Nutrition*, *22*(5), 302–310. DOI: 10.1177/0148607198022005302 PMID: 9739034

Saqui, O., Sinha, R., & Ethans, K. (2007). Telehealth in the management of home parenteral nutrition patients in rural Ontario: A five-year experience. *JPEN. Journal of Parenteral and Enteral Nutrition*, *31*(4), 300–305. DOI: 10.1177/0148607107031004300

Sasegbon, A., Dupont, C., Nguyen, T., & Martin, A. (2025). Telemedicine in Home Parenteral Nutrition: A Multinational Survey of Physician Perspectives During the COVID-19 Pandemic. *Clinical Nutrition ESPEN*, *57*, 112–119. DOI: 10.1016/j.clnesp.2025.03.006

Schneider, S. M., Raina, C., Pugliese, P., Pouget, I., Rampal, P., & Hebuterne, X. (2001). Outcome of patients treated with home enteral nutrition. *JPEN. Journal of Parenteral and Enteral Nutrition*, *25*(4), 203–209. DOI: 10.1177/0148607101025004203 PMID: 11434651

Schönenberger, K. A., Herren, L., Lutz, T., & Ballmer, P. E. (2022). Attitudes and expectations of patients receiving home parenteral nutrition towards eHealth: A Swiss multicenter survey study. *Clinical Nutrition ESPEN*, *47*, 314–320. DOI: 10.1016/j.clnesp.2022.01.025

Shah, N., Krupinski, E., Bernard, J., & Moyer, M. (2021). The evolution and utilization of telehealth in ambulatory nutrition practice. *Nutrition in Clinical Practice*, *36*(4), 739–749. DOI: 10.1002/ncp.10641 PMID: 33734469

Shamsabadi, A., Mehraeen, E., & Pashaei, Z. (2023). *Perspective chapter: telehealth technologies for the elderly people*. Geriatric Medicine and Healthy Aging., DOI: 10.5772/intechopen.105568

SINPE – Italian Society of Parenteral and Enteral Nutrition. (2014). Home artificial nutrition in Italy: Annual report and national registry data analysis (2005–2012). *Clinical Nutrition (Edinburgh, Lothian)*, *33*(5), 755–761. DOI: 10.1016/j.clnu.2014.01.012

Tewksbury, C., Deleener, M. E., Dumon, K. R., & Williams, N. N. (2021). Practical considerations of developing and conducting a successful telehealth practice in response to covid-19. *Nutrition in Clinical Practice*, *36*(4), 769–774. DOI: 10.1002/ncp.10742 PMID: 34156725

Turner, K., Bobonis Babilonia, M., Naso, C., Nguyen, O., Gonzalez, B. D., Oswald, L. B., Robinson, E., Elston Lafata, J., Ferguson, R. J., Alishahi Tabriz, A., Patel, K. B., Hallanger-Johnson, J., Aldawoodi, N., Hong, Y.-R., Jim, H. S. L., & Spiess, P. E. (2022). Health care providers' and professionals' experiences with telehealth oncology implementation during the COVID-19 pandemic: A qualitative study. *Journal of Medical Internet Research*, *24*(1), e29635. DOI: 10.2196/29635 PMID: 34907900

Wells Mulherin, D., Walker, R., Holcombe, B., & Guenter, P. (2020). ASPEN report on nutrition support practice processes with COVID-19: The first response. *Nutrition in Clinical Practice*, *35*(5), 783–791. DOI: 10.1002/ncp.10553 PMID: 32671870

Williams, K. S., Singh, M. J., Elumn, J. E., Threats, M., Sha, Y., McCall, T., Wang, K., Massey, B., Peng, M. L., & Wiley, K. (2024). Enhancing healthcare accessibility through telehealth for justice impacted individuals. *Frontiers in Public Health*, *12*, 1401950. DOI: 10.3389/fpubh.2024.1401950 PMID: 39175903

Wood, S., Khong, C., Dirlikov, B., & Shem, K. (2021). Nutrition counseling and monitoring via tele-nutrition for healthy diet for people with spinal cord injury: A case series analyses. *The Journal of Spinal Cord Medicine*, *45*(4), 547–555. DOI: 10.1080/10790268.2021.1871824 PMID: 33606588

Zagmutt, F. J., Pouzou, J. G., & Costard, S. (2020). The EAT-Lancet Commission's dietary composition may not prevent noncommunicable disease mortality. *The Journal of Nutrition*, *150*(5), 985–988. DOI: 10.1093/jn/nxaa020 PMID: 32061173

Zeevi, D., Korem, T., Zmora, N., Israeli, D., Rothschild, D., Weinberger, A., Ben-Yacov, O., Lador, D., Avnit-Sagi, T., Lotan-Pompan, M., Suez, J., Mahdi, J. A., Matot, E., Malka, G., Kosower, N., Rein, M., Zilberman-Schapira, G., Dohnalová, L., Pevsner-Fischer, M., & Segal, E. (2015). Personalized nutrition by prediction of glycemic responses. *Cell*, *163*(5), 1079–1094. DOI: 10.1016/j.cell.2015.11.001 PMID: 26590418

Zhai, S., Chu, F., Tan, M., Chi, N. C., Ward, T., & Yuwen, W. (2023). Digital health interventions to support family caregivers: An updated systematic review. *Digital Health*, *9*, 20552076231171967. DOI: 10.1177/20552076231171967 PMID: 37223775

Zheng, Y., Head, B. A., & Schapmire, T. J. (2016). A systematic review of telehealth in palliative care: Caregiver outcomes. *Telemedicine Journal and e-Health*, *22*(4), 288–294. DOI: 10.1089/tmj.2015.0090 PMID: 26360181

Chapter 7
The Importance of Home Healthcare Technologies in Disabled and Elderly Tourism

Çağla Çetinkaya
https://orcid.org/0000-0003-2039-7220
Istanbul Nisantasi University, Turkey

ABSTRACT

This chapter explores the increasing importance of home healthcare technologies in facilitating tourism participation among elderly and disabled populations. As the global aging demographic expands, the tourism sector must adapt to accommodate diverse accessibility needs. The chapter highlights how emerging technologies such as wearable healthcare devices, smart city infrastructure, and mobile navigation applications support greater autonomy and mobility for individuals with disabilities. Drawing on key statistical projections and academic literature, it addresses the concept of accessible tourism, the challenges disabled travelers face, and the role of inclusive technologies in overcoming physical and digital barriers. In doing so, this chapter emphasizes not only the social equity benefits but also the economic potential of integrating inclusive practices into tourism systems.

1. INTRODUCTION

The swift growth of the global aging population calls for incorporating older adults and those with disabilities into the social scene in a way that improves their quality of life. This change is evident not only in health services but also in areas

DOI: 10.4018/979-8-3373-3099-0.ch007

that enhance life quality, like tourism. The World Health Organization predicts that in 2050, individuals aged 60 years and older will constitute 22% of the world population. This projection emphasizes the need for new policies and technologies in tourism that are accessible and inclusive of older and disabled individuals (Ivanova & Senkiv, 2019).

New technologies have emerged as significant resources to respond to these challenges. Smart city infrastructure, wearable healthcare technologies, mobile applications that are designed to meet the needs of disabled individuals, and digital navigation technologies support older and disabled individuals to become more active participants in tourism. So, technology should be used to enhance not only individual comfort but also equity in society, sustainability, and economic benefits. Studies indicate that older travelers and people with disabilities tend to have a higher average expenditures (Domínguez et al., 2013).

2. THEORETICAL AND CONCEPTUAL FOUNDATIONS

The conceptual underpinning of accessible tourism, smart healthcare technologies are found within the nexus of aging, disability, social inclusion, and technological advancement. Altınay et al. (2019), advocate that accessibility in health tourism is more than a desire for access by individuals, it is also a policy initiative that strives to foster societal wellbeing (Altınay et al., 2019). The academic foundations of this subject are built upon primarily normative theories such as "Universal Design" and "Inclusive Tourism." The universal design approach aims to ensure that all users, without any discrimination. Zajadacz (2015) points out that geographic barriers are one of the most significant but often overlooked limitations in planning processes that hinder the participation of disabled individuals in tourism activities. This issue can theoretically be explained through the concept of a "barrier-free environment" (Zajadacz, 2015).

2.1 Universal Design and Inclusive Tourism

Universal design is predicated on the notion that all environments; physical and digital products and services should be accessible by everyone. This approach seeks to provide equal social participation regardless of age, gender, or disability. Poli (2019) emphasizes is that universal design goes beyond physical accessibility, and must include access to information and services. According to Poli, these principles support and improve the quality of tourism destinations, expand the customer base and promote inclusiveness (Poli, 2019). Singh et al. (2021) state that the incorporation of IoT technologies into universal design provides solutions that are more dynamic and functional. These also allow for the creation of "mainstream" products that are not for use exclusive to individuals with disabilities, but for all individuals (Singh et al., 2021).

Universal design is a critical approach to supporting basic accessibility, not just for disabled individuals but across a wider user profile, including the elderly, parents with babies, and pregnant individuals. This framework and theory need to be used for every facet of tourism, from the physical infrastructure to the digital platform used to book and participate in activities while continuing to evolve.

2.2 Smart Tourism and IoT-Enabled Accessibility

Smart tourism is the incorporation of information and communication technologies (ICT), big data and Internet of Things (IoT) into tourism. Through this integration, personalized, safe and accessible trip experiences are created, especially for an aging population and those with disabilities. Dias et al. (2021), contended smart city infrastructures are changing the tourism experience and improving accessibility in this arena, especially in transit, accommodation and guiding services. Smart technologies are used to help lessen inequalities of access (Dias et al., 2021). IoT based systems allow for elderly and disabled tourists to navigate destinations with increased independence. For example, smart walking paths could be supported by sensors and close to the user's location, could provide audio navigation.

The success of these applications would also rely upon data integrity and digital inclusiveness. Ercan (2022), reports that in Breda, the Netherlands digital maps, VR and mobile apps help the elderly explore the destination in advance and support travel decision making (Ercan, 2022). This suggests that smart tourism is included in both mobility and digital planning. However, ensuring the technological infrastructure is fully accessibly, is not the sole contributor to engaging with smart systems. The technology must be user-friendly, usable simplified language, and adaptable when needed by the user.

2.3 Smart Health and the Theory of Personalized Care

Smart health systems consist of digital solutions designed to personalize healthcare services, especially for elderly and disabled people. Similar to the more defined phrase, smart health systems include solutions such as telehealth, wearable devices, IoT-enabled remote monitoring systems, and artificial intelligence-based algorithms assessing one's health. In this way, the smart health system examines one's health status and subsequently provides a health care process that is deemed more proactive, preventative, and personalized. Personalized care creates a health model that takes into consideration one's daily routines, chronic conditions, and psychosocial health needs. Tuna and colleagues (2015) described a smart vest system that collects health parameters about someone's health status and then presents them in a smart home system. As a result, the smart vest system is deemed more efficient, as it not only permits elderly people living alone at home to manage their care with their family, it has the potential to alert appropriate authorities for medical attention in real time as necessary (Tuna et al., 2015).

Li and Borycki (2019) noted that health monitoring systems designed for smart home environments give not only clinical benefits, but social and psychological support. For example, systems designed for dementia patients with Alzheimer's disease or individuals with limited mobility, monitor one's routine behavior in real time and immediately identify variations from behavior, which may indicate potential risks. Thus, in this case, the application addresses independence and desire to live alone with awareness to a need for care (Li & Borycki, 2019). Smart health solutions can include being integrated into the tourism process. Accordingly, this can optimize holistic health tracking during travel (Hossain et al., 2015).

2.4 Accessible Smart City Theory

Smart cities represent a new model of urban development to promote quality of life through the use of digital infrastructure, artificial intelligence, and big data Technologies. Salha et al. (2020), claiming that smart city design can only be conceptualized by employing both strategies of "mainstreaming," and as a "targeted intervention," so that all communities have access to cities. For Salha et al., access should not be limited to ramps, instead, they include accessible smart building systems, audio guidance panels, accessible public transport stops, and emergency response infrastructure. Incorporating all of these systems during the design phase will incur relatively low costs now but will help contribute to a more holistic urban development in the future (Salha et al., 2020).

Alternatively, the second model proposed by Padrón Nápoles et al. (2021), the "Interactive Public Spaces," argues that the joining of digital and physical environments throughout smart city design will further promote the social participation of elder people. By using interactive systems existing in prepared spaces like parks, bus stops, or public squares, elder people can physically and cognitively engage themselves. Smart city technologies thus aid not only in mobility but in building social relationships. In this way, we can only achieve the theory of an accessible smart city, yes theory, through the simultaneous union of digital solutions with social, political, and spatial facets. Participatory models at the design stage need to be implemented to solve the everyday barriers faced by disabled and elderly population; the focus from the start needs to be the user experience and it is only through the proper theory can future cities be livable for everyone.

3. CURRENT STATE AND CHALLENGES IN ELDERLY AND DISABLED TOURISM

The participation of elderly and disabled individuals in tourism activities is not merely a personal experience but a strategic matter in terms of human rights, economic development, and social inclusion. However, on a global scale, this group continues to face significant barriers to accessing tourism. Saygılı and colleagues (2021) noted that health tourism for disabled individuals remains in a developmental phase in both Turkey and internationally, with multidimensional challenges including infrastructure, personnel, and costs (Saygılı et al., 2021). A 2016 study by Sarmento and colleagues in the Estoril region of Portugal concluded that five-star hotels' physical infrastructure was only accessible for particular impairments, highlighting the lack of integrated systems. This suggests that accessibility investment often remains fragmented and uncoordinated (Sarmento et al., 2016).

Transportation-related issues are ranked as one of the most considerable barriers to the tourism participation of the elderly and disabled. Similarly, Kamyabi and Alipour (2022) noted that even though North Cyprus is considered attractive in terms of its natural and cultural resources, any shortcomings in accommodation, transportation services, staff training for tourism, and awareness among the general public limited holiday opportunities for the disabled (Kamyabi & Alipour, 2022).

3.1 Global Overview of Accessibility

Accessible tourism has emerged at different stages in different parts of the world. European Union countries—especially France, Germany, and Sweden—have notable urban planning and infrastructure regulations prioritizing accessibility. Conversely, many developing countries continue to see accessibility as a "secondary issue" (Ivanova & Senkiv, 2019). Incentives such as the European Commission's Access City Award program have resulted in many cities renovating their infrastructures and being more inclusive in tourism. Nevertheless, accessibility standards are still insufficiently implemented in several Eastern European and Mediterranean countries. This lack of consistency threatens destination options for older people and people with disabilities when planning to travel. For instance, a study conducted in Spain found that most of the difficulties older people experienced accessing tourist sites stemmed from architectural and transportation infrastructures (Domínguez et al., 2013). Additionally, countries such as India and Brazil also have laws regarding accessibility; however, implementation failures which inhibit actual progress remain evident.

Most tourism businesses still only think of accessibility as "physical access", ignoring larger questions of information, communication, and service provision. The narrow view of accessibility has left many of these questions unanswered—questions that could have been answered through technological advancements. Furthermore, there is a misconception that accessibility can only be ensured through "assistive equipment". In reality, contemporary approaches seek to plan accessibility into design. Ultimately, awareness is often limited due to a lack of training and awareness among tourism professionals and decision-makers (Liasidou et al., 2018). Furthermore, on a global basis, the emergence of accessible tourism correlates to legal enforcement and civil society pressure. In some countries a disabled person's travel protection is regarded as a human right; in others, the rights of access are only recommendations, creating no binding obligations.

3.2 Transportation Challenges

Transportation is an essential aspect that influences the tourism experience of older and disabled individuals. More specifically, the inability to use public transportation system negatively affects their choice to travel. Rosa et al. (2020) conducted a study in the Algarve region of Portugal and revealed that older tourists only took buses, trams, and trains occasionally, and when they did, they found that the infrastructure was too inadequate and staff did not assist them enough (Rosa et al., 2020). Due to physical barriers (e.g., steps being high, the stop lacking access, feeling unstable inside the transport), older individuals often avoided public transport altogether. A study conducted by Rosa & Pinto (2020) noted that older individuals commonly complained about benches that were poorly designed, not being able to cross the street at pedestrian crossings, and limited space for wheelchair users (Rosa, Pinto & Assunção, 2020).

Most importantly, these issues are not just based on physical obstructions, as the relative absence of information is an equally significant barrier (Rosa, Pinto, & Assunção, 2020). A study by Ding et al. (2010) in Beijing indicated that the main reason disabled individuals avoid public transport is the lack of clear and accessible information about how transportation systems operate (Ding, Lin, & Liu, 2010). A similar situation was reported in Poland. Szewczyk (2020), in a study in the city of Szczyrk, noted that disabled individuals faced both physical and navigational deficiencies when trying to access bus stops, significantly restricting their mobility (Szewczyk, 2020).

The lack of accessible transportation not only discourages travel but also leads to loss of self-confidence and social isolation. Mahmoudzadeh and Sarjaz (2018), in their research in Tehran, found that the most frequently reported issue among disabled individuals was the unsuitability of the transportation infrastructure, which in turn limited the growth of tourism (Mahmoudzadeh & Sarjaz, 2018).

These problems cannot be resolved solely through infrastructure improvements; they must be supported by education and awareness among service providers. Rumetshofer and Wöß (2004) argue that tourism information systems integrated with transportation networks play a critical role in helping disabled individuals overcome travel planning difficulties (Rumetshofer & Wöß, 2004).

3.3 Barriers in Accommodation and Services

Accommodation facilities often fail to meet even the basic accessibility standards for elderly and disabled individuals. A study conducted in Poland revealed that most hotels lacked adequate infrastructure to serve these guests. The number of accessible rooms was low, navigation systems were confusing, and emergency exits were insufficient (Szewczyka & Zontek, 2018). In a study involving 995 participants in Brazil, accessibility was identified as the top priority for disabled individuals when choosing a hotel. When this criterion was met, customer loyalty significantly increased. Hotels lacking in accessibility received lower ratings, which directly affected their revenue (Ferst et al., 2023).

In New Zealand, a study found that accessibility information on hotel websites was limited and often misleading. This created serious information barriers for individuals with visual, hearing, or cognitive impairments, adding uncertainty to the booking process (Shetty & McIntosh, 2020). Moreover, many hotel managers perceive accessibility as a financial burden, leading to delays in necessary investments. Capitaine (2016), in a study from Canada, found that hotel managers underestimated the economic potential of the disabled customer segment and failed to assess accessibility as a marketing advantage (Capitaine, 2016).

3.4 Information and Digital Accessibility Deficiencies

One of the most significant challenges elderly and disabled individuals face in travel planning is the inability to access reliable and accessible information. Eichhorn and colleagues (2008) reported that accessible tourism information systems across Europe were highly fragmented, lacked comprehensive coverage, and suffered from poor reliability. This situation prevents many disabled individuals from actualizing their vacation plans (Eichhorn et al., 2008). Inadequate, incomplete, or incorrect information not only disrupts the planning process but also makes the entire travel experience risky and stressful.

Rumetshofer and Wöß (2004) made a notable point that conventional systems of tourism information do not consider people with disabilities. Thus, they advocated for resources that provide interactive and visually accessible information tailored to individual users (Rumetshofer & Wöß, 2004). Likewise, Achillas and colleagues

(2024) showed that providing digital information about routes and locations in Greece's Pieria region resulted in a direct improvement in a disabled individual's travel experience. Through the app, individuals selected routes based on their needs (Achillas et al., 2024). In general, digital maps and web-based systems do not meet accessibility standards. Hennig and colleagues (2015) noted that online maps used for tourism in natural areas do not actively indicate detailed, updated, or easy-to-follow maps. (Hennig et al., 2015).

3.5 Lack of Trained Personnel and Awareness

One of the major challenges elderly and disabled travelers encounter with tourism experiences is a lack of understanding and training among staff about their specific needs. Swanepoel and colleagues (2020) found in a study conducted at South African hotels that most of the front line employees had not had any practical training in relation to disability, which had an adverse effect on guest satisfaction (Swanepoel et al., 2020). In Egypt, Moris and colleagues (2019) found that many of the workers in the tourism sector were not familiar with the concept of accessible tourism and widespread lack of training. They indicated that training should not only provide awareness, but should also promote attitudinal change (Moris et al., 2019).

A study in Turkey reported that the majority of the problems encountered by hotel managers and staff assisting disabled guests were caused from a lack of knowledge. Sari and Ünüvar (2019) found that personnel with higher levels of education had a better total understanding of accessibility (Sari & Ünüvar, 2019). A study in Brazil by Ferst and Coutinho (2021) found that training programs enhanced personnel attitudes towards accessibility and developed behavioral awareness. A comparison of data from before and after training demonstrated a significant and positive change (Ferst & Coutinho, 2021).

Putri and Taufik (2024) identified trained personnel as being among the critical aspects of disability-friendly tourism infrastructure. In the case of trained staff, tourist's needs are discussed in terms of not only providing physical assistance, but also providing assurance and creating a perception of value as a customer, which builds loyalty and commitment (Putri & Taufik, 2024).

Trained personnel provide guests with more than just physical support; they also provide psychological comfort. Fortuna and colleagues (2024) examined staff at museums, and determined that training in disability improved staff ability to communicate and support participant experience. They implied adaptations of the model could be easily made into the context of hotel and tourism staff (Fortuna et al., 2024). Psychological and social barriers are equally important as physical barriers in a disabled person's participation in tourism. Popiel (2016) indicated that psychological barriers included both internal and external barriers, and were not limited to architecture or financial issues (Popiel, 2016). Common barriers include denial or rejection of requests for support or assistance while traveling, misunderstanding of social judgements when in public, and overall pressure or fear of possible judgements.

Disabled individuals often feel and expect judgement while traveling, overall denial of their requests for help and/or support, and a general reduction in social value when in public. Fraser (2017) framed his study within the social model, and found prejudice and discrimination in broader society can sometimes be directly tied to travel decisions of the disabled, which can create psychological stress through a sense of "loss of control" (Fraser, 2017). This is particularly relevant and easily observed in historical or cultural destinations. Zahari and colleagues (2023) determined that disabled individuals' interest in cultural heritage tourism is diminished by fear of social exclusion (Zahari et al., 2023). Kastenholz and colleagues (2015) found feelings of social exclusion among those with mental and psychosocial disabilities was intense and one of the reasons why group travel was not approached (Kastenholz et al., 2015). Feeling either socially excluded or intentionally isolated from the social group of tourism experiences those companies actively facilitated leads to inequity, both for disabled individuals and social groups overall. In their study in Poland, Kaganek and colleagues (2017) identified anxiety, fear of failure, and feelings of social incompatibility as the most important internal factors limiting the tourism participation of elderly and disabled individuals. These psychological barriers were found to be especially common among older adults (Kaganek et al., 2017).

4. AGE-FRIENDLY TOURISM AND THE ROLE OF TECHNOLOGY

Web 2.0–based platforms also enable elderly and disabled users to access reliable information during the travel planning stage. The "nobatravel.at" platform, developed by Drews (2008), allows users to explore accessible hotels, restaurants, and museums, as well as share their experiences with others. Such digital communities enhance information exchange among travelers and support informed, safe decision-making (Drews, 2008). Info-mobility systems aim to reduce accessibility barriers encountered during transportation. In the ASK-IT project, Bekiaris et al. analyzed the types of information elderly and disabled individuals need throughout their travel and tourism experiences. The results revealed that when designed accessibly, digital maps, stop information systems, and personal journey planners significantly improve travel comfort (Bekiaris et al., 2007).

Accessibility applications not only provide physical navigation but also promote social inclusion. The GIS-based application developed by Rosa and Pereira (2021) enables users to discover accessible tourist spots and leave community feedback on these locations. The app is available on Google Play and, through its open data policy, contributes to municipal-level planning (Rosa & Pereira, 2021). Websites and apps developed specifically for individuals with hearing impairments also help make tourism more inclusive. Luccio and Beltrame (2018) analyzed an app designed for visitors in Venice and found that it served as an effective tourism guide for the hearing impaired through sign language translation, subtitle support, and written navigation instructions (Luccio & Beltrame, 2018).

4.1 Data Collection and Integration of Digital Health Systems in Tourism

In tourism, the ability for elderly and disabled individuals to have safe, sustainable, and personalized experiences depends critically on the systematic collection of health data and its integration with digital health systems. The study by Altınay et al. (2019) emphasizes that integrating healthcare and tourism services through technology not only improves individuals' quality of life but also enhances social welfare as a strategic policy (Altınay et al., 2019). Smart monitoring systems and mobile health applications used in tourism areas simultaneously analyze users' location, health data (such as heart rate, temperature, oxygen levels), and emergency responses, and share this information with relevant institutions.

Digital health systems are important not only for immediate interventions but also for long-term analysis and health planning. The research by Haghi et al. (2022) demonstrated that multi-layered sensor systems installed in smart homes collected environmental, behavioral, and physiological data, contributing to both event detection and disease prevention processes (Haghi et al., 2022). Data security and privacy are among the main ethical concerns when sharing health information. As emphasized in the article by Saif et al. (2019), blockchain-based solutions and advanced encryption protocols can be used to maintain data integrity when health data is shared among multiple stakeholders (e.g., doctors, patients, insurers, researchers) (Saif et al., 2019). All these data-driven systems not only facilitate individual health monitoring but also contribute to the planning of tourism destinations, the development of elderly- and disability-friendly cities, and the improvement of health tourism policies. Ping Wang (2024) elaborated on how big data integration in smart tourism management provides advantages in resource planning, customer expectation analysis, and service quality enhancement (Wang, 2024).

5. TECHNOLOGY-SUPPORTED TOURISM APPLICATIONS FOR ELDERLY AND DISABLED INDIVIDUALS

For elderly and disabled individuals, tourism is not only about physical mobility—it also plays a critical role in social participation, psychological well-being, and a sense of belonging. Technology-supported tourism solutions encompass a variety of solutions from mobile apps, to virtual reality, artificial intelligence navigation systems, and voice-activated digital assistants. In doing this, technology provides solutions for physical barriers, but also cognitive, psychological and informational barriers to access (Ribeiro et al., 2018). Applications designed with older users in mind, for example have, simplified interfaces with large buttons and icons where possible, and voice feedback which all lead to improved usability. Similarity, voice activated systems, such as digital assistants, provide older individuals with an easier way to access information (Remillard & Rogers, 2019). The intent of utilizing technology is not replacing the individual, but supporting them. Thus, wired technology supported solutions should not be considered "alternatives to travel" but "tools enabling access" (Johnson & Kent, 2007).

5.1 Mobile Applications and Digital Assistants

Mobile technologies play a significant role in facilitating the participation of elderly and disabled individuals in tourism activities. Digital assistants also provide great convenience for these groups. Remillard and Rogers (2019) demonstrated that elderly individuals could perform tasks such as making reservations, obtaining information, and navigating more easily using voice-activated digital assistants like Amazon Alexa. This also had a positive effect on their social integration (Remillard & Rogers, 2019). Personalized content in applications allows disabled individuals to receive recommendations tailored to their needs. Ribeiro et al. (2018) revealed that some mobile apps suggest travel routes based on the user's type of disability, thereby expanding the travel freedom of those with physical impairments (Ribeiro et al., 2018).

However, many of these applications are still limited in terms of accessibility. Richards et al. (2021) reported that visually impaired users faced major issues in travel apps due to complex interfaces, insufficient voice guidance, and low contrast levels (Richards et al., 2021). Given the widespread use of digital technologies, inclusive design principles must become standard in all mobile applications. Johnson and Kent (2007) showed that applications developed for elderly and disabled individuals also enhance usability for younger and non-disabled users, proving that universal design is valuable for all (Johnson & Kent, 2007).

6. GLOBAL STANDARDS AND POLICIES

Accessible tourism policies are framed by international documents such as the United Nations Convention on the Rights of People with Disabilities (UNCRPD). This convention defines access to tourism—regardless of age, gender, or disability status—as a fundamental human right (Ivanova & Senkiv, 2019). It is often emphasized that accessibility must be achieved through universal design principles. (Ambrose et al., 2012).These global policies are not limited to normative frameworks. They are also reflected in development priorities and investment agendas. The European Commission's Access City Awards are a good example of this, recognizing cities that improve their infrastructure to become more inclusive (Ivanova & Senkiv, 2019).

However, in many countries, accessibility standards remain only on paper, and implementation falls short. Therefore, these policies must be backed by monitoring and The European Union views accessible tourism not only as a human rights issue but also as an economic development strategy. The European Accessibility Act covers a broad range of areas—from digital services to transportation systems (Anca, 2010). Cities like Lyon, Ljubljana, and Barcelona are included on the EU's list of accessible cities and prioritize these standards in their infrastructure investments. These cities serve as models for shaping future projects (Ivanova & Senkiv, 2019). Under the European Disability Strategy (2021–2030), the integration of accessibility with digital transformation in the tourism sector has become a key objective. In this context, web accessibility, mobile application design, and remote information systems play a critical role (Altinay, 2021). For national policies to be effective, local governments must be actively involved in the process. Local-scale examples enable central regulations to be implemented at the grassroots level (Shanimon & Hameedu, 2013).

7. THE ECONOMIC POTENTIAL OF ACCESSIBLE TOURISM

Accessible tourism is an economic market that should not be underestimated. In Europe, its direct and indirect contributions are estimated to reach €400 billion annually (Mihaela, 2019). Elderly and disabled individuals tend to stay longer at destinations and increase their spending capacity by traveling with family members. Ferst et al. (2021) emphasize that accessibility increases the competitiveness of destinations. Regions with strong access infrastructure are preferred significantly more than others, which underscores the importance of indirect returns on infrastructure investments. Sanz et al. (2013) evaluated accessibility not only as a matter of social responsibility but also as a model that can be integrated with environmental sustainability and energy efficiency. This approach allows investments to yield multiple benefits.

There is a direct correlation between service quality and return on investment in the tourism industry. In a study conducted in Brazil, Ferst et al. (2021) found that destinations with high accessibility had a significant competitive advantage. One of the greatest challenges for investors is the lack of information. Therefore, expanding accessibility consultancy services within the framework of public–private sector collaborations is strongly recommended (Mihaela, 2019). Additionally, international brands can lead the market by developing accessibility practices that comply with global standards. This not only strengthens brand reputation but also accelerates return on investment (Shanimon & Hameedu, 2013).

8. CONCLUSION

Accessible tourism is not merely a matter of social responsibility for contemporary societies; it is a necessity for ensuring social inclusion. The freedom of elderly and disabled individuals to travel must be recognized as an extension of their fundamental human rights. Denying this right contradicts the inclusive nature of tourism. Therefore, structural transformations in the tourism sector are essential. Although numerous legal regulations have been implemented across countries, their impact at the practical level remains limited. Legislation alone is not sufficient; what matters is its visibility and enforceability in the field. This gap between policy and practice is particularly evident in developing countries. Accessibility must be experienced in practice-not just acknowledged in theory.

At the core of the tourism experience for disabled individuals lies independence. These individuals demand the right to travel without dependence on others. However, accessibility is often viewed as a “support service,” undermining autonomy. A truly inclusive system must empower independence.

Accessibility cannot be confined to physical structures. Websites, booking systems, signage, and information tools must all be designed with accessibility in mind. Especially in this age of rapid digitalization, access to information has become one of the greatest challenges for disabled individuals. Thus, accessibility requires a holistic approach. The level of knowledge tourism staff have about accessibility directly affects service quality. Unfortunately, there is often a lack of training in this area. Uninformed staff may cause disabled individuals to feel excluded. To prevent this, systematic in-service training must be implemented.

Accessibility investments benefit not only disabled individuals but also families with children, the elderly, and people with temporary health conditions. This proves that accessibility is a design principle that serves society as a whole. The philosophy of "design for all" is highly valuable in this regard. Every investment that prioritizes social benefit yields long-term returns. Accessibility is often perceived as a costly endeavor. However, research shows that these investments offer high returns. Factors such as customer satisfaction, repeat visitation, and brand reputation are tangible indicators of this return. Short-term cost concerns should not hinder long-term benefits.

Local governments are among the most effective actors in advancing accessibility. While central authorities provide budgets and legal frameworks, implementation is usually driven by municipal efforts. The proactive stance of municipalities fosters public awareness and encourages private sector investment. Therefore, the active role of local governments is vital. Disabled individuals frequently express that tourism facilities are inadequate and that they are excluded from planning processes. This not only harms the inclusive nature of tourism but also results in financial losses for service providers. Including user experience in planning is one of the most effective strategies for problem-solving. User feedback forms the foundation of viable strategies.

The lack of accessibility practices in rural areas limits the potential of rural development and tourism strategies. Yet, rural areas offer unique advantages such as proximity to nature and cultural authenticity. Unless accessible rural tourism models are developed, these advantages remain untapped. Accessibility investments focused on rural areas must be supported through public–private partnerships. Civil society organizations play a critical role in promoting accessible tourism. They can advocate for users' needs and pressure policymakers. Through awareness campaigns and public education, NGOs accelerate the transformation of public perception. In doing so, they increase the visibility of disabled individuals and foster societal acceptance. Certification and labeling of accessible tourism facilities is a positive development. However, the practical applicability of these certifications must be verified. Merely possessing a certificate does not guarantee actual accessibility. Without strong inspection mechanisms, such certifications remain symbolic.

Digital transformation has introduced numerous innovations that facilitate tourism accessibility. Mobile apps, augmented reality, and virtual tours significantly ease access to information for disabled individuals. However, if these digital tools are not designed accessibly, they can become exclusionary. Therefore, accessibility principles must be integrated into digital services from the outset. The travel experiences of disabled women are shaped by the intersection of gender inequality and disability. These individuals face both physical access issues and social prejudice. Ignoring the needs of women in tourism contradicts principles of gender equality and human rights. Thus, inclusive tourism must be reimagined from a gender-sensitive perspective. Educational institutions—especially tourism faculties—must make accessibility education mandatory. The lack of knowledge in this area not only leads to individual errors but also increases institutional risk. If future tourism professionals are not equipped with knowledge of accessibility, sectoral transformation will progress slowly. Education is one of the most powerful levers for systemic change.

Data-driven policy making is essential for the development of accessible tourism. Yet, there is still a shortage of data on the travel habits of disabled individuals. This lack of information leads to misdiagnoses and poor policy choices. Government agencies must improve data collection and analysis processes in collaboration with industry stakeholders. The financial dimension of accessibility is often overlooked. However, accessibility investments generate both direct and indirect economic benefits. These investments increase customer satisfaction and loyalty, thereby enhancing brand value. Therefore, the private sector should regard accessibility not only as social responsibility, but also as a strategic investment. Enhancing cultural events and heritage site accessibility is an important way to enrich tourism experiences. Services such as sign language interpretation, audio descriptions and the provision of subtitles in museums are useful ways to create better access to culture. These measures enable people with disabilities to participate in culture, which leads to a more inclusive society. When culture and the arts are made accessible, it creates a sense of community.

Destination management organizations (DMOs) need to create disability access policies and advise local businesses on how to be more accessible. DMOs are the organizations closest to local knowledge and have a strategic position with the potential to influence access to a wider amount of local culture. With good idea of what to do, investments by both public and private sectors will be optimized. Exemplary local examples may also influence national policy. Travel safety is one of the top concerns for elderly travelers. Accessibility is not just about providing a service—it's also about ensuring that service can be used safely. Sidewalk conditions, bus step heights, and emergency call systems in hotel rooms should all be evaluated within this context. A sense of safety is a psychological threshold that directly influences travel decisions.

The sustainability of accessible tourism depends not only on structural arrangements but also on raising awareness throughout society. This awareness can be fostered through media campaigns and public service announcements. Visibility is the first step toward raising awareness. As public consciousness grows, accessibility becomes not a privilege, but a norm. Accessibility investments should cover not just accommodation, but also transportation infrastructure. Barriers in transportation can negatively affect the entire travel experience. Low-floor buses, elevators at train stations, and clearly marked help points at airports are essential elements. A destination that is not accessible cannot be marketed effectively.

Accessibility standards vary widely between countries, causing additional challenges for international travel. Although efforts are being made—particularly in the EU—to harmonize these norms, major discrepancies still exist. These variations can discourage disabled individuals from traveling across borders. International accessibility standards must be established. The development of rural tourism presents a major opportunity for sustainable development. However, to seize this opportunity, accessibility standards must be extended to rural areas. Guesthouses, village homes, and hiking trails often lack accessible features. Access to nature is a right for everyone; thus, accessibility must be designed in an environmentally conscious way.

The needs of elderly travelers differ from those of younger ones. Physical comfort, medical support, quiet environments, and less intense schedules are important to this demographic. Planning products and services that cater to these needs is critical for creating age-friendly tourism destinations. Accessibility must reflect these specific sensitivities. Viewing disabled individuals merely as a group "in need of help" poses a psychological barrier to accessible tourism. These individuals are independent, active, and capable decision-makers—and services must be planned with this perspective in mind. Participation, not assistance, should be the guiding principle. A participation-centered approach encourages service delivery based on equality.

Voluntary accessibility practices alone are insufficient. Mechanisms such as monitoring, incentives, and—when necessary—sanctions must be implemented together. Without enforcement, regulations remain optional privileges rather than obligatory standards. A destination's level of accessibility also affects its international competitiveness. In developed countries, tourists increasingly value not only natural beauty or affordability, but also ease of access. This highlights the need for national tourism strategies to include accessibility dimensions. Successful destinations incorporate these strategies into their long-term planning.

The tourism experience is measured not just by service quality, but also by its psychological impact on the individual. A person who does not feel comfortable, free, and respected is unlikely to return. This makes respect and a sense of security essential components of accessible services. Accessibility principles must not be forgotten in disaster and crisis situations. As witnessed during the pandemic, some disabled individuals were overlooked during public health measures. For future emergencies, the accessibility dimension must be integrated into planning. Disaster management and accessibility must intersect.

Accessible tourism is not solely a matter of national policy—it can also develop through international collaboration and knowledge exchange. Adapting successful models from other countries can accelerate progress. The EU encourages such cooperation through various projects. Turkey and similar nations should actively participate in these programs. Accessibility efforts must include not only end-users but also service providers, decision-makers, architects, and software developers. When all stakeholders converge around a shared vision, more feasible solutions emerge. Stakeholder-based governance is the foundation of sustainable accessibility systems. A system shaped by collective contributions is more enduring.

Public policies in the tourism sector must address accessibility in a comprehensive manner. From environmental regulations to incentive systems, from educational programs to monitoring processes, accessibility standards must be developed in all areas. Without a systematic approach, fragmented practices fall short. Defining accessibility as a state policy is crucial in this regard. Variables such as gender, age, and type of disability shape accessibility needs in diverse ways. Therefore, accessibility cannot rely on one-size-fits-all solutions. Instead, it requires flexible approaches that accommodate diversity. Services tailored to specific types of disabilities must be developed. Rather than a "one solution for all" mindset, the principle of "different solutions for everyone" should be embraced. In conclusion, accessible tourism is a multidisciplinary field encompassing ethical, economic, administrative, and technological dimensions. Its development enhances not only service quality, but also social cohesion and well-being. Accessibility is directly linked to human dignity, equality, and sustainability. Therefore, all stakeholders must act with determination.

REFERENCES

Abdelmaksoud, N. S. A. (2022). Universal design approach to a smart, sustainable, safe, and accessible city. *WIT Transactions on Ecology and the Environment, 260*, 259–270. DOI: 10.2495/SC220211

Achillas, C., Aidonis, D., Folinas, D., & Vlachokostas, C. (2024). Empowering tourism accessibility: A digital revolution in Pieria, Greece. *Applied Sciences (Basel, Switzerland), 14*(23), 11136. DOI: 10.3390/app142311136

Aldousari, A., Alotaibi, M., Khajah, F., Jaafar, A., Alshebli, M., & Kanj, H. (2023). A wearable IoT-based healthcare monitoring system for elderly people. In *2023 International Conference on BioSMART (BioSMART)* (pp. 1–4). IEEE. DOI: 10.1109/BioSMART58455.2023.10162041

Altınay, F., Dagli, G., Altinay, M., & Altınay, Z. (2019). The role of technology in tourism and health services for accessibility in service management. *Postmodern Openings, 10*(4), 1–7. DOI: 10.18662/po/90

Altınay, Z., Saner, T., Bahçelerli, N. M., & Altınay, F. (2016). The role of social media tools: Accessible tourism for disabled citizens. *Journal of Educational Technology & Society, 19*(1), 89–99. https://www.jstor.org/stable/jeductechsoci.19.1.89

Altinay Ozdemir, M. (2021). Virtual reality (VR) and augmented reality (AR) technologies for accessibility and marketing in the tourism industry. In M. C. tom Dieck & T. Jung (Eds.), *Virtual and augmented reality in tourism marketing* (pp. 277–301). IGI Global. DOI: 10.4018/978-1-7998-7539-0.ch014

Ambrose, I., Darcy, S., & Buhalis, D. (2012). *Best practice in accessible tourism: Inclusion, disability, ageing population and tourism* (Aspects of Tourism, Vol. 53). Channel View Publications.

Anca, G. (2010). European Union policy on accessible tourism as millstones for future development of worldwide accessibility standards for tourism. In *TRANSED 2010: 12th International Conference on Mobility and Transport for Elderly and Disabled People*. Hong Kong Society for Rehabilitation; S. K. Yee Medical Foundation; Transportation Research Board.

Bekiaris, E., Panou, M., & Mousadakou, A. (2007). Elderly and disabled travelers' needs in infomobility services. In Stephanidis, C. (Ed.), Lecture Notes in Computer Science: Vol. 4554. *Universal access in human computer interaction: Coping with diversity* (pp. 853–860). Springer., DOI: 10.1007/978-3-540-73279-2_95

Capitaine, V. (2016). Inciting tourist accommodation managers to make their establishments accessible to people with disabilities. *Journal of Tourism Futures*, *2*(2), 196–205. DOI: 10.1108/JTF-03-2015-0010

Cortés, U., Annicchiarico, R., Campana, F., Vázquez-Salceda, J., Urdiales, C., Cañamero, L., López, M., Sànchez-Marrè, M., Di Vincenzo, S., & Caltagirone, C. (2004). Artificial intelligence in medicine: Project of a mobile platform in an intelligent environment for the care of disabled and elderly people. *Recenti Progressi in Medicina*, *95*(4), 190–195. PMID: 15147063

Darrat, M., & Flaherty, G. T. (2019). Retrospective analysis of older travellers attending a specialist travel health clinic. *Tropical Diseases, Travel Medicine and Vaccines*, *5*(1), 17. DOI: 10.1186/s40794-019-0094-8 PMID: 31548898

Dias, A., Santinha, G., Rodrigues, M., Queirós, A., Rodrigues, C., & Rocha, N. P. (2021). Smart cities and accessible tourism. In Augusto, J. C. (Ed.), *Handbook of smart cities* (pp. 96–114). Springer., DOI: 10.1007/978-3-030-69698-6_45

Ding, Y., Lin, Y., & Liu, Q. (2010). Developing an accessible transport network for accessible tourism in Beijing. In *TRANSED 2010: 12th International Conference on Mobility and Transport for Elderly and Disabled People*. Hong Kong Society for Rehabilitation; S. K. Yee Medical Foundation; Transportation Research Board.

Domínguez, J. A., Fraiz, J. A., & Alén, E. (2013). Economic profitability of accessible tourism for the tourism industry. *Journal of Tourism and Hospitality Management*, *1*(3), 84–100.

Drews, W. (2008). A Web 2.0 tourism information system for accessible tourism. In P. O'Connor, W. Höpken, & U. Gretzel (Eds.), *Information and communication technologies in tourism 2008* (pp. 164–174). Springer. DOI: 10.1007/978-3-211-77280-5_15

Eichhorn, V., Miller, G., Michopoulou, E., & Buhalis, D. (2008). Enabling disabled tourists? Accessibility tourism information schemes. *Annals of Tourism Research*, *35*(1), 189–210. DOI: 10.1016/j.annals.2007.07.005

Ercan, F. (2022). Accessible tourism experiences in smart destinations: The case of Breda (Netherlands). In Öztürk, I. E. (Ed.), *Planning and managing the experience economy in tourism* (pp. 274–300). IGI Global., DOI: 10.4018/978-1-7998-8775-1.ch014

Ferràs, X., Hitchen, E. L., Tarrats-Pons, E., & Serrat, N. (2020). Smart tourism empowered by artificial intelligence: The case of Lanzarote. *Journal of Cases on Information Technology*, *22*(1), 1–13. DOI: 10.4018/JCIT.2020010101

Ferst, M. D. C., & Coutinho, H. R. M. (2021). Impacts of training on perceptions of accessibility in tourism. *Revista Turismo em Análise*, *32*(1), 27–35. DOI: 10.14210/at.v6n1.p27-35

Ferst, M. D. C., dos Anjos, S. J. G., & Kuhn, V. (2023). Valuing accessibility in hospitality and the loyalty of tourists with disabilities. *Turismo: Visão e Ação*, *25*(2), 243–262. DOI: 10.14210/rtva.v25n2.p243-262

Fortuna, J., Cantwell-Jurkovic, L., Dean, J., Fry, H., & Ross, S. (2024). Staff training on disability awareness in museum settings: A scoping review. *The American Journal of Occupational Therapy*, *78*(5, Supplement_2), 7805205060. DOI: 10.5014/ajot.2024.78S2-PO119 PMID: 39133619

Fraser, D. A. (2017). *Perceptions of risks and barriers to participation in tourism for the disabled* [Unpublished master's thesis]. University of Plymouth.

Haghi, M., Spicher, N., Wang, J., & Deserno, T. M. (2022). Integrated sensing devices for disease prevention and health alerts in smart homes. *Studies in Health Technology and Informatics*, *291*, 39–61. DOI: 10.3233/SHTI220007 PMID: 35593757

Hasan, N., & Ahmed, M. F. (2024). Wearable technology for elderly care: Integrating health monitoring and emergency alerts. *Journal of Computer Networks and Communications*, *2024*(1), 5593708. DOI: 10.1155/jcnc/5593708

Helal, S., Mokhtari, M., & Abdulrazak, B. (Eds.). (2008). *The engineering handbook of smart technology for aging, disability, and independence*. John Wiley & Sons., DOI: 10.1002/9780470379424

Hennig, S., Sattler, T., Wasserburger, W., & Wasserburger, M. (2015). How to improve accessibility of natural areas: About the relevance of providing information on accessible services and facilities in natural areas. In M. Schrenk, V. V. Popovich, P. Zeile, P. Elisei, & C. Beyer (Eds.), *PLANNING TIMES – You better keep planning or you get in trouble: Proceedings of 19th International Conference on Urban Planning, Regional Development and Information Society* (pp. 803–812). CORP.

Hossain, M. N. A., Pal, A., & Hossain, S. K. A. (2015). A wearable sensor based elderly home care system in a smart environment. In *2015 18th International Conference on Computer and Information Technology (ICCIT)* (pp. 329–334). IEEE. DOI: 10.1109/ICCITechn.2015.7488091

Ivanova, M., & Senkiv, G. (2019). Accessible tourism for all in the European Union. *International Journal of Scientific Research and Management*, *7*(2), 87–93. DOI: 10.17721/1728-2721.2019.74.12

Johnson, R., & Kent, S. (2007). Designing universal access: Web-applications for the elderly and disabled. *Cognition Technology and Work*, *9*(4), 209–218. DOI: 10.1007/s10111-007-0063-2

Kaganek, K., Ambroży, T., Mucha, D., Jurczak, A., Bornikowska, A., Ostrowski, A., Janiszewska, R., & Mucha, T. (2017). Barriers to participation in tourism in the disabled. *Polish Journal of Sport and Tourism*, *24*(3), 121–129. DOI: 10.1515/pjst-2017-0013

Kamanzi, G. N. (2024). Improved access to healthcare, remote monitoring of joint function, and increased patient engagement in managing arthritis symptoms: The role of telehealth in arthritis care. *IDOSR Journal of Scientific Research*, *9*(1), 12–24. DOI: 10.59298/IDOSRJSR/2024/9.3.434700

Kamyabi, M., & Alipour, H. (2022). An investigation of the challenges faced by the disabled population and the implications for accessible tourism. *Sustainability (Basel)*, *14*(8), 4702. DOI: 10.3390/su14084702

Kastenholz, E., Eusébio, C., & Figueiredo, E. (2015). Contributions of tourism to social inclusion of people with disability. *Disability & Society*, *30*(8), 1259–1281. DOI: 10.1080/09687599.2015.1075868

Ko, M., Azzopardi, M., Loizou, C., Logeswaran, A., Ng, B., Pacho, A., & Chong, Y. J. (2025). Telehealth and people with disabilities in the United Kingdom: A scoping review. *Frontiers in Public Health*, *13*, 1433755. DOI: 10.3389/fpubh.2025.1504318 PMID: 40013026

Ku, W., Lim, S. S., Look, K. S., & Tan, W. H. (2019). Investigating tourists' behavioral intentions using stimulus-organism-response theory. *Asia Pacific Journal of Tourism Research*, *24*(7), 689–702. DOI: 10.1080/10941665.2019.1622638

Kyung, R., & Park, C. S. (2020). How artificial intelligence and virtual reality benefit the elderly and individuals with disabilities. *Journal of Gerontology and Medicine*, *1*(2), 1–7. DOI: 10.30564/jgm.v1i2.1824

Li, C. Z., & Borycki, E. M.Li Cindy ZhiruiBorycki Elizabeth M. (2019). Smart homes for healthcare. *Studies in Health Technology and Informatics*, *257*, 283–287. DOI: 10.3233/978-1-61499-951-5-283 PMID: 30741210

Li, K. F. (2013). Smart home technology for telemedicine and emergency management. *Journal of Ambient Intelligence and Humanized Computing*, *4*(5), 535–546. DOI: 10.1007/s12652-012-0129-8 PMID: 32218875

Li, Y., Zhang, Y., & Lv, B. (2017). A health monitoring system based on wearable equipment. *MATEC Web of Conferences, 139*, Article 00164. DOI: 10.1051/matecconf/201713900164

Liasidou, S., Umbelino, J., & Panão, M. J. (2019). Revisiting tourism studies curriculum to highlight accessible tourism issues. *European Journal of Tourism Research, 21*, 103–106. DOI: 10.54055/ejtr.v21i.357

Luccio, F. L., & Beltrame, L. (2018). Accessible tourism for users with hearing loss. In *Proceedings of the 4th EAI International Conference on Smart Objects and Technologies for Social Good* (pp. 243–248). ACM. DOI: 10.1145/3284869.3284909

Mahmoudzadeh, M., & Sarjaz, M. B. (2018). Environmental barriers to tourism development for people with disabilities. *Tourism Planning & Development, 15*(3), 288–305. DOI: 10.1080/21568316.2017.1331252

Marwah, K., & Hajati, F. (2021). A survey on Internet of Things in telehealth. In *Lecture notes in networks and systems* (Vol. 204, pp. 235–248). Springer., DOI: 10.1007/978-3-030-75025-1_22

Marwah, R., Thakur, J. S., & Tanwar, P. (2024). Augmented reality assistive technologies for disabled individuals. *arXiv*. /arXiv.2402.17256DOI: 10.48550

Mihaela, D. (2019). Accessibility in tourism – Need and opportunity. *Journal of Tourism Research, 21*, 12–18.

Moris, M. I., Alakhras, H., Eid, N. G., & Higazy, M. (2019). Human resources capacity building in accessible tourism in Egypt. *Journal of Association of Arab Universities for Tourism and Hospitality, 17*(3), 82–89. DOI: 10.21608/jaauth.2019.92004

Nasr, M. M., Islam, M. M., Shehata, S., Karray, F., & Quintana, Y. (2021). Smart healthcare in the age of AI: Recent advances, challenges, and future prospects. *IEEE Access : Practical Innovations, Open Solutions, 9*, 145248–145270. DOI: 10.1109/ACCESS.2021.3118960

Odeh, B., Philip, N., & Kayyali, R. (2014). Acceptability of telehealth by elderly patients. *Age and Ageing, 43*(Suppl_2), ii13. DOI: 10.1093/ageing/afu036.4

Padrón Nápoles, V. M., Gachet Páez, D., Esteban Penelas, J. L., García Pérez, O., Martín de Pablos, F., & Muñoz Gil, R. (2021). Social inclusion in smart cities. In Augusto, J. C. (Ed.), *Handbook of smart cities* (pp. 159–190). Springer., DOI: 10.1007/978-3-030-69698-6_42

Panyadee, C., Krajangchom, S., Sangkakorn, K., & Intawong, K. (2023). Smart wellness technology for tourism destination. *TEM Journal, 12*(2), 456–467. DOI: 10.18421/TEM122-03

Poli, M. (2019). Tourism, design and disability? In D. Gursoy & R. Nunkoo (Eds.), *Strategic innovative marketing and tourism: 7th ICSIMAT, Athenian Riviera, Greece, 2018* (pp. 603–611). Springer. DOI: 10.1007/978-3-030-12453-3_69

Popiel, M. (2016). Barriers in undertaking tourist activity by disabled people. *Journal of Kinesiology and Exercise Sciences, 15*(74), 103–110.

Putri, D., & Taufik, D. N. (2024). Development of disabled-friendly tourism infrastructure. *SocioVoyage: International Journal of Social Dynamics in Tourism, 1*(3), 26–35. DOI: 10.56910/sociovoyage.v1i3.4

Ramlee, R., Tang, D. H., & Ismail, M. M. (2012). Smart home system for disabled people via wireless Bluetooth. In *2012 International Conference on System Engineering and Technology (ICSET)* (pp. 1–4). IEEE. DOI: 10.1109/ICSEngT.2012.6339347

Remillard, E. T., Rogers, W. A., & Ruiz, S. (2019). Utilizing technology networks to support social networks for people aging with disability. *Innovation in Aging, 3*(Suppl_1), S758–S759. DOI: 10.1093/geroni/igz038.2787

Ribeiro, F., Metrôlho, J., Leal, J., Martins, H., & Bastos, P. (2018). A mobile application to provide personalized information for mobility impaired tourists. In *ICT tools and applications for accessible tourism* (pp. 171–191). IGI Global., DOI: 10.4018/978-1-7998-6428-8.ch008

Richards, V., Matthews, N., Williams, O. J., & Khan, Z. (2021). The challenges of accessible tourism information systems for tourists with vision impairment. In Michopoulou, E., Swain, S., & Buhalis, D. (Eds.), *ICT tools and applications for accessible tourism* (pp. 154–171). IGI Global., DOI: 10.4018/978-1-7998-6428-8.ch002

Rosa, M., Gameiro, C., Sousa, C., & Pinto, P. (2020). An analysis of elderly tourists' constraints in the use of public transport. *Transport Development and Integration, 4*(2), 163–178. DOI: 10.2495/TDI-V4-N2-163-178

Rosa, M., Pinto, A., & Assunção, P. (2020). An evaluation of the universal accessibility of bus stop infrastructure. *International Journal of Sustainable Development and Planning, 15*(6), 835–840. DOI: 10.18280/ijsdp.150606

Rosa, M. P., & Lopes, J. D. C. (2019). Senior tourists' perceptions of bus stop environments used in collaborative design. *WIT Transactions on the Built Environment, 186*, 121–132. DOI: 10.2495/UT190111

Rumetshofer, H., & Wöß, W. (2004). Tourism information systems promoting barrier-free tourism. In *ICCSA 2004: International Conference on Computer Science and its Applications* (pp. 280–286). Springer. DOI: 10.1007/978-3-540-24707-4_35

Saif, S., Biswas, S., & Chattopadhyay, S. (2020). Intelligent, secure big health data management using deep learning and blockchain technology: An overview. In Dash, S., Acharya, B. R., Mittal, M., Abraham, A., & Kelemen, A. (Eds.), *Deep learning techniques for biomedical and health informatics* (pp. 187–209). Springer., DOI: 10.1007/978-3-030-33966-1_10

Salha, R. A., Jawabrah, M. Q., Badawy, U., Jarada, A., & Alastal, A. I. (2020). Towards smart, sustainable, accessible and inclusive city for people with disability by taking into account checklists tools. *Journal of Geographic Information System, 12*(4), 348–371. DOI: 10.4236/jgis.2020.124022

Sancho-Esper, F., Ostrovskaya, L., Rodriguez-Sanchez, C., & Campayo-Sanchez, F. (2022). Virtual reality in retirement communities: Technology acceptance and tourist destination recommendation. *Journal of Vacation Marketing, 28*(4), 370–385. DOI: 10.1177/13567667211066387

Sanz, M. F., Ferrandis, E. D., & Ferrer, J. G. (2013). Involving elderly and disabled tourists as active participants in energy savings. *Journal of Sustainable Tourism, 21*(2), 256–272. DOI: 10.1080/09669582.2012.709211

Sari, S., & Ünüvar, Ş. (2019). Hotel managers and staff's attitudes towards accessible tourism. *Journal of Tourism and Gastronomy Studies, 7*(4), 3060–3087. DOI: 10.21325/jotags.2019.516

Sarmento, E., Brás, C., & Vargas de Oliveira, C. (2016). Issues and challenges of accessibility for senior tourism. *European Journal of Tourism Research, 14*, 7–26. DOI: 10.54055/ejtr.v14i.251

Saygılı, T., Oymak Yalçın, S., & Özsarı, H. (2021). Advanced age and disabled health tourism: Concept, problems and solution suggestions. *International Journal of Health Management and Tourism, 6*(2), 492–514. DOI: 10.31201/ijhmt.918595

Shanimon, S., & Hameedu, M. S. (2013). Foreign direct investment and accessible tourism in India. *International Journal of Scientific and Research Publications, 3*(12), 1–5.

Shetty, E. A., & McIntosh, A. (2020). Online communications of accessibility in hotel restaurants. *Hospitality Insights, 4*(2), 7–8. DOI: 10.24135/hi.v4i2.87

Shidende, D., Kessel, T., Treydte, A., & Moebs, S. (2023). A systematic literature review of accessibility evaluation methods for augmented reality applications. *Studies in Health Technology and Informatics*, *306*, 575–582. DOI: 10.3233/SHTI230681 PMID: 37638964

Singh, R., Seniaray, S., & Das, P. (2022). Role of IoT in universal design. In Kumar, A., Maurer, J. L., & Kadry, S. (Eds.), *Handbook of smart materials, technologies, and devices* (pp. 709–728). Springer., DOI: 10.1007/978-3-030-84205-5_128

Soussi, O., Lemiere, P., Millot, S., & others. (2024). Beyond telehealth in heart failure: How a nurse-led mobile team unit improves management. *European Heart Journal, 45*(Suppl_1), Article ehae758.2623. DOI: 10.1093/eurheartj/ehae758.2623

Stock, S. E., Davies, D. K., Herold, R. G., & Wehmeyer, M. L. (2019). Technology to support transportation needs assessment, training, and pre-trip planning by people with intellectual disability. *Advances in Neurodevelopmental Disorders*, *3*(3), 319–324. DOI: 10.1007/s41252-019-00117-x

Swanepoel, L., Spencer, J., & Draper, D. (2020). Education and training for disability awareness of hospitality staff. *African Journal of Hospitality, Tourism and Leisure*, *9*(4), 402–417. DOI: 10.46222/ajhtl.19770720-36

Szewczyk, I. (2020). Problems of collective transport management – Obstacles to access for disabled people. *Transportation Research Procedia*, *45*, 78–86. DOI: 10.1016/j.trpro.2020.02.064

Szewczyka, I., & Zontek, E. L. (2018). Adjustment for elderly and disabled tourists in Polish hotels. *New Trends and Issues Proceedings on Humanities and Social Sciences*, *5*(2), 160–170. DOI: 10.18844/prosoc.v5i2.3667

Thomas, A., & Wee, H. (2022). Educational tourist motivations, destination image, and destination selection behavior in an extended S-O-R model. *International Journal of Academic Research in Business & Social Sciences*, *12*(10), 2198–2210. DOI: 10.6007/IJARBSS/v12-i10/14849

tom Dieck, M. C., Jung, T., & Michopoulou, E. (2019). Experiencing virtual reality in heritage attractions: Perceptions of elderly users. In tom Dieck, M. C., & Jung, T. (Eds.), *Augmented reality and virtual reality* (pp. 89–98). Springer., DOI: 10.1007/978-3-030-06246-0_7

Tuna, A., Das, R., & Tuna, G. (2015). Integrated smart home services and smart wearable technology for the disabled and elderly. In *Proceedings of the 7th International Conference on Computer Supported Education* (pp. 173–177). SCITEPRESS. DOI: 10.5220/0005552001730177

Wai-leung, B. C. (2004). Accessible tourism in Hong Kong: An untapped market. In *10th International Conference on Mobility and Transport for Elderly and Disabled People*. Japan Society of Civil Engineers; Transportation Research Board.

Wang, P. (2024). The integration and innovation of smart tourism management and big data technology. In *2023 3rd International Conference on Artificial Intelligence, Automation, and High-Performance Computing (AIAHPC)* (pp. 45–51). IEEE. DOI: 10.1109/AIARS63200.2024.00118

Wu, S., & Wang, S. (2025). Exploring the impact of AI-enhanced virtual tourism on tourists' pro-environmental behavior: A stimulus-organism-response model perspective. *Acta Psychologica, 253*, 104773. DOI: 10.1016/j.actpsy.2025.104773 PMID: 39904230

Wu, X., & Lai, I. K. W. (2022). The use of 360-degree virtual tours to promote mountain walking tourism: Stimulus–organism–response model. *Information Technology & Tourism, 24*(1), 85–107. DOI: 10.1007/s40558-021-00218-1

Xu, M. (2023). Research on smart tourism system based on artificial intelligence. In *2023 IEEE 3rd International Conference on Information Technology, Big Data and Artificial Intelligence (ICIBA)* (pp. 201–205). IEEE. DOI: 10.1109/ICIBA56860.2023.10165293

Yu, J., Kim, S., Hailu, T. B., Park, J., & Han, H. (2024). The effects of virtual reality (VR) and augmented reality (AR) on senior tourists' experiential quality. *Current Issues in Tourism, 27*(3), 464–478. DOI: 10.1080/13683500.2023.2165483

Zahari, N. F., Kamarudin, H., Zawawi, Z. A., Rashid, R. B. A., & Bahari, M. M. (2023). Heritage tourism: A disabled person's rights to engage in social activity. *Planning Malaysia, 21*(5), 484–494. DOI: 10.21837/pm.v21i25.1252

Zajadacz, A. (2015). The contribution of the geography of disability to the development of accessible tourism. *Turyzm (Lódz), 25*(1), 19–27. DOI: 10.2478/tour-2014-0016

Chapter 8
Management of Home Healthcare in the Technological Era and Implications

Yiğit Kerem Yıldız
https://orcid.org/0000-0002-2976-9169
Istanbul Nisantasi University, Turkey

ABSTRACT

Nowadays countries are entering a period where their social profiles are increasingly dominated by the elderly population. Due to increasing demand and limited personnel resources, home healthcare services are becoming increasingly difficult to manage. Technological applications are used to prevent disruptions that mentioned here. This section evaluates the effects of technological applications on home healthcare services and management. In order to make this assessment, studies on home healthcare services and technologies which emerged with Health 4.0 were examined. All technologies that used in home healthcare services have effects in terms of saving costs and resources, as well as providing convenience to people who have difficulty accessing services, and increasing patients' quality of life. When these are considered in terms of healthcare management, they will provide savings in the health economics, efficient use of limited resources and the provision of accessible, patient-focused services with no boundaries.

DOI: 10.4018/979-8-3373-3099-0.ch008

INTRODUCTION

Home healthcare services are a continuous and comprehensive service type that allows individuals to receive health services in their own houses. Home healthcare services are known for contributing to cost management by reducing occupancy rates in hospitals which has been proven in some studies (Güdük, 2025; Lawrence et al., 2023; Roberts et al., 2023). These services which improve health and prioritize the independence of the individuals are provided by public, private, and non-profit organizations (Chen et al., 2022). These healthcare services are especially preferred by the elderly people who have chronic diseases and need palliative care (Fang et al., 2022; Oelschlägel et al. 2023, Steindal et al. 2020).

Home healthcare services have evolved due to the influence of technologies. The factors that have caused this evolution are various. One of the most important factor is the aging of the population. This increase especially in developed countries puts great strain on their healthcare systems (Senillosa et al., 2022). The excessive demand for health services challenges the management of health services both strategically and operationally (İnaç & Ekmekçi, 2023). In healthcare services where resources are limited and demand is high, technology is the savior for healthcare systems. Technological developments made to solve the limitations have accelerated the change and development of the concept of healthcare delivery (Şimşir & Mete, 2021). Gradual decrease in the number of healthcare professionals is another reason for the technological transformation. What is mentioned here is not about general decrease in healthcare professionals but rather a decrease in the number of staff who working in home healthcare services. Healthcare personnel have high turnover rates especially in home healthcare services (Chua et al., 2022; Güdük, 2025; Oelschlägel et al. 2024; Roberts et al., 2023). The third factor that caused the technological transformation is Covid-19. During the Covid-19 period, countries focused on remote healthcare services to manage the high demands on hospitals caused by Covid-19 (Brocard et al., 2021; Mundi et al., 2021). This helped individuals with chronic health conditions to overcome the pandemic safely. In addition, these developments have increased the trust in home healthcare services.

Despite the decrease in the number of professionals which providing home healthcare services, health institutions are directing patients and professionals to home healthcare services using technological applications due to the aging society, the increase of the life expectancy at birth and increasing burden on the healthcare budget (Álvarez-Castañón et al., 2022). In order to successfully provide these services and prevent possible negativities that may arise from limited resources, health systems have positioned technology at the center of home healthcare services. In these periods when technology is dominant, information about home healthcare services and their effects as well as the technologies which used are quite diverse. This section evaluates the effects of technological applications on home healthcare services and management. In order to make this assessment, studies on home healthcare services and technologies which emerged with Health 4.0 were examined.

HOME HEALTHCARE SERVICES MANAGEMENT

Home healthcare services can be defined as primary and rehabilitation nursing care, intermediate care with in-home assistance, and care providing care at home to patients (Genet et al., 2011; Vaartio-Rajalin et al., 2019). Nowadays, institutions which provide healthcare services prefer to provide home healthcare services especially to patients in need of palliative care (Vaartio-Rajalin et al., 2019; Vaartio-Rajali & Fagerström, 2019). The main purpose of home healthcare services is to help people who have difficulties accessing services and to manage health resources efficiently. The purposes of using these services can be summarized as follows (Merih et al., 2021):

- Reducing the length of stay and minimizing hospital-acquired infection risks
- Increasing bed turnover rate and ensure that more patients receive service from hospitals
- Providing socio-psychological support by providing the service in a family environment
- Improving patients' quality of life
- Reducing healthcare expenditures

Home healthcare services management can be defined as a comprehensive management style which addresses individuals' who have advanced chronic illnesses and functional impairments. The main focus of this type of management approach is to provide service at the patient's address (Shurson et al., 2019). The goal of home healthcare services and management is to reduce the impact of illness and disability by providing the most suitable treatment with minimal disruption to daily life while simultaneously enhancing the patient's quality of life (İnaç & Ekmekçi, 2023; Munyewende et al., 2014). There are some advantages of home healthcare services management approach and these can be explained as follows (Shurson et al., 2019):

- Reducing readmission rates
- Reducing excessive emergency room visits
- Reducing costs resulting from unnecessary use of healthcare services
- Ensuring appropriate hospitalization of patients

In order to benefit from the advantages that mentioned here by integrating digital health applications into home healthcare services, health systems need to prepare themselves for possible obstacles which may affect home healthcare services management. If the obstacles are not overcome they will break the trust in both home healthcare services management and digitalization in healthcare. Possible obstacles that may affect home healthcare services management are explained in detail as follows (Sabetsarvestani et al., 2022):

- **Lack of Effective and Comprehensive Standards:** Patients may have doubts about the scientific nature of the home healthcare service or technology used and which steps to follow. Because patients do not have the same level of knowledge as healthcare professionals. Therefore information needs to be provided. Apart from this, there may not be any auditing mechanisms that can monitor the performance and standards of the professional who providing the service. This makes it difficult to evaluate and manage the effective provision of home healthcare services. Doubts that mentioned here can be resolved through inspections by official authorities.
- **Unproductive Interaction:** Patients may be dissatisfied with health professionals due to reasons such as indifference and poor quality service delivery as in all areas of health. The important point here is the decision that the unit managers. If managers are as indifferent to the issue as the staff, this will be a serious problem. There may be problems regarding employees not being at the same point of communication with patients and their families from the perspective of healthcare professionals. To resolve such miscommunications, communication management needs to be implemented.
- **Sociocultural Inappropriate Situations:** Although some patients are open to the home healthcare services, some of them approach with caution. The reason for their cautious approach is the idea that it will invade their privacy. Apart from this, some countries' health systems may not have fully defined the basic dimensions of home healthcare services such as their scope and purpose. Due to such situations, patients cannot fully trust institutions which provide home healthcare services. Some countries may not prefer to provide home healthcare services to patients because they see these services as costly. Access to healthcare services differs based on the patient's location. This is unfortunately also true for home healthcare services. Because institutions which can provide home healthcare services are generally located in big cities. In rural areas, this opportunity is quite limited. Another difficulty in access is financial conditions. A certain number of patients can meet the financial obligations of home healthcare services. In addition to financial capacity, the availability of resources is another criterion for access. Access problems

resulting from insufficient equipment or staff negatively affect the quality of home healthcare services.

- **Occupational Problems:** Violence in healthcare is a problem which not only in home healthcare services but also in all dimensions of healthcare. Some healthcare professionals even consider quitting their jobs due to the negative experiences such as insults and violence. Another point among occupational problems is burnout among staff who working in home healthcare services. These employees experience difficulties because they do not work in a fixed location and cannot find a colleague who can immediately reach when a problem occurs.

TECHNOLOGICAL DEVELOPMENTS AND THEIR EFFECTS ON HOME HEALTHCARE SERVICES

With the development of technology approaches to remote healthcare services have become increasingly positive. Remote monitoring and real-time communication between healthcare professionals and patients are now feasible with the advent of 5G technology. In addition, developments in wearable technology in particular have led to extraordinary developments (Bijalwan et al., 2021; Cheng et al., 2024; Huang et al., 2009).

The ability to provide remote healthcare services has enabled individuals to receive these services comfortably at home. Providing this comfort which is also the focal point of home healthcare services is especially critical for the elderly and individuals with chronic health problems (Gilmour, 2018). Some advantages that make home healthcare services attractive as well as some points that should be taken into consideration have emerged with the developments in healthcare technology. These advantages can be listed as follows (Avcı & Gözüm, 2024, p. 64):

- **Access to Services:** Individuals who have difficulty accessing healthcare institutions have easier access to services, and thus their quality of life increases thanks to telehealth/telemedicine applications.
- **Cost-Effectiveness:** The use of technology in home healthcare services reduces costs by reducing long-term care and hospitalization rates.
- **Real-Time Tracking:** In case of an emergency situation, the ability to intervene immediately with technology makes the job of healthcare professionals easier.
- **Personalized Care:** Technologic health applications can develop special programs to meet the needs of patients who may have different needs.

- **Reducing Carbon Footprint:** Patients do not have to pay transportation costs to go to healthcare institutions thanks to technological applications. This also reduces carbon emissions that harm the environment.

In addition to the beautiful features that mentioned above, there are some points to consider. These dimensions which we can describe as difficulties, can be listed as follows (Avcı & Gözüm, 2024, p. 64):

- **Security and Privacy:** Concerns such as cybersecurity threats and data breaches still persist.
- **Technology Adoption:** It takes a long time for patients and healthcare professionals to accept some technologies.
- **Costs:** For some institutions and patients, accessing or using such technologies can be quite costly.
- **The Impact of Human Touch:** Patients generally seek human touch in healthcare. Besides some patients may have negative thoughts about these technologies because of the view that machines cannot replace the sense of empathy that exists in humans.

The world which is in the Health 4.0 era that is a tool for the digitalization of health is moving towards Health 5.0. Health 5.0 is a movement which adopts a patient-centered, comprehensive approach to healthcare services and aims to integrate the latest technologies, patient participation, personalized care and proactive healthcare management. The main focus of this movement is to address patient needs, personalize care, improve diagnoses, and provide patients with access to data-driven insights (Naureen et al., 2024, p.1-3). The technologies which emerge with this trend should reflect dimensions that will increase the quality of healthcare services, reduce costs and improve benefits, address the satisfaction of all healthcare stakeholders (Basulo-Ribeiro & Teixeira, 2024). Technologies such as telemedicine, artificial intelligence have emerged and are frequently used in healthcare along with technological trends. Patients can access information and services regarding their health status more easily with these technologies. In terms of healthcare management, higher quality service is provided as the workload of the staff decreases. Thus, healthcare costs are reduced (Koçaş, 2022, p. 24). The technologies that are prominent in home healthcare management today can be listed below (Merih et al., 2021):

- Artifical Intelligence (AI)
- Big Data
- Internet of Things (IoT)
- Virtual Reality (VR)

- Wearable Technologies

Apart from the technologies which mentioned above, blockchain, drone and robotic technologies can also be used in home healthcare services. In this section, this topic will be explained through the technologies that used in home healthcare services today in order to look at the effects of technological applications on home healthcare services.

BIG DATA AND HOME HEALTHCARE SERVICES

Big data is a term that covers technologies developed in recent years to process and transform unusable data created in computers and internet into something useful in a way that can create value (Merih et al., 2021). It is fair to say that the concept of big data has played a key role in the development of technologies like virtual reality and artificial intelligence. Because the data processed in these applications are big data. When considering home healthcare services and big data, this technology does not mean anything on its own. However, big data technology gains meaning with applications that bring big data together in a meaningful way, such as telemedicine. Data that gains meaning makes home healthcare services more visible, legal and a source that can produce value for scientific studies (Merih et al., 2021).

In summary, big data is a concept that is at the core of technological applications used in home healthcare services. If the data is not designed to create value and benefit, it is not possible to manage and provide healthcare services from home with technological applications.

VIRTUAL REALITY AND HOME HEALTHCARE SERVICES

Virtual reality can be defined as an alternative world in which a person can move with the help of fiber optic data, gloves and video glasses (Merih et al., 2021; Önder, 2021; Stavropoulos et al., 2020). Virtual reality is basically a technological application that makes a person's experiences in a virtual environment feel as if they were real. The main feature of virtual reality is that it reflects the individual's feeling of being there.

Virtual reality technologies can be used in many areas such as surgery, diagnosing diseases by healthcare professionals, training other professionals in medicine or healthcare services, patient education, patient rehabilitation, exercise (Merih, et al., 2021; Önder, 2021; Whende, 2019).

When the use of virtual reality in healthcare is examined, it is seen that these technologies is known for its benefits especially in the field of physiotherapy. In studies on home healthcare, it is generally seen that the literature is about home based rehabilitation. The study of Funoa et al. (2024) found that such technologies will alleviate chronic pain caused by exercise and patients who cannot leave their homes can psychologically recover thanks to the experience of nature scenery provided by virtual reality. Kraśnik et al. (2024) suggested that rehabilitation with virtual reality support has similar effects to traditional rehabilitation services, but that certain conditions must be met. First, the therapy must be patient-specific and appropriately designed. Second, safety concerns, especially for elderly with visual or sensory impairments should be prioritized. Finally, interaction methodology selection is necessary to insure safe implementation for individuals with cognitive limitations. It can be seen from latest studies on virtual reality usage in home healthcare services that it improves the health status of individuals and helps them receive remote services from their homes. However, it should not be forgotten that individuals have security concerns and patient-specific programming is required.

TELEMEDICINE AND HOME HEALTHCARE SERVICES

Telemedicine is a technology that includes many technologies, such as digital X-rays and remote surgery. Telehealth is an application that provides remote access between citizens and healthcare personnel for the purpose of disease diagnosis, treatment and prevention, and continuous improvement of healthcare services, used by all healthcare professionals. Telehealth can be seen as a broader version of telemedicine. Telemedicine and telehealth are used under a single heading called telemedicine in this section because of their similar functions. The critical point in all these services is patient satisfaction and the effectiveness of the service provided. The slightest deficiency in these two factors can cause both serious financial losses and problems that endanger the patient's life. The areas of use of telemedicine in health systems are quite wide. Tele surgery, tele monitoring, tele consultation are the main ones (Dilbaz et al., 2020).

Telemedicine is the most well-known applications in digitalization in health. Studies on telemedicine and home healthcare services are common in the literature. Muñoz-Bonet et al. (2020) stated that telemedicine applications in home healthcare services is useful in disease diagnosis and first aid. Heratanti et al. (2021) stated that telemedicine usage in home healthcare services improves patients quality of life, reduces costs, increases patient satisfaction, reduces the waiting time for re-admission to the hospital, and makes it easier for individuals to manage their own health. Besides satisfactions which identified here include consumer-focused satisfaction, adherence to patient-centered care, empathy toward healthcare providers and patients relationship to quality of care, support for home healthcare providers, emotional support, professionalism, and cultural competence of healthcare providers. Onofori et al. (2025) developed a telemedicine application called TytoHome. They have been determined that this application significantly reduces the number of examinations performed with the classic stethoscope. The team working on the study concluded that a standardized anamnesis assessment in home healthcare could serve as a valuable qualitative tool to evaluate a patient's health status and identify potential needs prior to the objective examination. This led reducing hospitalization rates. The strength of the application is that it can reach patients who are difficult to reach and that it makes it easier to exchange information with other healthcare professionals. They stated that the weakness was that despite the ease of use, there were patients who had access problems. Another benefit which emphasized by studies in the literature is cost (Chua et al., 2022; Güdük, 2025; Lawrence et al., 2023; Megido et al., 2023). Such applications reduce costs by saving on transportation for healthcare professionals and patients. Thus, patients can manage their own health more comfortably (Güdük, 2025; Snoswell et al., 2020). Another positive effect, apart from cost is patient satisfaction. Studies in the literature show that this technology allows patients who especially need palliative care to receive the service they want at home. This also increases the quality of service and life (Güdük, 2025; Oelschlägel et al., 2023). It has been observed in the literature that telemedicine applications also have positive effects on healthcare professionals. In particular, healthcare professionals may need to quickly get support from their colleagues when providing home healthcare services. The opportunity that these applications provide services such as training, counseling and psychological support to home healthcare service professionals (Adashek & Subbiah, 2020; Güdük, 2025; Klimova, 2019; Scott et al. 2022; Sitges-Maciá et al., 2021).

INTERNET OF THINGS (IoT) AND HOME HEALTHCARE SERVICES

Internet of Things enables objects/devices to communicate with each other and fulfill their assigned tasks by sharing the information available in objects/devices using technologies such as embedded devices, sensors and sensor networks, and advanced internet protocols. Internet of Things usage in home healthcare services offers several advantages. These benefits can be summarized as follows (Şimşir & Mete, 2021):

- Remote patient care

- Patient monitoring
- Diagnosis and treatment management
- Medicine control
- Monitoring of medical staff and equipment
- Reducing of medical care errors (wrong drug/dose/time/procedure)
- Wireless body area network systems consisting of physiological sensors (Electrocardiography, oximetry, thermometer, pulse, blood glucose, etc.) and collecting biological signals from the human body

Home healthcare services are known to be services provided from home by healthcare professionals who are experts in their fields. In order to provide services successfully, it should be in an environment where the patient is accustomed and comfortable. This increases patients' quality of life. However in some cases, healthcare professionals have problems accessing patients health information remotely. Internet of Things can solve exactly this problem. Data is sent directly to information systems through communication networks in Internet of Things applications. As a result, it reduces the necessity for healthcare professionals to make frequent hospital visits (Mansour et al., 2024). It has enabled the establishment of measurement tracking systems that allow for the remote monitoring of chronic diseases with Internet of Things making health systems smart. Thus, patients and healthcare professionals can instantly monitor the situation and thus enable immediate intervention in an emergency. In addition, it can enable individuals with functional losses such as hearing and vision to participate in social life (Koçaş, 2022, p. 24). Due to these benefits use of Internet of Things are quite diverse. These areas of use can be listed as follows (Shirvanian et al., 2025):

- Electrodiagram monitoring
- Blood pressure monitoring
- Glucose level monitoring
- Fever monitoring
- Oxygen saturation monitoring
- Medication Monitoring
- Remote surgery opportunity

In order for home healthcare services to be successfully provided with Internet of Things, the technology must meet certain criterias. These criteria also apply to other technology applications. For the success of the home healthcare services provided using the Internet of Things, the technology must have the following features (Iqbal et al., 2022):

- Performance
- Reliability
- Good interface
- Security
- Privacy
- Hosting principles and rules
- Interoperability with other technologies
- Measurability

Internet of Things which links devices through the Internet to grant access to data centers, has a significant influence on home healthcare services. These devices allow for continuous data collection from elderly people and chronically ill patients who lives at home, while also allowing them to be monitored from locations remotely. Internet of Things enables individuals to communicate more easily with healthcare professionals about their basic health indicators, helping individuals make independent decisions about their own health (Avcı & Gözüm, 2024, p. 70).

Most of the studies in the literature on home healthcare services with the Internet of Things consist of model and prototype tests. In the model which developed by Mansour et al. (2024), it was stated that home healthcare service systems integrated with the Internet of Things will increase patient satisfaction and reducing transportation costs due to service provision from home. Guo et al. (2015) stated that information about individuals' basic health indicators such as blood pressure and oxygen level, ECG status can be stored and analyzed via the Internet of Things and users can control these with smart devices such as phones and wristbands. In another study which conducted on the remote biomedical control system model that can provide benefits in home healthcare services through Internet of Things stated that this model can benefit the development of accessible and adaptable technological solutions tailored to the increasing demands for remote health monitoring, especially in the context of chronic disease management, home healthcare, emergency response (Rabearison et al., 2025). Raja et al. (2025) found that the monitoring system using the Internet of Things has potential to help people with chronic illnesses manage their illnesses and reduce the number of hospital visits, despite concerns about data security, the need for reliable wireless connectivity, and possible limitations in sensor accuracy during physical activity or long-term use. Puja et al. (2023) stated that Internet of Things has the potential to enable remote monitoring for elderly individuals who require constant medication supervision.

In the studies conducted in the literature, most of the studies have positive views on providing healthcare services from home with the Internet of Things. However, there are also studies that express some concerns. For example, Shirvanian et al. (2025) stated that although technologies will increase quality of life and reduce health costs, there are concerns about standardization, data security, performance and validity, big data management, cost and measurability. The concerns here also apply to technologies such as virtual reality, artificial intelligence. Despite many concerns, it is expected that prototypes and models of the Internet of Things will become more widespread in the future thanks to big data and artificial intelligence (Iqbal et al., 2022).

ARTIFICIAL INTELLIGENCE AND HOME HEALTHCARE SERVICES

Artificial intelligence is an application that has emerged with the aim of copying people's thinking ability through computers and providing computers with the ability to learn to a certain extent. From the standpoint of home healthcare services, artificial intelligence provides numerous opportunities in areas like telemedicine applications. Artificial intelligence is widely used in care services and education, from electronic health records to mobile health, remote patient monitoring and patient tracking sensors in home healthcare services. Apart from this, artificial intelligence can be used in decision-support systems which ensures the prevention of errors and effective guidance in service processes (Merih et al., 2021; Önder, 2021; Whende, 2019).

It can be seen that various applications supported by artificial intelligence are used in various dimensions of home healthcare services. Like big data, artificial intelligence does not make sense when used alone in home healthcare services. It makes sense when used with another technology such as wearable technologies. Technologies commonly used with artificial intelligence support in home health services are as follows (Avcı & Gözüm 2024, p. 68-69):

- **Machine Learning:** This technology particularly helps individuals to receive personalized healthcare services. In addition, artificial intelligence-supported monitoring systems have been developed thanks to machine learning. In this way, the patient can send information about patients' health situation to doctors at home, thus making faster treatment decisions (Davenport & Kalakota, 2019). Basic medical images captured at home can undergo advanced analysis using deep learning techniques in specialized fields like radiology. Furthermore, these technologies enable healthcare professionals to enhance communication with their patients using voice commands (Hosny et al., 2018).
- **Natural Language Processing (NLP):** This technology offers effective resolutions speech recognition, text analysis areas. Natural Language Processing

allows health professionals to quickly analyze clinical notes to get information about patient's health situation and treatment plan. This approach could enable them to make more informed decisions in real time based on their patients' needs. In addition, this technology not only reduce healthcare professionals workload, but also provide a more effective home care experience by personalizing services for patients (Woo et al., 2022).

- **Clinical Decision Support Systems:** This systems can provide data and analysis to assist healthcare personnel in their treatment plans. In home healthcare services, a care environment that includes many variables such as chronic diseases in addition to the different needs of patients is required. Clinical decision support systems allow multiple variables to be managed within a single framework. These systems also help home healthcare providers predict potential complications and determine appropriate treatment options with real-time assessment tools. This allows providers to take timely action and develop a proactive care plan. However, these systems need continuous updates and adjustments to integrate effectively due to the personalized nature of home healthcare (Nibbelink & Brewer, 2018).
- **Physical Robots:** This technology is employed to carry out a range of tasks across industries, including healthcare and the growing capabilities of artificial intelligence are enabling the management of more complex processes. When used in conjunction with technologies like mobile health, this technology can enable health professionals to monitor their patients remotely. Especially these robots can improve elderly persons' quality of life and enable healthcare personnel to manage home healthcare service procedure more effectively (Yang et al., 2020).
- **Care Planning:** Artificial intelligence enables treatment planning by analyzing with past medical records of patients. Artificial intelligence has the potential to support the creation of healthcare plans that are centered around the patient. Patients can live more comfortably thanks to integrated home automation systems which can personalize plans (Hosny et al., 2018). Artificial intelligence can reduce healthcare professionals' workload and increase patients quality of life of patients by organizing care plans (Xu et al., 2021).

There are also studies that reporting concerns about artificial intelligence. Pruszyński et al. (2022) stated that although patients can manage the exercise and treatment processes required for rehabilitation and transfer the results to professionals thanks to robotic technologies developed with artificial intelligence, the elderly are not ready to directly transfer the entire process in healthcare to technology. In another study, patients have concerns that using AI-supported robotic technologies will make them more dependent (EPTA, 2019, p. 13).

WEARABLE TECHNOLOGIES AND HOME HEALTHCARE SERVICES

Wearable technology is the general name for technological devices that people wear. However, there is a clear distinction here. These devices can receive data from a person through sensors and provide personalized feedback. Wearable technologies can be defined as jewelry, clothes and products that can carry on or that are invasively placed on which will protect health, give pre-disease alarms, monitor the treatment process. Internet of Things has played important role especially in wearable technologies' development process. Biometric sensors, wearable sensors have emerged thanks to Internet of Things (Merih et al., 2021; Stavropoulos et al., 2020). These devices can be used especially in home healthcare of people with cardiovascular diseases in pre and post-operative patient follow-up. In addition, mood and sleep disorders can also be measured in relation to general elderly care (Chwistek, 2020; Merih et al., 2021; Stavropoulos et al., 2020).

Wearable health technologies especially when modified with technologies like artificial intelligence become very useful for health systems. Wearable technologies have become capable of analyzing the data they have obtained with these modifications. This has greatly expanded the areas of use in healthcare. All areas of use of wearable technologies are also valid for different technologies which used in home healthcare services. These areas of use can be listed as follows (Vo & Trinh, 2024):

- **Monitoring Vital Health Indicators:** Applications of wearable technologies can monitor patients' vitals such as glucose, heart rate, blood pressure.
- **Non-Invasive Detection:** Traditional blood draw vital status analysis is increasingly being replaced by painless, non-invasive methods of measuring vital signs using body fluids such as saliva, sweat on the skin thanks to advances in technology.
- **Providing Health Recommendations:** Wearable technologies can collect and analyze health-related data of individuals and make predictions about their health status. With these predictions, it can offer suggestions about future health status.
- **Remote Patient Monitoring:** It has become easier to monitor patients remotely with telemedicine. Wearable technologies are used in telemedicine applications, especially as a means of monitoring patients remotely. Patient data which received through wearable technologies helps healthcare professionals make treatment plans before providing services at home.

Wearable technologies have various benefits in home healthcare services and are directly related to their areas of use. These benefits can be summarized as follows (Merih et al., 2021):

- Smart watches, bracelets and necklaces are used for cases of missing and falling.
- Smart bracelets, bands and watches that can measure ECG, calculate heart rate and show blood oxygen saturation are used for monitoring Cardiovascular Diseases.
- Suitable fork and spoon designs are used especially for Parkinson's patients who cannot perform independent eating and drinking activities due to tremors.
- There are bone conduction headphones with sensors for individuals with hearing impairments.
- There are air cushion vests for individuals with back and pressure sores.
- Smart bracelets can help obese patients manage their nutritional activities.
- There are devices that can analyze the respiratory status of patients with respiratory system disorders.
- There are wearable support systems for patients with balance problems.
- There are technologies such as smart socks that can measure glucose levels in diabetic patients and transmit these to mobile devices such as phones, and can diagnose diabetes in advance.

Despite the benefits of wearable technologies, there are studies that contain various concerns and negative thoughts about such technologies. Tanak et al. (2024) stated that wearable technologies help to increase the health levels and quality of life of older adults who want to receive service at home, but individuals do not know very well what to do about technical problems that may occur in such technologies. Goldrick & Gethin (2021) reported that despite technological advances and benefits, some individuals may not easily adopt such technologies. Despite all these negative views, it is predicted that wearable technologies will become more prevalent in whole healthcare system in the future. Besides individuals quality of life will increase and healthcare costs will decrease with these technologies (Vo & Trinh, 2024).

BLOCKCHAIN AND HOME HEALTHCARE SERVICES

Blockchain represents a shared, immutable data structure containing cryptographically linked blocks of information. Each block is connected to the one before it, ensuring that the data is stored in a highly secure system where unauthorized actions cannot alter it (Avcı & Gözüm, 2024, p. 65; Mustafa et al., 2022).

Blockchain makes treatment processes easier and more adaptable for monitoring in healthcare. Besides all steps in a patient's treatment plan can be tracked and recorded. This will help healthcare professionals manage treatment plans and track the patient's response to this plan. Automated contracts which stored on blockchains enable to improve home healthcare services. This improvement can enable more effective healthcare service provisions including a range of useful services like appointment reminders (Avcı & Gözüm, 2024, p. 72; Wylde et al., 2022). The application of blockchain technology in healthcare can be outlined as follows (Gökalp et al., 2018):

- **Storage and Access of Personal Health Records:** Blockchain technology enables flawless communication and data exchange between institutions and application vendors in the healthcare industry.
- **Genomic Datas of Patients:** This technology can assist in combining DNA data from various owners and sources without the need to store it in a centralized database while also enabling the backup of an individual's DNA and distributing their genetic information across multiple computers globally.
- **Supply Chain Management for Hospital Resources:** This technology can also be applied in supply chain systems to oversee hospital inventories and optimize the buying and selling processes.
- **Smart Contract Automation Technology:** This technology has the capability to minimize insurance fraud, from fund management to individual claims. It also does all of this at a lower cost. Fundamentally, it functions as a digital legal intermediary to create and store contracts, facilitating real-time data exchange through blockchain architecture.
- **Private Blockchain Systems:** Private blockchain networks require authorization to access information. This defines which entities are allowed to conduct transactions on the blockchain and add new blocks. Patients grant health professionals to access their records. There are some various levels of access. Access levels can be established to regulate who can view records, who can modify them, and who holds final authority within the system. Security combinations and flexibility are adequate in healthcare.
- **Health Data Research Commons:** Genome files and core quantitative data stored in an encrypted and pseudonymous blockchain format, enable analysis while ensuring confidentiality when integrating patient medical records. Datas which have diversity, value, accuracy are valuable for researchers who study in health to drive innovations to improve health system.
- **Notarization Services:** One possible application of blockchain technology is its role as a notary, securely encoding critical documents such as ID cards and

passports. Certain documents require verification, including medical results, treatment plans and proof of insurance in healthcare. These documents are verified within seconds through encryption as opposed to the hours or days required with traditional methods in the proposed system.

- **Service Management:** Blockchain-based approach can provide improvements for healthcare services provided by healthcare professionals. These improvements include automatic listing of services provided and management of payment processes. Improvements like these make it easier to manage healthcare services.

Considering blockchain technology usage in home healthcare services, it is not at the same level as technologies such as artificial intelligence, wearable technologies. However, investments in blockchain technology are increasing. The primary motivation for the investments is the potential that blockchain technology offers. These potentials can be listed as follows (Gökalp et al., 2018):

- **Transparency:** Blockchain technology can allow to create objective data sources where people can access informations such as evaluations about providers. Ensuring transparency allows patients to share their data with healthcare professionals without any concerns in a patient-centered service approach. Thus, individuals can obtain the services they want from any institution, personnel or even remotely. The ability to share data transparently strengthens healthcare professionals' decision-making in the face of cases.
- **Accountability:** Reimbursement is a complex issue in the healthcare industry that increases the likelihood of many unethical incidents. Because insurance companies do not want to face fraudulent bills from unnecessary medical procedures performed by organizations and physicians. Blockchain makes documentation and sharing much easier. As health information becomes increasingly transparent and verifiable, all parties involved in healthcare must be held to a higher standard of accountability.
- **Record Accuracy:** Patients might experience inconsistencies in their records. Hence data consistencies among healthcare professionals is challenging in traditional healthcare information management technology applications. Patient health records can be stored in separate systems, with each participant in the chain linked to one another, allowing data to be updated simultaneously across all computers through blockchain technology. Enhanced communication and more accurate record-keeping can greatly minimize frequent problems, such as medication errors. Patients are more likely to trust their healthcare providers when accurate and current information is available to all participants in the healthcare blockchain.

- **Protected Transactions:** This technology encourages the use of sophisticated decryption techniques with both public and private key pairs to ensure security and protect against intermediary attacks. It improves data security while reducing the cost, time and resources required to establish a secure framework for sharing medical records and processing payments.
- **Interoperability:** This technology enables the standardization of data from multiple sources including wearable devices into a unified format. As a result, blockchain facilitates the interoperability of health information by granting both patients and providers access to data from diverse systems including organ donation and blood bank records. This feature also accelerates the retrieval of data from various sources enhancing both the volume and quality of information available for healthcare research. Emerging technologies such as big data analytics and deep learning can be utilized on blockchain data to analyze various datasets including genetic markers and demographic patterns for continuous research and development.
- **Low Cost:** Blockchain provides patients with accurate information thus increasing their ability to make decisions regarding the financial aspects of their treatment services. This technology enables patients to track their expenses and gain a clearer understanding of their spending on services. Additionally, the use of Blockchain lowers the costs related to operating and maintaining transaction systems for providers.
- **Partnership:** Blockchain enables collaboration between manufacturers, suppliers, customers for collecting historical actions across the chain so that patients and healthcare service providers can transparently access information about items such as drugs, surgical supplies. In short, blockchain technology plays significant role in the fight against fraud and unethical practices in the healthcare field.
- **Agility:** The time limit for collecting health records from patients has been eliminated with the availability of wearable devices and mobile health devices. This allows personalized diagnoses and treatments to be produced.

Given the advantages of blockchain technology which outlined above, it serves as a complementary tool that can address the shortcomings or gaps of other technologies, particularly when integrated with them. However despite this knowledge, healthcare systems that have achieved successful results or experienced similar positive developments with blockchain technology are rare. This is because the conditions that need to be met for the implementation of such technologies are many. If these qualifications are not met, blockchain technology cannot be applied in healthcare. Compelling factors that could cause such an effect include (Gökalp et al., 2018):

- **Governance:** Blockchain technology requires public and private collaboration, especially in areas where society is sensitive such as healthcare. In short, it requires public and private interoperability. This creates a need for globally coordinated standards and agreements across international borders and jurisdictions.
- **Lack of Regulations:** Global regulations concerning property rights in medical procedures are crucial for the successful implementation of a blockchain-based healthcare system. Developing suitable regulations is challenging because of the numerous stakeholders involved. Furthermore, it is crucial to clearly define the ownership of blockchain records, the access permissions granted and the decentralized storage framework.
- **Sustainability:** The encryption key plays a vital role in the operation of the blockchain. The private encryption key cannot be recovered once lost. This introduces complexity in healthcare data, as it involves long-term opportunities and challenges in analysis. Missing information in a patient's health record significantly reduces its reliability and worth. Additionally, if a user's private encryption key is compromised or taken, it provides access to all the stored information.
- **Scalability:** As users add data the structure of the blockchain grows more. This causes storage and computational demands to increase. If this need is not fulfilled, there is a greater risk of increased centralization and slower data verification and validation. This makes it difficult to optimize processes.
- **Adoption:** Blockchain technology depends on a network of connected computers to supply the computational power necessary for creating transaction blocks. Consequently, the effectiveness of blockchain technology grows with the number of participants. Participants should be motivated through reward systems to adopt technologies. Furthermore, healthcare organizations may need to be incentivized to adopt blockchain technology and participate in the shared network.
- **Cost:** Developing, maintaining and operating the proposed blockchain-based integrated healthcare system entails specific costs to guarantee the ongoing availability of resources for functions like troubleshooting, updates, backups, and reporting.

There is a great feature that blockchain technology can provide. In fact, this feature is related to data security, which is usually mentioned in home healthcare service technologies. One of the most fundamental concerns in almost all technological applications is security and privacy. Health data is a very sensitive issue due to the fact that it contains private information. Blockchain technology offers a robust security framework designed to block unauthorized access. It plays a pivotal role in maintaining security and access control particularly in home healthcare where multiple caregivers or healthcare professionals are involved in an individual's care. The transparency and integration provided by blockchain improve the security and quality of patient data storage. This technology enhances the quality of home healthcare services by ensuring that all records are consistently stored in an unchangeable and permanent manner (Avcı & Gözüm, 2024, p. 65; Kumar & Mallick, 2018; Wang, et al., 2020).

Studies on the use of blockchain technology in home healthcare are less common in the literature than other types of technologies. However, there are studies that provide important information. Aujla & Jindal (2020) stated that blockchain technology protects the data in the health monitoring sensor with a certain security chain while it is being transmitted. Besides blockchain technology can manage the data more effectively as a result of the design of a tensor-based evaluation chain for the secure use of the same data more than once and technology has the potential to solve security problems. Ali & Dhanaraj (2024) stated that although the benefits obtained by using the technology are similar to the literature, however there are some security concerns. But technology has potential to solve security problems. Besides this technology can also ensure availability and integrity of the data.

DRONE AND HOME HEALTHCARE SERVICES

Unmanned aerial vehicles or drones are technological innovations used by a remote-controlled pilot to fly in airspace in accordance with the guidelines set by the country's Civil Aviation Ministry or Transportation Ministries. Drones are known for providing basic medical and food needs especially for those who cannot meet their basic needs due to situations such as war and disaster. Due to the aerial imaging capability and high transmission speed of drones, there are demands for vaccines, medicines, blood and food package deliveries and the collection of samples for testing (Haidari et al., 2016; Sharma et al., 2021; Thiels et al., 2015; Van de Voorde et al., 2017). Drones are a technology frequently used in healthcare, especially in first aid. In particular, life-saving medicines that cannot be replaced play an important role in delivering medical aid to areas where the area is inaccessible. Sharma et al. (2021) estimated that the delivery of medicines, samples via drones is efficient and takes a quarter of the time spent by road travelers. According to this statement, drones can be seen as an important part of healthcare logistics and supply chain. However, drones carry the risk of falling due to a possible malfunction. This risk results in material loss. There is also the risk of a falling drone falling into residential areas and onto cars.

Drones on their own are not an effective technology. To expand their use in healthcare and maximize their potential, drones should be combined with technologies such as artificial intelligence, Internet of Things, and big data. Drones integrated with such technologies are very useful for the healthcare sector. The areas of use of an integrated drone device in the healthcare field and its advantages can be summarized as follows (Lakhwani et al., 2025):

- **Emergency Response:** Such technologies are especially suitable for emergency response in cases such as any natural disaster or epidemic. Drones facilitate the swift delivery of critical supplies including food, water, medical equipment, first aid to areas which affected by disasters (Erdelj et al., 2017).
- **Vaccine Distribution:** Drones were used in some places as a distribution channel for urgent vaccine needs that arose during the pandemic period (Fathollahi-Fard et al., 2022).

In order to gain certain advantages by using such technologies, certain requirements are needed. Since it is not easy to meet those requirements, healthcare systems may turn to other technologies. These requirements which cause other technologies to be used more frequently in drones, can be seen as an obstacle to the success of these technologies by some. These factors can be listed as follows (Lakhwani et al., 2025):

- **Technical Difficulties:** Especially in rural areas, the connection quality is lower than in other places. Therefore, quality data is not received. Poor quality data also prevents consistent decisions. In addition, since the materials to be transported are products that must be preserved in storage conditions, such as vaccines, it is costly to establish temperature-balancing mechanisms and storage areas. Apart from this, drones are devices with limited carrying capacity, range and battery life. Although advancements like durable batteries, solar-powered charging stations, and modular drones with interchangeable batteries have been made they remain expensive.
- **Regulatory Challenges:** Drone use in healthcare requires compliance with aviation and healthcare standards. The regulatory environment is quite challenging, especially in areas with high population density, due to the risk of accidents. However, there is a solution to this issue. It is possible to prevent this problem thanks to the route planning frequently used in aviation.
- **Infrastructure Requirements:** For high-tech drones to be used especially in rural areas a serious infrastructure investment is needed. Reliable operations depend on consistent power sources, robust internet connectivity and

designated drone hubs for takeoff and landing (Sivakumar et al., 2023). Unfortunately, limited infrastructure in rural areas limits the effective operation of drones. Innovative solutions like mobile charging stations and temporary logistics hubs can address infrastructure gaps in remote or disaster-prone regions.

- **Data Protection and Privacy:** Real-time monitoring and transmission of healthcare data via Internet of Things (IoT) systems pose significant security risks. Leaks of sensitive information such as patient details and the condition of medical supplies can undermine trust and disrupt operational effectiveness (Dash et al., 2019). Compliance with health privacy regulations, such as strict data encryption protocols and secure cloud storage is critical. Taking a proactive approach to cybersecurity guarantees that the IoT-Drone framework meets regulatory requirements and helps build trust among stakeholders.
- **Extreme Weather Conditions:** Severe weather conditions can interfere with drone operations and cause delays in essential deliveries. These risks are especially significant in regions that are prone to frequent severe weather conditions. Real-time tracking systems combined with IoT sensors and AI-powered predictive analytics allow drones to adjust their paths in response to dangerous conditions. Non-urgent deliveries can be postponed strategically while priority is given to critical operations.
- **Infrastructure Dependency:** The reliance on infrastructure restricts the use of the IoT-Drone framework in less developed areas (Graboyes et al., 2020). To ensure seamless operations reliable communication between drones, logistic commons and healthcare institutions is crucial.

Despite the challenges which mentioned above healthcare systems still prefer to use drones and produce prototypes. The main reason for this is that it can reach individuals who have difficulty accessing services. When it comes to the use of drones in home healthcare services, this technology is used less frequently than the other technologies. Munawar et al. (2023) stated that AI-driven drones can transport self-testing kits, collect samples, and provide online support from healthcare personnel. It also reduce the carbon footprint. Besides they think that the suggested approach is a flexible enhancement to the existing rules and regulations aimed at controlling the spread of an epidemic, and a step forward in advancing smart healthcare systems. Kim et al. (2017) mentioned that the drone-based home healthcare service model will lower out-of-pocket healthcare costs, ease the workload of healthcare providers, and offer access to services for people in remote areas. Some studies state that drones can easily reach hard-to-reach areas and reduce human contact (Euchi, 2021; Hapsari et al., 2024). Based on the information that mentioned here, it can be said that drone usage in home healthcare services is more useful especially for the elderly in rural areas who have serious difficulties in accessing the service. It cannot be said to be a widely used technology because it is difficult to implement compared to other technologies.

ROBOTIC TECHNOLOGIES AND HOME HEALTHCARE SERVICES

Another type of technology which emerged with digitalization in healthcare is robotic technologies. Robotic technologies are a fundamental resource and widely used especially for organizations operating in sectors that require mass production such as industry and retail. Nowadays, robotic technologies have entered the healthcare sector with the digitalization. Robotic technologies in healthcare are systems that can perform coordinated mechatronic actions based on the processing of information obtained through sensor technology to support individuals with medical interventions, patient care, rehabilitation, treatment and preventive services. Robotic technologies have changed the functioning of both the medical and general healthcare systems. Potential features such as improving treatment alternatives for diseases, facilitating access to services and making it easier for healthcare professionals to do their jobs can be given as examples of the changes which mentioned here. Robotic technologies in healthcare are divided into three main categories. These can be listed as follows (Fosch-Villaronga, & Drukarch, 2021):

- **Surgical Robots:** These are technologies that emerge to support surgeons during surgical procedures.
- **Assistive Robots:** These devices are divided into two groups according to their scope of usage. These are socially assistive robots which help users through social interaction and physically assistive robots which support users through physical interaction.
- **Healthcare Service Robots:** Technologies that support the successful fulfillment of responsibilities of facilities and personnel in healthcare institutions.

Assistive robots technologies are seen to be more suitable for home health services, among the types of robotic technologies. The reason for this is that assistive robot technology can provide support through social and physical interaction, which is critical for home healthcare services. Studies in the literature provide various information on the use of robotic technologies in home healthcare services.

Su et al. (2024) examined the expectations of stakeholders regarding the use of assistive robotics in home healthcare services. As a result of their examination, it is stated that the elderly who are one of the groups that demand home healthcare services the most have certain expectations from assistive robotics. The most important of these expectations are the ability to detect falls and to provide this information to the healthcare professionals. Apart from these, it also requires functions that support daily life such as medication tracking and appointment reminders. In particular, the medication reminder dimension is the top priority expectation of healthcare professionals who provide services. The authors also state that it would be more effective to use this technology together with other technological applications such as telehealth for individuals living in rural areas to benefit from home healthcare services. However, the study also highlighted some aspects that healthcare professionals are concerned about. The main concerns are data security and inadequate infrastructure in rural areas. In addition, some elderly people may have low levels of skills and adoption of technological applications. This situation has also been reported to reduce the chance of success of technology.

Kosinski et al. (2025) stated that robotic assistants are pleased with the fact that they remind elderly people who want to receive home healthcare services about their medication doses at the right time. The authors also stated that robotics could provide a financially sound solution for the future of healthcare by encouraging independent living for the elderly and helping with chronic disease management. Besides these technologies have some administrative benefits. The benefits stated in the study include; providing cost savings in various dimensions, preventing unnecessary use of healthcare professionals and emergency services thanks to the services provided by the technology.

Lin et al. (2025) stated that robotic technologies are important for elderly people who living alone. Because this technology provides not just home healthcare services, but also provides companionship. Elderly people stated that the feeling of companionship is a priority and that they do not have much concern about the functions which robotic technology carries. It has been also revealed that another criterion which the elderly care about is the affordability of the technology, while the cost savings it provides are not a priority. The opinions of elderly individuals from their acquaintances indicate that the adoption of robotic technologies in home healthcare services is more important than the external social perception. Besides they have different expectations regarding home healthcare services. These expectations also apply to robotic technologies which used in providing services. The study found that adapting to the different needs of older individuals is more important than other features.

Badr & Dankar (2022) stated that assistive robotics when used in home healthcare services has many benefits such as making services more accessible, providing cost-effectiveness, increasing satisfaction with services and reducing the burden of providing services on healthcare professionals. However, the same study also highlighted some potential risks that this technology carries. These risks include;

the risk of harm to patients due to reasons such as lack of maintenance, psychological risks arising from the decrease in human interaction due to the use of robotic technology, ethical risks as in other technologies and the cost of maintenance and procurement of such technologies.

FACTORS NEGATIVELY AFFECTING TECHNOLOGICAL EFFICIENCY

In order to successfully manage home healthcare services with technological applications and benefit from the positive effects, it is necessary to mention the possible difficulties and obstacles that the health system may face. Because if there is no environment to use technology effectively, we cannot benefit from the positive effects of technology on home healthcare services. The possible obstacles that may affect the success of home healthcare services management in the technological era can be listed as follows (Galavi et al., 2022):

- **Technical Problems:** The first criterion for technological applications usage in healthcare is the adequacy of the technical infrastructure. If the technical infrastructure is not sufficient, the technical problems that will arise here will affect the delivery of health services. The technical problems that will be listed below are not impossible to solve. User opinions can be obtained to ensure that applications are user-friendly. Technical problems can be listed as follows:
    - Low usability
    - Non-functional equipment
    - Difficulties in accessing data on time and easily
    - Lack of integration
    - Internet access problems
- **Adoption of Technological Applications:** One of the obstacles that comes to the fore after technical problems is that individuals do not adopt such technologies. The reasons for non-adoption can be listed as follows:
    - Technological applications which use in home healthcare services may not appropriate treatment methods
    - Uncertainty of the advantages of technologies such as telemedicine
    - Lack of relative advantage
    - Reluctance of health professionals to adopt technologic applications
- **Knowledge and Skills:** There may be deficiencies in the knowledge and skills of both patients and health professionals regarding the use of technologic applications. User training can be provided for end-user awareness.

- **Legal Regulations:** Concerns about the disclosure of personal data is the most prominent obstacle to legal regulation. Beyond concerns related to personal data, the absence of a legal framework such as ambiguous laws and policies regarding technology usage in healthcare and privacy issues also hinders the effective implementation of technology in the healthcare sector. In order to solve such problems, it is recommended to create a set of legal plans and a well-functioning audit mechanism, and to develop practices that give confidence to patients and healthcare personnel that the security of their data is protected.
- **Motivation for Change:** Individuals have concerns about technology usage in home healthcare services due to their fear of having a worse experience than the current process they have experienced while using health services as technology becomes more active. The following activities can be carried out to address the concerns which stated here:
    - Determining the value of services according to the patient profile
    - Governments should work to raise public awareness
    - Sharing the experiences of family members who were pleased with the services they had received in the past

Tian et al. (2024) identified the factors which prevent the successful technology usage in home healthcare services in their systematic literature review study, apart from the factors which mentioned above. At the same time, these factors which may negatively affect service delivery if not eliminated are classified as follows:

- **Usability:** Individuals who requesting home healthcare care services state that the technologies used are complex and some have fear of technology. Apart from these, technical problems such as lack of integration of technologies, internet connection and infrastructure are other obstacles to the efficient use of technologies in home healthcare services.
- **Social Adoption:** Studies have shown that if technologies are prepared to truly meet the needs of home healthcare services, the adoption process will be easier and if they are not compatible with the needs, the adoption process will be difficult. The main reason is that individuals find such technologies valuable and potential for home healthcare services. In addition to the masses that are positive about technology, there is also a mass that is hesitant. The reasons for their hesitations are that this technology is difficult for some users and it is not easy to learn, that there is a negative attitude towards technology because it gives warnings too often, and that family members have negative attitudes towards the use of technology.

- **Cost:** The use of technologies not only reduces healthcare professionals' workload but also reduces costs such as transportation to healthcare institutions for individuals that receiving healthcare services from home. However, technology is costly especially maintenance, consultancy services, and integration. Access levels vary due to this cost. This is exactly where individuals living in rural areas experience problems. For this reason, technology must be made accessible to everyone.
- **Increased Loneliness:** There are various opinions on this subject. Service providers believe that the technologies used will befriend the elderly rather than increasing their loneliness in social life. However, those receiving the service do not think this way. They feel that technological devices will cause losses in their social connectedness.
- **Increased Workload:** Some healthcare professionals believe that technology increases rather than reduces workload. The reason they say this is that healthcare professionals spend time training individuals on the technology used, overcoming the language barrier between the device and the patient, processing and responding to the warnings given by the devices.

One of the most important dimensions of providing home healthcare services through technologies is patients. Patients' attitudes towards technologies are critical in reflecting the success of healthcare systems in providing services effectively with digitalization. Bertolazzi et al. (2024) summarized the difficulties faced by elderly people who widely use home healthcare services in adopting technologies which used in healthcare realizing the importance here. They summarized the topics that can make it difficult to provide home healthcare services using technology as follows:

- **Demographic and Socioeconomic Factors:** Especially the elderly's attitudes towards these technologies progress negatively as they age. Elderly people with a good level of education accept and use such technologies more comfortably. Individuals with a low socioeconomic profile and those who do not have access to the internet also have more negative perspectives on technology than others.
- **Health Related Factors:** Some elderly people may have physical limitations. Individuals who cannot fully perform basic life functions such as these cannot be provided with effective services provided by technologies compared to others. Individuals who are especially at the early stages of their illnesses are more positive about providing health services through technologies. Individuals who struggle with diseases such as cancer, which affect both the physical and mental health of individuals, may have a negative attitude towards technologies.

- **Dispositional Factors:** Some elderly people may have a traditional mindset or a character structure that does not want to get out of their daily routine. People with this type of profile will also have negative attitudes towards technologies. In addition, low motivation and desire to learn new techniques and technologies in managing their own health conditions is a critical factor. For some individuals, change is a concept that increases feelings of anxiety and fear. This also applies to health technologies. The anxiety and fear mentioned here are also negative factors.
- **Social Factors:** If a technology facilitates communication between healthcare professionals and patients, patients' willingness to use the technology increases. Older adults' attitude towards using and adopting technology shifted towards being more positive, especially when there was someone around who encouraged the use of technology. The increasing presence of technology in today's life is changing the way individuals communicate. The change which mentioned here has caused the communication between elderly and healthcare professionals to evolve from face-to-face to online communication. Some elderly people have concerns that technology will end the concept of receiving face-to-face services. Due to this concern, their attitudes towards technology are negative.

CONCLUSION

The global increase in the aging population and the changing disease profiles are directing healthcare systems towards home healthcare services. In addition, the economic developments and resource constraints experienced by countries have directed the healthcare field towards technological solutions. With the combination of these, home healthcare services like other areas of healthcare have been affected by technology.

The technologies which used in home healthcare services and their effects are diverse. Despite the different technologies that used in the delivery of services, it has been understood that they have similar effects on home healthcare services and management. One of the main impact of technological applications on home healthcare services is reducing costs. Reducing costs has an impact on many areas of healthcare management such as facility management and disease management. Limited resources in the health sector will be used efficiently and excessive demand for hospitals will be balanced owing to this positive impact. The use of home healthcare services with technology allows the diagnosis, treatment and rehabilitation period of diseases to be shortened and managed more easily. This reduces care costs. The reduction in costs also creates resources for the necessary expenses for technology updates, investments and infrastructure improvements.

Home healthcare services which integrated with technology increase access to health services especially for elderly people that lives in rural area. The treatment and rehabilitation activities of people who living in rural areas and has chronic diseases can be monitored remotely through advanced and modified technologies. This increases the quality of life of patients and saves healthcare professionals both cost and time. In terms of health systems, technology makes it easier to manage the health status of the society who especially live in rural areas and efficient use of limited resources.

Advanced technologies have made it easier to provide healthcare services to individuals based on their health problems rather than providing standard healthcare services to everyone. This also applies to home healthcare services. Providing personalized home health services with technology enables; increased patient satisfaction, evidence-based clinical decisions, successful implementation of patient-centered service approach and the implementation of disease management processes for early diagnosis and prevention of diseases. The outcomes which listed here are the factors that improve the community health status and system. However, some of the studies in the literature report that some technological home healthcare services are not patient-centered. Technological home healthcare services are not successful due to reasons such as digital inequality caused by the differences between rural and urban life, cost-focused approaches of healthcare systems, healthcare professionals do not want to adopt technological applications and technologies not reflecting patient needs. In order to fully understand the factors that cause home healthcare services not to be patient-centered, studies are needed to adoption of technology use in these services and to explain the expectations of patients.

Services are being developed to increase the living standards of individuals receiving home health services with the diversification of technological alternatives. This not only reduces the length of time patients are waiting in hospital and the rate of readmission, but also improves their quality of life. Reducing waiting times and readmission rates provide advantages to healthcare systems such as more effective management of hospital resources, reducing workload on healthcare personnel and ensuring the financial sustainability of healthcare institutions. Increasing the quality of life of patients enables them to manage their own health and thus be more active in using services. This facilitates acceptance of a patient-focused health approach and preventive health services thereby improving health status.

When home healthcare services were implemented using traditional methods, healthcare professionals had difficulties communicating with their colleagues in case of a specific emergency or need for consultation. Healthcare professionals can now communicate with their colleagues more quickly in home healthcare services with technologic developments. Ensuring this communication improves communication between patients and healthcare professionals. It also supports employees who are exhausted or have low morale psychologically. Other improvements are; improving communication with patients, ensuring that services are more comprehensive and of higher quality. These help reduce the workload on healthcare systems and create a productive work environment.

Positive thoughts about home healthcare services that have developed with technology are predominant. However, there are some points to be concerned about in technology-integrated home healthcare services. One of the main concern is security. If a security system that protects and processes the private information of patients and healthcare professionals is not available or inadequate when providing technology-integrated home healthcare services, it will be difficult for individuals to adopt and trust technologies. Security gaps cause patients information to be misused and healthcare professionals to use incorrect data to perform incorrect treatment practices. Problems in security also raise performance and validity which is also a concern in all technological applications. If a technology is not integrated into health systems and its interface is not understandable, critical situations cannot be detected in time while providing services and serious errors occur with incorrect data. The validity of technologies that are not secure and perform well becomes debatable. Because the final result of security and performance-related situations is invalid technologies. Invalid technologies make adoption difficult which is another concern. The process of adopting technologies is long and carries the possibility of being damaged immediately by the slightest problem that may arise during this process. Because trust and adoption of technologies do not occur quickly however trust and adoption of technologies that are achieved under difficult conditions have the possibility of being eliminated at the slightest hitch.

It is estimated that technology-centered home healthcare services will diversify in the future depending on the variety of technologies to be used. Besides many studies will be conducted by implementing technological prototypes and models that contribute to home healthcare services. It is anticipated that technologies like Blockchain could help address concerns related to home healthcare services in the future. In order to successfully provide home healthcare services in the technological era and benefit from their positive effects, it is necessary to examine the expectations of patients and healthcare professionals regarding the technologies which they use at regular intervals, conduct research on the adoption of technologies, and analyze patients requests and needs regarding home healthcare services.

REFERENCES

Adashek, J. J., & Subbiah, I. M. (2020). Caring for the caregiver: A systematic review characterising the experience of caregivers of older adults with advanced cancers. *ESMO Open*, *5*(5), e000862. DOI: 10.1136/esmoopen-2020-000862 PMID: 32963088

Ali, M. A., & Dhanaraj, R. K. (2024). IoMT and blockchain oriented smart healthcare monitoring system. In *AIP Conference Proceedings* (Vol. 2919, Article 020008). AIP Publishing. DOI: 10.1063/5.0184364

Álvarez-Castañón, L. D. C., Arroyo, P., Contreras-Cruz, M. A., & Villaseñor-Mora, C. (2022). Health 4.0 and its potential adoption and contribution to the Mexican health system. In *2022 Portland International Conference on Management of Engineering and Technology (PICMET)* (pp. 1–10). IEEE. DOI: 10.23919/PICMET53225.2022.9882603

Aujla, G. S., & Jindal, A. (2021). A decoupled blockchain approach for edge-envisioned IoT-based healthcare monitoring. *IEEE Journal on Selected Areas in Communications*, *39*(2), 491–499. DOI: 10.1109/JSAC.2020.3020655

Avcı, Y. D., & Gözüm, S. (2024). The impact of Industry 5.0: The artificial intelligence, IoT and blockchain revolution in home healthcare. In Zafar, S., Kumar, S. N., Ahilan, A., & Cakir, G. K. (Eds.), *Industry 5.0 for smart healthcare technologies* (pp. 62–76). CRC Press., DOI: 10.1201/9781032632223-6

Badr, N. G., & Dankar, M. (2022). Assistive healthcare robotics—Challenges in nursing service innovation: Critical review. In *ITM Web of Conferences* (Vol. 41, Article 02002). EDP Sciences. DOI: 10.1051/itmconf/20224102002

Basulo-Ribeiro, J., & Teixeira, L. (2024). The future of healthcare with Industry 5.0: Preliminary interview-based qualitative analysis. *Future Internet*, *16*(3), 68. DOI: 10.3390/fi16030068

Bertolazzi, A., Quaglia, V., & Bongelli, R. (2024). Barriers and facilitators to health technology adoption by older adults with chronic diseases: An integrative systematic review. *BMC Public Health*, *24*(1), 506. DOI: 10.1186/s12889-024-18036-5 PMID: 38365698

Bijalwan, V., Semwal, V. B., & Mandal, T. K. (2021). Fusion of multi-sensor-based biomechanical gait analysis using vision and wearable sensor. *IEEE Sensors Journal*, *21*(13), 14213–14220. DOI: 10.1109/JSEN.2021.3066473

Brocard, E., Antoine, P., Mélihan-Cheinin, P., & Rusch, E. (2021). COVID-19's impact on home health services, caregivers and patients: Lessons from the French experience. *The Lancet Regional Health. Europe*, *8*, 100197. DOI: 10.1016/j.lanepe.2021.100197 PMID: 34423328

Chen, P.-J., Smits, L., Miranda, R., Liao, J.-Y., Petersen, I., Van den Block, L., & Sampson, E. L. (2022). Impact of home healthcare on end-of-life outcomes for people with dementia: A systematic review. *BMC Geriatrics*, *22*(1), 80. DOI: 10.1186/s12877-022-02768-3 PMID: 35081914

Cheng, W., Cao, X., Lian, W., & Tian, J. (2024). An introduction to smart home ward–based hospital-at-home care in China. *JMIR mHealth and uHealth*, *12*, e44422. DOI: 10.2196/44422 PMID: 38298026

Chua, C. M. S., Ko, S. Q., Lai, Y. F., Lim, Y. W., & Shorey, S. (2022). Perceptions of hospital-at-home among stakeholders: A metasynthesis. *Journal of General Internal Medicine*, *37*(3), 637–650. DOI: 10.1007/s11606-021-07065-0 PMID: 34363185

Chwistek, M. (2020). "Are you wearing your white coat?": Telemedicine in the time of pandemic. *Journal of the American Medical Association*, *324*(2), 149–150. DOI: 10.1001/jama.2020.10619 PMID: 32584375

Dash, S., Shakyawar, S. K., Sharma, M., & Kaushik, S. (2019). Big data in healthcare: Management, analysis and future prospects. *Journal of Big Data*, *6*(1), 54. DOI: 10.1186/s40537-019-0217-0

Davenport, T., & Kalakota, R. (2019). The potential for artificial intelligence in healthcare. *Future Healthcare Journal*, *6*(2), 94–98. DOI: 10.7861/futurehosp.6-2-94 PMID: 31363513

Dilbaz, B., Kaplanoğlu, M., & Kaya, D. (2020). Teletıp ve telesağlık: Geçmiş, bugün ve gelecek. *Eurasian Journal of Health Technology Assessment*, *4*(1), 40–56. DOI: 10.5281/zenodo.4321472

Erdelj, M., Król, M., & Natalizio, E. (2017). Wireless sensor networks and multi-UAV systems for natural disaster management. *Computer Networks*, *124*, 72–86. DOI: 10.1016/j.comnet.2017.05.021

Euchi, J. (2021). Do drones have a realistic place in a pandemic fight for delivering medical supplies in healthcare systems problems? *Chinese Journal of Aeronautics*, *34*(2), 182–190. DOI: 10.1016/j.cja.2020.06.006

European Parliamentary Technology Assessment. (2019). *Technologies in care for older people*. https://www.europarl.europa.eu/stoa/en/document/EPTA_Report_2019

Fang, K. Y., Ginige, J. A., Basilakis, J., Bjering, H., & Javadi, B. (2022). Smart homecare research translation into broader practice: Enablers, barriers and directions. *IEEE Access : Practical Innovations, Open Solutions*, *10*, 134726–134743. DOI: 10.1109/ACCESS.2022.3229871

Fathollahi-Fard, A. M., Ahmadi, A., & Karimi, B. (2022). Sustainable and robust home healthcare logistics: A response to the COVID-19 pandemic. *Symmetry*, *14*(2), 193. DOI: 10.3390/sym14020193

Fosch-Villaronga, E., & Drukarch, H. (2021). On healthcare robots: Concepts, definitions, and considerations for healthcare robot governance. *arXiv*. /arXiv.2106.03468DOI: 10.48550

Funao, H., Momosaki, R., Tsujikawa, M., Kawamoto, E., Esumi, R., & Shimaoka, M. (2024). Virtual reality–applied home-visit rehabilitation for patients with chronic pain: Protocol for single-arm pre-post comparison study. *JMIR Research Protocols*, *13*, e58734. DOI: 10.2196/58734 PMID: 39753216

Galavi, Z., Montazeri, M., & Ahmadian, L. (2022). Barriers and challenges of using health information technology in home care: A systematic review. *The International Journal of Health Planning and Management*, *37*(5), 2542–2568. DOI: 10.1002/hpm.3492 PMID: 35643906

Genet, N., Boerma, W. G. W., Kringos, D. S., Bouman, A., Francke, A. L., Fagerström, C., Melchiorre, M. G., Greco, C., & Devillé, W. (2011). Home care in Europe: A systematic literature review. *BMC Health Services Research*, *11*(1), 207. DOI: 10.1186/1472-6963-11-207 PMID: 21878111

Gilmour, H. (2018). Unmet home care needs in Canada. *Health Reports*, *29*(11), 3–11. PMID: 30485384

Gökalp, E., Gökalp, M. O., Çoban, S., & Eren, P. E. (2018). Analysing opportunities and challenges of integrated blockchain technologies in healthcare. In S. Wrycza & J. Maślankowski (Eds.), *Information systems: Research, development, applications, education: 11th SIGSAND/PLAIS EuroSymposium 2018* (Lecture Notes in Business Information Processing, Vol. 333, pp. 174–183). Springer. DOI: 10.1007/978-3-030-00060-8_13

Goldrick, M. R., & Gethin, G. T. (2021). Patients' perceptions of, and acceptance toward, using wearable sensor technology in wound care. *Journal of Wound Management*, *22*(1), 13–26. DOI: 10.35279/jowm2021.22.01.04

Graboyes, R. F., Bryan, D. S., & Coglianese, J. (2020). Overcoming technological and policy challenges to medical uses of unmanned aerial vehicles. *Mercatus Research Paper*. DOI: 10.2139/ssrn.3561743

Güdük, Ö. (2025). Telehealth applications in home health services: A bibliometric analysis. *Türkiye Aile Hekimligi Dergisi*, *29*(1), 20–35. DOI: 10.54308/turkjfampract.2025.811

Guo, B., Dong, B., Zhang, X., Yang, J., & Wang, Z. (2015). Research on home healthcare management system based on the improved Internet of Things architecture. *International Journal of Smart Home*, *9*(9), 51–62. DOI: 10.14257/ijsh.2015.9.9.06

Haidari, L. A., Brown, S. T., Ferguson, M., Bancroft, E., Spiker, M., Wilcox, A., Ambikapathi, R., Sampath, V., Connor, D. L., & Lee, B. Y. (2016). The economic and operational value of using drones to transport vaccines. *Vaccine*, *34*(34), 4062–4067. DOI: 10.1016/j.vaccine.2016.06.022 PMID: 27340098

Hapsari, A. A., Vresdian, D. J., Dionova, B. W., Zuhriyah, H., Pratama, L. P., & Islami, A. Y. (2024). A systematic review of drone development and innovation helps handling during a pandemic and its challenges for health technology. *Jurnal Teknologi dan Manajemen, 22*(2), 1–10. DOI: 10.52330/jtm.v22i2.246

Heratanti, N., Rambi, A. P., & Syarifurrahman, I. (2021). The telehealth effectiveness in home care services: A systematic review. *STRADA Jurnal Ilmiah Kesehatan*, *10*(1), 1057–1065. DOI: 10.30994/sjik.v10i1.761

Hosny, A., Parmar, C., Quackenbush, J., Schwartz, L. H., & Aerts, H. J. W. L. (2018). Artificial intelligence in radiology. *Nature Reviews. Cancer*, *18*(8), 500–510. DOI: 10.1038/s41568-018-0016-5 PMID: 29777175

Huang, Y., Hsieh, M.-Y., Chao, H.-C., Hung, S.-H., & Park, J. H. (2009). Pervasive, secure access to a hierarchical sensor-based healthcare monitoring architecture in wireless heterogeneous networks. *IEEE Journal on Selected Areas in Communications*, *27*(4), 400–411. DOI: 10.1109/JSAC.2009.090505

İnaç, R. Ç., & Ekmekçi, İ. (2023). Analysis of home healthcare practice to improve service quality: Case study of megacity Istanbul. *Health Care*, *11*(3), 319. DOI: 10.3390/healthcare11030319 PMID: 36766894

Iqbal, O., Iftakhar, T., & Ahmad, S. Z. (2022). Internet of Things for in-home health based monitoring system: Modern advances, challenges and future directions. *Journal on Internet of Things*, *4*(1), 35–55. DOI: 10.32604/jiot.2022.022256

Kim, S. J., Lim, G. J., Cho, J., & Côté, M. J. (2017). Drone-aided healthcare services for patients with chronic diseases in rural areas. *Journal of Intelligent & Robotic Systems*, *88*(1), 163–180. DOI: 10.1007/s10846-017-0548-z

Klimova, B. (2019). Exploring eLearning for dementia care. In J. J. Park, L. T. Yang, Y. S. Jeong, & F. Hao (Eds.), *Advanced multimedia and ubiquitous engineering* (Lecture Notes in Electrical Engineering, Vol. 518, pp. 341–346). Springer. DOI: 10.1007/978-981-13-1328-8_44

Koçaş, M. (2022). Sağlık hizmetleri ve yönetiminde Nesnelerin İnterneti. In Yeşilyurt, Ö. (Ed.), *Sağlık yönetiminde yenilikçi yaklaşımlar* (pp. 19–37). Efeakademi Yayınları.

Kosinski, K., Bucher, G., Szczerba, P., Weiss, E., Burch, C., & Chan, P. (2025). Exploring robotic solutions for home health care: A research study on robot assistants in home health-care delivery. *Mental Health and Digital Technologies*. DOI: 10.1108/MHDT-12-2024-0083

Kraśnik, W., Jankowska, O., Kurzeja, J., Piotrowicz, K., Piotrowicz, H., Bajkacz, A., Rogala, A., & Osmólska, J. (2024). The benefits and challenges of virtual reality application in rehabilitation for chronic conditions. *Journal of Education, Health and Sport*, *75*, 56379–56379. DOI: 10.12775/JEHS.2024.75.56379

Kumar, N. M., & Mallick, P. K. (2018). Blockchain technology for security issues and challenges in IoT. *Procedia Computer Science*, *132*, 1815–1823. DOI: 10.1016/j.procs.2018.05.140

Lakhwani, T. S., Sinjana, Y., & Kapoor, A. P. (2025). Beyond numbers: A novel IoT and drone framework for enhancing healthcare logistics. *Discover Health Systems*, *4*(1), 19. DOI: 10.1007/s44250-025-00187-w

Lawrence, J., Truong, D., Dao, A., & Bryant, P. A. (2023). Virtual hospital-level care—Feasibility, acceptability, safety and impact of a pilot hospital-in-the-home model for COVID-19 infection. *Frontiers in Digital Health*, *5*, 1068444. DOI: 10.3389/fdgth.2023.1068444 PMID: 37090066

Lin, K. Y., Chang, K. H., Lin, Y. W., & Wu, M. J. (2025). Exploring key considerations for artificial intelligence robots in home healthcare using the unified theory of acceptance and use of technology and the fuzzy analytical hierarchy process method. *Systems*, *13*(1), 25. DOI: 10.3390/systems13010025

Mansour, M. B., Ayman, A., & Yehia, M. (2024). E-healthcare system using IoT-based wearable device. *International Journal of Fuzzy Logic and Intelligent Systems*, *24*(3), 295–305. DOI: 10.5391/IJFIS.2024.24.3.295

Megido, I., Sela, Y., & Grinberg, K. (2023). Cost effectiveness of home care versus hospital care: A retrospective analysis. *Cost Effectiveness and Resource Allocation : C/E*, *21*(1), 13. DOI: 10.1186/s12962-023-00424-0 PMID: 36732792

Merih, Y. D., Ertürk, N., Yemenici, M., & Satman, İ. (2021). Evde sağlık hizmetlerinde teknoloji kullanımı. *Journal of Health Institutes of Türkiye*, *4*(3), 76–89. DOI: 10.54537/tusebdergisi.1037224

Munawar, H. S., Akram, J., Khan, S. I., Ullah, F., & Choi, B. J. (2023). Drone-as-a-service (DaaS) for COVID-19 self-testing kits delivery in smart healthcare setups: A technological perspective. *ICT Express*, *9*(4), 748–753. DOI: 10.1016/j.icte.2022.09.008

Mundi, M. S., Mohamed Elfadil, O., Bonnes, S. L., Salonen, B. R., & Hurt, R. T. (2021). Use of telehealth in home nutrition support: Challenges and advantages. *Nutrition in Clinical Practice*, *36*(4), 775–784. DOI: 10.1002/ncp.10736 PMID: 34245465

Muñoz-Bonet, J. I., López-Prats, J. L., Flor-Macián, E. M., Cantavella, T., Domínguez, A., Vidal, Y., & Brines, J. (2020). Medical complications in a telemedicine home care programme for paediatric ventilated patients. *Journal of Telemedicine and Telecare*, *26*(7–8), 462–473. DOI: 10.1177/1357633X19843761 PMID: 31023136

Munyewende, P. O., Rispel, L. C., & Chirwa, T. (2014). Positive practice environments influence job satisfaction of primary health care clinic nursing managers in two South African provinces. *Human Resources for Health*, *12*(1), 27. DOI: 10.1186/1478-4491-12-27 PMID: 24885785

Mustafa, M., Alshare, M., Bhargava, D., Neware, R., Singh, B., & Ngulube, P. (2022). Perceived security risk based on moderating factors for blockchain technology applications in cloud storage to achieve secure healthcare systems. *Computational and Mathematical Methods in Medicine*, *2022*, 6112815. DOI: 10.1155/2022/6112815 PMID: 35096132

Naureen, A., Vamshi, K., Krishna, K. C., & Hussain, M. M. (2024). Healthcare 5.0 fundamentals. In Hassan, A., Prasad, V. K., Bhattacharya, P., Dutta, P., & Damaševičius, R. (Eds.), *Federated learning and AI for Healthcare 5.0* (pp. 1–33). IGI Global., DOI: 10.4018/978-1-6684-9510-0.ch001

Nibbelink, C. W., & Brewer, B. B. (2018). Decision-making in nursing practice: An integrative literature review. *Journal of Clinical Nursing*, *27*(5–6), 917–928. DOI: 10.1111/jocn.14151 PMID: 29098746

Oelschlägel, L., Christensen, V. L., Moen, A., Heggdal, K., Österlind, J., Dihle, A., & Steindal, S. A. (2023). Patients' experiences with a welfare technology application for remote home care: A longitudinal study. *Journal of Clinical Nursing*, *32*(17–18), 6545–6558. DOI: 10.1111/jocn.16592 PMID: 36437490

Oelschlägel, L., Moen, A., Dihle, A., Christensen, V. L., Heggdal, K., Österlind, J., & Steindal, S. A. (2024). Implementation of remote home care: Assessment guided by the RE-AIM framework. *BMC Health Services Research*, *24*(1), 145. DOI: 10.1186/s12913-024-10625-9 PMID: 38287394

Önder, E. (2021). Geçmişten günümüze evde sağlık hizmetleri. In Özaydın, Ö., & Güdük, Ö. (Eds.), *Evde sağlık hizmetlerinde teknoloji kullanımı* (pp. 203–224). Nobel Akademik Yayıncılık.

Onofri, A., Ullmann, N., Verrillo, E., Paglietti, M. G., Pavone, M., & Cutrera, R. (2025). Televisit with TytoHome™ device in medically complex child in long-term mechanical ventilation: A pilot study. *Italian Journal of Pediatrics*, *51*(1), 45. DOI: 10.1186/s13052-025-01885-0 PMID: 39939975

Pruszyński, J., Jasik, A., Marcinowska-Suchowierska, E., Puzianowska-Kuźnicka, M., & Zgliczyński, W. S. (2022). New technologies in elderly care. *Wiedza Medyczna*, *4*(1), 43–52. DOI: 10.36553/wm.131

Puja, D., Upadhyay, S., Agrawal, S., Goswami, J. K., & Singh, S. K. (2023). A healthcare system for patients based on IoT. *Scandinavian Journal of Information Systems*, *35*(1), 446–456. DOI: 10.5281/SJIS.7752846

Rabearison, H. M., Razafison, F., Razafimanjato, N., Zafintsalama, M., & Andriatsihoarana, H. (2025). Architecture and organizational protocol of a connected medical monitoring device. *International Journal of Scientific Research and Technology*, *2*(4), 204–216. DOI: 10.5281/zenodo.15191781

Raja, A., Lakshmi, K. U., Chaitanya, K., Kavya, M., Mahammed, N., & Palankaiah, C. C. (2025). IoT based wearable ECG monitoring system for patient emergency condition. *International Journal for Modern Trends in Science and Technology*, *11*(3), 136–142. DOI: 10.5281/zenodo.15084903

Roberts, N., Carrigan, A., Hibbert, P., Williams, R. C., Austin, E., Pulido, D. F., Meulenbroeks, I., Nguyen, H. M., Hatem, S., Maka, K., Loy, G., & Braithwaite, J. (2023). Consumer and provider perspectives on hospital in the home: A qualitative study. *Health & Social Care in the Community*, *2023*, 7105751. DOI: 10.1155/2023/7105751

Sabetsarvestani, P., Mohammadi, F., Tehranineshat, B., Bijani, M., & Fereidouni, Z. (2022). Barriers to efficient management of in-home care: A qualitative content analysis. *Nursing Open*, *9*(2), 1200–1209. DOI: 10.1002/nop2.1161 PMID: 34908248

Scott, A. F., Ayers, S., Pluye, P., Grad, R., Sztramko, R., Marr, S., Papaioannou, A., Clark, S., Gerantonis, P., & Levinson, A. J. (2022). Impact and perceived value of iGeriCare e-learning among dementia care partners and others: Pilot evaluation using the IAM4all questionnaire. *JMIR Aging*, *5*(4), e40357. DOI: 10.2196/40357 PMID: 36150051

Senillosa, M. B., Saimovici, J., Mandirola Brieux, H. F., Rabinovich, D., Galván, C., Jauregui, O. I., Rizzato Lede, D. A., Otero, C. M., & Luna, D. R. (2022). Mobile application for home healthcare: Physician's expectations and perceptions. *Studies in Health Technology and Informatics*, *290*, 197–199. DOI: 10.3233/SHTI220060 PMID: 35672999

Sharma, K., Singh, H., Sharma, D. K., Kumar, A., Nayyar, A., & Krishnamurthi, R. (2021). Dynamic models and control techniques for drone delivery of medications and other healthcare items in COVID-19 hotspots. In Gupta, B. B., Agrawal, P., Hassanien, A. E., & Abraham, A. (Eds.), *Emerging technologies for battling COVID-19: Applications and innovations* (pp. 1–34). Springer., DOI: 10.1007/978-3-030-60039-6_1

Shirvanian, N., Shams, M., Rahmani, A. M., Lansky, J., Mildeova, S., & Hosseinzadeh, M. (2025). The Internet of Things in elderly healthcare applications: A systematic review and future directions. *IEEE Access : Practical Innovations, Open Solutions*, *13*, 71335–71373. DOI: 10.1109/ACCESS.2025.3562147

Shurson, L., Pilon, B., Ketel, C., & Anthamatten, A. (2019). Development of an interprofessional home healthcare management service within an urban housing development. *Home Healthcare Now*, *37*(5), 285–291. DOI: 10.1097/NHH.0000000000000817 PMID: 31483361

Şimşir, İ., & Mete, B. (2021). Sağlık hizmetlerinin geleceği: Dijital sağlık teknolojileri. *Journal of Innovative Healthcare Practices*, *2*(1), 33–39.

Sitges-Maciá, E., Bonete-López, B., Sánchez-Cabaco, A., & Oltra-Cucarella, J. (2021). Effects of e-health training and social support interventions for informal caregivers of people with dementia—A narrative review. *International Journal of Environmental Research and Public Health*, *18*(15), 7728. DOI: 10.3390/ijerph18157728 PMID: 34360020

Sivakumar, V. G., Baskar, V. V., Vadivel, M., Vimal, S. P., & Murugan, S. (2023). IoT and GIS integration for real-time monitoring of soil health and nutrient status. In *2023 International Conference on Self Sustainable Artificial Intelligence Systems (ICSSAS)* (pp. 1265–1270). IEEE. DOI: 10.1109/ICSSAS57918.2023.10331694

Snoswell, C. L., Taylor, M. L., Comans, T. A., Smith, A. C., Gray, L. C., & Caffery, L. J. (2020). Determining if telehealth can reduce health system costs: Scoping review. *Journal of Medical Internet Research*, *22*(10), e17298. DOI: 10.2196/17298 PMID: 33074157

Stavropoulos, T. G., Papastergiou, A., Mpaltadoros, L., Nikolopoulos, S., & Kompatsiaris, I. (2020). IoT wearable sensors and devices in elderly care: A literature review. *Sensors (Basel)*, *20*(10), 2826. DOI: 10.3390/s20102826 PMID: 32429331

Steindal, S. A., Nes, A. A. G., Godskesen, T. E., Dihle, A., Lind, S., Winger, A., & Klarare, A. (2020). Patients' experiences of telehealth in palliative home care: Scoping review. *Journal of Medical Internet Research*, *22*(5), e16218. DOI: 10.2196/16218 PMID: 32369037

Su, Z., Liang, F., Sheng, W., & Bishop, A. (2024). Robot-assisted homecare for older adults: A user study on needs and challenges. *Cobot*, *2*, 100013. DOI: 10.12688/cobot.17644.2

Tanaka, M., Ishii, S., Matsuoka, A., Tanabe, S., Matsunaga, S., Rahmani, A., Dutt, N., Rasouli, M., & Nyamathi, A. (2024). Perspectives of Japanese elders and their healthcare providers on use of wearable technology to monitor their health at home: A qualitative exploration. *International Journal of Nursing Studies*, *152*, 104691. DOI: 10.1016/j.ijnurstu.2024.104691 PMID: 38262231

Thiels, C. A., Aho, J. M., Zietlow, S. P., & Jenkins, D. H. (2015). Use of unmanned aerial vehicles for medical product transport. *Air Medical Journal*, *34*(2), 104–108. DOI: 10.1016/j.amj.2014.10.011 PMID: 25733117

Tian, Y. J., Felber, N. A., Pageau, F., Schwab, D. R., & Wangmo, T. (2024). Benefits and barriers associated with the use of smart home health technologies in the care of older persons: A systematic review. *BMC Geriatrics*, *24*(1), 152. DOI: 10.1186/s12877-024-04702-1 PMID: 38355464

Vaartio-Rajalin, H., & Fagerström, L. (2019). Professional care at home: Patient-centeredness, interprofessionality and effectivity? A scoping review. *Health & Social Care in the Community*, *27*(4), e270–e288. DOI: 10.1111/hsc.12731 PMID: 30843316

Vaartio-Rajalin, H., Näsman, Y., Santamäki-Fischer, R., & Hemberg, J. (2019). Working in home healthcare and suggestions for development. *Home Health Care Services Quarterly*, *38*(4), 257–269. DOI: 10.1080/01621424.2019.1641450 PMID: 31295058

Van de Voorde, P., Gautama, S., Momont, A., Ionescu, C. M., De Paepe, P., & Fraeyman, N. (2017). The drone ambulance [A-UAS]: Golden bullet or just a blank? *Resuscitation*, *116*, 46–48. DOI: 10.1016/j.resuscitation.2017.04.037 PMID: 28487253

Vo, D. K., & Trinh, K. T. L. (2024). Advances in wearable biosensors for healthcare: Current trends, applications, and future perspectives. *Biosensors (Basel)*, *14*(11), 560. DOI: 10.3390/bios14110560 PMID: 39590019

Wang, J., Chen, W., Wang, L., Ren, Y., & Sherratt, R. S. (2020). Blockchain-based data storage mechanism for industrial Internet of Things. *Intelligent Automation & Soft Computing*, *26*(5), 1157–1172. DOI: 10.32604/iasc.2020.012174

Whende, M. C. (2019). Artificial intelligence, critical thinking and the nursing process. *On-Line Journal of Nursing Informatics*, *23*(1).

Woo, K., Song, J., Adams, V., Block, L. J., Currie, L. M., Shang, J., & Topaz, M. (2022). Exploring prevalence of wound infections and related patient characteristics in homecare using natural language processing. *International Wound Journal*, *19*(1), 211–221. DOI: 10.1111/iwj.13623 PMID: 34105873

Wylde, V., Rawindaran, N., Lawrence, J., Balasubramanian, R., Prakash, E., Jayal, A., Khan, I., Hewage, C., & Platts, J. (2022). Cybersecurity, data privacy and blockchain: A review. *SN Computer Science*, *3*(2), 127. DOI: 10.1007/s42979-022-01020-4 PMID: 35036930

Xu, X., Lu, Y., Vogel-Heuser, B., & Wang, L. (2021). Industry 4.0 and Industry 5.0—Inception, conception and perception. *Journal of Manufacturing Systems*, *61*, 530–535. DOI: 10.1016/j.jmsy.2021.10.006

Yang, G., Pang, Z., Jamal Deen, M., Dong, M., Zhang, Y.-T., Lovell, N., & Rahmani, A. M. (2020). Homecare robotic systems for Healthcare 4.0: Visions and enabling technologies. *IEEE Journal of Biomedical and Health Informatics*, *24*(9), 2535–2549. DOI: 10.1109/JBHI.2020.2990529 PMID: 32340971

Compilation of References

Aalaei, S., Firouraghi, N., Aalaei, M., Karbin, K., Bararbakhti, H., Nematy, M., & Rezvani, R. (2025). Feasibility of Mobile Telehealth for Health Literacy Enhancement via Nutritional Counseling during COVID-19. Journal of Nutrition. *Fasting and Health*, *13*(1), 24–34.

Abdaoui, N., Khalifa, I., & Faiz, S. (2023). Creating a personalized recommendation framework in smart shopping by using IoT devices. In *Proceedings of the 8th International Conference on Internet of Things, Big Data and Security* (pp. 200–207). SCITEPRESS. DOI: 10.5220/0011969400003482

Abdellatif, M. M., & Mohamed, W. (2020). Telemedicine: An IoT based remote healthcare system. *International Journal of Online and Biomedical Engineering*, *16*(6), 72–85. DOI: 10.3991/ijoe.v16i06.13651

Abdelmaksoud, N. S. A. (2022). Universal design approach to a smart, sustainable, safe, and accessible city. *WIT Transactions on Ecology and the Environment*, *260*, 259–270. DOI: 10.2495/SC220211

Abràmoff, M. D., Lavin, P. T., Birch, M., Shah, N., & Folk, J. C. (2018). Pivotal trial of an autonomous AI-based diagnostic system for detection of diabetic retinopathy in primary care offices. *NPJ Digital Medicine*, *1*(1), 39. DOI: 10.1038/s41746-018-0040-6 PMID: 31304320

Achillas, C., Aidonis, D., Folinas, D., & Vlachokostas, C. (2024). Empowering tourism accessibility: A digital revolution in Pieria, Greece. *Applied Sciences (Basel, Switzerland)*, *14*(23), 11136. DOI: 10.3390/app142311136

Acumen Research and Consulting. (2024). *Remote healthcare market*. https://www.acumenresearchandconsulting.com/press-releases/remote-healthcare-market

Adashek, J. J., & Subbiah, I. M. (2020). Caring for the caregiver: A systematic review characterising the experience of caregivers of older adults with advanced cancers. *ESMO Open*, *5*(5), e000862. DOI: 10.1136/esmoopen-2020-000862 PMID: 32963088

Adner, R., & Kapoor, R. (2010). Value creation in innovation ecosystems: How the structure of technological interdependence affects firm performance in new technology generations. *Strategic Management Journal, 31*(3), 306–333. DOI: 10.1002/smj.821

Ahmad, I., Asghar, Z., Kumar, T., Li, G., Manzoor, A., Mikhaylov, K., Shah, S. A., Höyhtyä, M., Reponen, J., Huusko, J., & Harjula, E. (2022). Emerging technologies for next generation remote health care and assisted living. *IEEE Access : Practical Innovations, Open Solutions, 10*, 56094–56132. DOI: 10.1109/ACCESS.2022.3177278

Ahmadi, A. (2024). Digital health transformation: Leveraging ai for monitoring and disease management. [IJBLS]. *International Journal of BioLife Sciences, 3*(1), 10–24.

Akgün, Z. (2021). Evaluation of the regulation on providing remote healthcare services. *Türkiye Biyoetik Dergisi, 8*(4), 194–198. DOI: 10.5505/tjob.2021.49344

Akter, S., Motamarri, S., Hani, U., Shams, R., Fernando, M., Mohiuddin Babu, M., & Shen, K. N. (2020). Building dynamic service analytics capabilities for the digital marketplace. *Journal of Business Research, 118*, 177–188. DOI: 10.1016/j.jbusres.2020.06.016

Aldousari, A., Alotaibi, M., Khajah, F., Jaafar, A., Alshebli, M., & Kanj, H. (2023). A wearable IoT-based healthcare monitoring system for elderly people. In *2023 International Conference on BioSMART (BioSMART)* (pp. 1–4). IEEE. DOI: 10.1109/BioSMART58455.2023.10162041

Ali, M. A., & Dhanaraj, R. K. (2024). IoMT and blockchain oriented smart healthcare monitoring system. In *AIP Conference Proceedings* (Vol. 2919, Article 020008). AIP Publishing. DOI: 10.1063/5.0184364

Allan, R. (2006, June 15). *A brief history of telemedicine*. Electronic Design. https://www.electronicdesign.com/technologies/components/article/21770508/a-brief-history-of-telemedicine

Allee, V. (2000). Reconfiguring the value network. *The Journal of Business Strategy, 21*(4), 36–39. DOI: 10.1108/eb040103

Allee, V. (2008). Value network analysis and value conversion of tangible and intangible assets. *Journal of Intellectual Capital, 9*(1), 5–24. DOI: 10.1108/14691930810845777

Allifah, N. M., & Zualkernan, I. A. (2022). Ranking security of IoT-based smart home consumer devices. *IEEE Access : Practical Innovations, Open Solutions, 10*, 18352–18369. DOI: 10.1109/ACCESS.2022.3148140

Almathami, H. K. Y., Win, K. T., & Vlahu-Gjorgievska, E. (2020). Barriers and facilitators that influence telemedicine-based, real-time, online consultation at patients' homes: Systematic literature review. *Journal of Medical Internet Research, 22*(2), e16407. DOI: 10.2196/16407 PMID: 32130131

Almunawar, M. N., Anshari, M., de Pablos, P. O., & Fauzi, A. M. (2025). Embracing digital business ecosystem: Transforming traditional marketplaces. *Journal of Science and Technology Policy Management*. DOI: 10.1108/JSTPM-09-2022-0144

Almunawar, M. N., & Anshari, M. (2020). Multi-sided networks of digital platform ecosystem: The case of ride-hailing in Indonesia. *Asia Pacific Journal of Information Systems, 30*(4), 803–825. DOI: 10.14329/apjis.2020.30.4.808

Almunawar, M. N., & Anshari, M. (2022). Digital enabler and value integration: Revealing the expansion engine of digital marketplace. *Technology Analysis and Strategic Management, 34*(7), 847–857. DOI: 10.1080/09537325.2021.1926967

Almunawar, M. N., Anshari, M., & Lim, S. A. (2021). Value network view on digital marketplace. In Khosrow-Pour, M. (Ed.), *Encyclopedia of organizational knowledge, administration, and technology* (pp. 1349–1363). IGI Global., DOI: 10.4018/978-1-7998-3473-1.ch091

Almunawar, M. N., Anshari, M., Susanto, H., & Chen, C. K. (2015). Revealing customer behavior on smartphones. *International Journal of Asian Business and Information Management, 6*(2), 33–49. DOI: 10.4018/IJABIM.2015040103

Alpert, J. M. (2020). Secondary care provider attitudes towards patient-generated health data from smartwatches. npj. *Digital Medicine, 3*(1), 1–7. PMID: 32140569

Altinay Ozdemir, M. (2021). Virtual reality (VR) and augmented reality (AR) technologies for accessibility and marketing in the tourism industry. In M. C. tom Dieck & T. Jung (Eds.), *Virtual and augmented reality in tourism marketing* (pp. 277–301). IGI Global. DOI: 10.4018/978-1-7998-7539-0.ch014

Altınay, F., Dagli, G., Altinay, M., & Altınay, Z. (2019). The role of technology in tourism and health services for accessibility in service management. *Postmodern Openings, 10*(4), 1–7. DOI: 10.18662/po/90

Altınay, Z., Saner, T., Bahçelerli, N. M., & Altınay, F. (2016). The role of social media tools: Accessible tourism for disabled citizens. *Journal of Educational Technology & Society, 19*(1), 89–99. https://www.jstor.org/stable/jeductechsoci.19.1.89

Álvarez-Castañón, L. D. C., Arroyo, P., Contreras-Cruz, M. A., & Villaseñor-Mora, C. (2022). Health 4.0 and its potential adoption and contribution to the Mexican health system. In *2022 Portland International Conference on Management of Engineering and Technology (PICMET)* (pp. 1–10). IEEE. DOI: 10.23919/PICMET53225.2022.9882603

Ambrose, I., Darcy, S., & Buhalis, D. (2012). *Best practice in accessible tourism: Inclusion, disability, ageing population and tourism* (Aspects of Tourism, Vol. 53). Channel View Publications.

Anca, G. (2010). European Union policy on accessible tourism as millstones for future development of worldwide accessibility standards for tourism. In *TRANSED 2010: 12th International Conference on Mobility and Transport for Elderly and Disabled People*. Hong Kong Society for Rehabilitation; S. K. Yee Medical Foundation; Transportation Research Board.

Anderson, J. W., & Visweswaran, S. (2025). Algorithmic individual fairness and healthcare: A scoping review. *JAMIA Open*, *8*(1), ooae149. DOI: 10.1093/jamiaopen/ooae149 PMID: 39737346

Anggraeni, E., den Hartigh, E., & Zegveld, M. (2007). Business ecosystem as a perspective for studying the relations between firms and their business networks. In *ECCON 2007 Annual meeting* (pp. 1–21). Netherlands Organisation for Scientific Research.

Antona, M., & Stephanidis, C. (Eds.). (2020). *Universal access in human-computer interaction. Design approaches and supporting technologies: 14th International Conference, UAHCI 2020, Held as Part of the 22nd HCI International Conference, HCII 2020, Copenhagen, Denmark, July 19–24, 2020, Proceedings, Part I* (Vol. 12188). Springer. DOI: 10.1007/978-3-030-49282-3

Ardila, D., Kiraly, A. P., Bharadwaj, S., Choi, B., Reicher, J. J., Peng, L., Tse, D., Etemadi, M., Ye, W., Corrado, G., Naidich, D. P., & Shetty, S. (2019). End-to-end lung cancer screening with three-dimensional deep learning on low-dose chest computed tomography. *Nature Medicine*, *25*(6), 954–961. DOI: 10.1038/s41591-019-0447-x PMID: 31110349

Arem, H., Moses, J., Cisneros, C., Blondeau, B., Nekhlyudov, L., Killackey, M., & Pratt-Chapman, M. L. (2022). Cancer provider and survivor experiences with telehealth during the COVID-19 pandemic. *JCO Oncology Practice*, *18*(4), e452–e461. DOI: 10.1200/OP.21.00401 PMID: 34714706

Arık, Y. (2023). Evaluation of telemedicine applications within the scope of healthcare marketing. *Hacettepe Journal of Health Administration*, *26*(2), 511–534.

Armbrust, M., Stoica, I., Zaharia, M., Fox, A., Griffith, R., Joseph, A. D., Katz, R., Konwinski, A., Lee, G., Patterson, D., & Rabkin, A. (2010). A view of cloud computing. *Communications of the ACM*, *53*(4), 50–58. DOI: 10.1145/1721654.1721672

Asare-Bediako, B., Kling, W. L., & Ribeiro, P. F. (2013). Integrated agent-based home energy management system for smart grids applications. In *2013 IEEE PES Innovative Smart Grid Technologies Conference (ISGT)* (pp. 1–5). IEEE. DOI: 10.1109/ISGTEurope.2013.6695332

Ashley, E. A. (2015). The precision medicine initiative: A new national effort. *Journal of the American Medical Association*, *313*(21), 2119–2120. DOI: 10.1001/jama.2015.3595 PMID: 25928209

Ashraf, Z., Sohail, A., & Yousaf, M. (2019). Performance analysis of network applications on IPv6 cloud connected virtual machine. *International Journal of Computer Network and Information Security*, *11*(12), 1–9. DOI: 10.5815/ijcnis.2019.12.01

Assaad, M., Chamma, N., Mateev, M., & Rizk, R. (2024). Telehealth during and beyond the covid-19 pandemic: evidence from licensed dietitians in an emerging economy. DOI: 10.1101/2024.09.19.24314030

Atluri, H., & Thummisetti, B. S. P. (2022). A holistic examination of patient outcomes, healthcare accessibility, and technological integration in remote healthcare delivery. *Transactions on Latest Trends in Health Sector*, *14*(14), 1–14.

Aujla, G. S., & Jindal, A. (2021). A decoupled blockchain approach for edge-envisioned IoT-based healthcare monitoring. *IEEE Journal on Selected Areas in Communications*, *39*(2), 491–499. DOI: 10.1109/JSAC.2020.3020655

Avcı, Y. D., & Gözüm, S. (2024). The impact of Industry 5.0: The artificial intelligence, IoT and blockchain revolution in home healthcare. In Zafar, S., Kumar, S. N., Ahilan, A., & Cakir, G. K. (Eds.), *Industry 5.0 for smart healthcare technologies* (pp. 62–76). CRC Press., DOI: 10.1201/9781032632223-6

Avis, J. (2018). Socio-technical imaginary of the fourth industrial revolution and its implications for vocational education and training: A literature review. *Journal of Vocational Education and Training*, *70*(3), 337–363. DOI: 10.1080/13636820.2018.1498907

Awotunde, J. B., Oluwabukonla, S., Chakraborty, C., Bhoi, A. K., & Ajamu, G. J. (2022). Application of artificial intelligence and big data for fighting COVID-19 pandemic. In Mishra, S., Suanpang, H. S., Wu, Y.-S., & Nagar, A. K. (Eds.), *Decision sciences for COVID-19: Learning through case studies* (pp. 3–26). Springer., DOI: 10.1007/978-3-030-87019-5_1

Badr, N. G., & Dankar, M. (2022). Assistive healthcare robotics—Challenges in nursing service innovation: Critical review. In *ITM Web of Conferences* (Vol. 41, Article 02002). EDP Sciences. DOI: 10.1051/itmconf/20224102002

Baker, L. C., Johnson, S. J., Macaulay, D., & Birnbaum, H. (2011). Integrated telehealth and care management program for Medicare beneficiaries with chronic disease linked to savings. *Health Affairs, 30*(9), 1689–1697. DOI: 10.1377/hlthaff.2011.0216 PMID: 21900660

Barazzoni, R., Bischoff, S. C., Breda, J., Wickramasinghe, K., Krznaric, Z., Nitzan, D., Pirlich, M., & Singer, P. (2020). ESPEN expert statements and practical guidance for nutritional management of individuals with SARS-CoV-2 infection. *Clinical Nutrition (Edinburgh, Lothian), 39*(6), 1631–1638. DOI: 10.1016/j.clnu.2020.03.022 PMID: 32305181

Barclay, A. R., McGuckin, C., Hill, S., Protheroe, S., & Batra, A. (2021). Exit strategies from the COVID-19 lockdown for children and young people receiving home parenteral nutrition (HPN): Lessons from the BSPGHAN Intestinal Failure Working Group experience. *Frontline Gastroenterology, 12*(4), 348–353. DOI: 10.1136/flgastro-2020-101598 PMID: 34249323

Bashshur, R. L., Doarn, C. R., Frenk, J., Kvedar, J. C., Shannon, G. W., & Woolliscroft, J. O. (2020). Beyond the covid pandemic, telemedicine, and health care. *Telemedicine Journal and e-Health, 26*(11), 1310–1313. DOI: 10.1089/tmj.2020.0328 PMID: 32809913

Bashshur, R. L., & Shannon, G. W. (2009). *History of telemedicine: Evolution, context, and transformation*. Mary Ann Liebert.

Bashshur, R. L., Shannon, G. W., Krupinski, E. A., & Grigsby, J. (2011). The taxonomy of telemedicine. *Telemedicine Journal and e-Health, 17*(6), 484–494. DOI: 10.1089/tmj.2011.0103 PMID: 21718114

Bashshur, R. L., Shannon, G. W., Smith, B. R., Alverson, D. C., Antoniotti, N., Barsan, W. G., Bashshur, N., Brown, E. M., Coye, M. J., Doarn, C. R., Ferguson, S., Grigsby, J., Krupinski, E. A., Kvedar, J. C., Linkous, J., Merrell, R. C., Nesbitt, T., Poropatich, R., Rheuban, K. S., & Yellowlees, P. (2014). The empirical foundations of telemedicine interventions for chronic disease management. *Telemedicine Journal and e-Health, 20*(9), 769–800. DOI: 10.1089/tmj.2014.9981 PMID: 24968105

Bashshur, R., Doarn, C. R., Frenk, J. M., Kvedar, J. C., & Woolliscroft, J. O. (2020). Telemedicine and the COVID-19 pandemic, lessons for the future. *Telemedicine Journal and e-Health, 26*(5), 571–573. DOI: 10.1089/tmj.2020.29040.rb PMID: 32275485

Basulo-Ribeiro, J., & Teixeira, L. (2024). The future of healthcare with Industry 5.0: Preliminary interview-based qualitative analysis. *Future Internet, 16*(3), 68. DOI: 10.3390/fi16030068

Beard, N. (1993, March 1). *Wired doctors*. Wired. https://www.wired.com/1993/03/wired-doctors/

Bekiaris, E., Panou, M., & Mousadakou, A. (2007). Elderly and disabled travelers' needs in infomobility services. In Stephanidis, C. (Ed.), Lecture Notes in Computer Science: Vol. 4554. *Universal access in human computer interaction: Coping with diversity* (pp. 853–860). Springer., DOI: 10.1007/978-3-540-73279-2_95

Bender, D., & Sartipi, K. (2013). HL7 FHIR: An agile and RESTful approach to healthcare information exchange. In *2013 IEEE 26th International Symposium on Computer-Based Medical Systems (CBMS)* (pp. 326–331). IEEE. DOI: 10.1109/CBMS.2013.6627810

Benmansour, A., Bouchachia, A., & Feham, M. (2016). Multioccupant activity recognition in pervasive smart home environments. *ACM Computing Surveys, 48*(3), 34. DOI: 10.1145/2835372

Bergerot, C. D., Bergerot, P. G., Philip, E. J., Ferrari, R., Peixoto, R. M., Crane, T. E., Schmitz, K. H., & Soto-Pérez-de-Celis, E. (2024). Enhancing cancer supportive care: Integrating psychosocial support, nutrition, and physical activity using telehealth solutions. *JCO Global Oncology*, (10), e2400333. DOI: 10.1200/GO-24-00333 PMID: 39509661

Bertolazzi, A., Quaglia, V., & Bongelli, R. (2024). Barriers and facilitators to health technology adoption by older adults with chronic diseases: An integrative systematic review. *BMC Public Health, 24*(1), 506. DOI: 10.1186/s12889-024-18036-5 PMID: 38365698

Bestsennyy, O., Gilbert, G., Harris, A., & Rost, J. (2021a). *Telehealth: A quarter-trillion-dollar post-COVID-19 reality?* McKinsey & Company. https://www.mckinsey.com/industries/healthcare/our-insights/telehealth-a-quarter-trillion-dollar-post-covid-19-reality

Bestsennyy, O., Gilbert, G., Harris, A., & Rost, J. (2021b). *Telehealth: A quarter-trillion-dollar post-COVID-19 reality?* Connect with Care. https://connectwithcare.org/wp-content/uploads/2021/07/telehealth-a-quarter-trillion-dollar-post-covid-19-reality.pdf

Bhalotia, N., Kumar, M., Alameen, A., Mohapatra, H., & Kolhar, M. (2023). A helping hand to the elderly: Securing their freedom through the HAIE framework. *Applied Sciences (Basel, Switzerland)*, *13*(11), 6797. DOI: 10.3390/app13116797

Bijalwan, V., Semwal, V. B., & Mandal, T. K. (2021). Fusion of multi-sensor-based biomechanical gait analysis using vision and wearable sensor. *IEEE Sensors Journal*, *21*(13), 14213–14220. DOI: 10.1109/JSEN.2021.3066473

Bodenheimer, T. S., & Grumbach, K. (2020). *Understanding health policy: A clinical approach* (8th ed.). McGraw Hill.

Boric-Lubecke, O., Gao, X., Yavari, E., Baboli, M., Singh, A., & Lubecke, V. M. (2014). E-healthcare: Remote monitoring, privacy, and security. In *2014 IEEE MTT-S International Microwave Symposium (IMS2014)* (pp. 1–3). IEEE. DOI: 10.1109/MWSYM.2014.6848595

Bouabida, K., Lebouché, B., & Pomey, M.-P. (2022). Telehealth and COVID-19 pandemic: An overview of the telehealth use, advantages, challenges, and opportunities during COVID-19 pandemic. *Health Care*, *10*(11), 2293. DOI: 10.3390/healthcare10112293 PMID: 36421617

Bowles, K. H., McDonald, M., Barron, Y., Kennedy, E., O'Connor, M., & Mikkelsen, M. (2021). Surviving COVID-19 after hospital discharge: Symptom, functional, and adverse outcomes of home health recipients. *Annals of Internal Medicine*, *174*(3), 316–325. DOI: 10.7326/M20-5206 PMID: 33226861

Brahman, F., Honarmand, M., & Jadid, S. (2015). Optimal electrical and thermal energy management of a residential energy hub, integrating demand response and energy storage system. *Energy and Building*, *90*, 65–75. DOI: 10.1016/j.enbuild.2014.12.039

Broadbent, E., Stafford, R., & MacDonald, B. (2009). Acceptance of healthcare robots for the older population: Review and future directions. *International Journal of Social Robotics*, *1*(4), 319–330. DOI: 10.1007/s12369-009-0030-6

Brocard, E., Antoine, P., Mélihan-Cheinin, P., & Rusch, E. (2021). COVID-19's impact on home health services, caregivers and patients: Lessons from the French experience. *The Lancet Regional Health. Europe*, *8*, 100197. DOI: 10.1016/j.lanepe.2021.100197 PMID: 34423328

Brown, T. B., Mann, B., Ryder, N., Subbiah, M., Kaplan, J. D., Dhariwal, P., Neelakantan, A., Shyam, P., Sastry, G., Askell, A., Agarwal, S., Herbert-Voss, A., Krueger, G., Henighan, T., Child, R., Ramesh, A., Ziegler, D. M., Wu, J., Winter, C., & Amodei, D. (2020). Language models are few-shot learners. *Advances in Neural Information Processing Systems*, *33*, 1877–1901.

Brunton, C., Arensberg, M., Drawert, S., Badaracco, C., Everett, W., & McCauley, S. (2021). Perspectives of registered dietitian nutritionists on adoption of telehealth for nutrition care during the covid-19 pandemic. *Health Care*, *9*(2), 235. DOI: 10.3390/healthcare9020235 PMID: 33672179

Buchanan, B., & Feigenbaum, E. (1993). DENDRAL and Meta-DENDRAL: Roots of knowledge systems and expert system applications. *Artificial Intelligence*, *59*(1–2), 233–240. DOI: 10.1016/0004-3702(93)90010-M

Butzner, M., & Cuffee, Y. (2021). Telehealth interventions and outcomes across rural communities in the United States: Narrative review. *Journal of Medical Internet Research*, *23*(8), e29575. DOI: 10.2196/29575 PMID: 34435965

Cannan, J., & Hu, H. (2011). *Human-machine interaction (HMI): A survey* (Technical Report CES-508). University of Essex.

Capitaine, V. (2016). Inciting tourist accommodation managers to make their establishments accessible to people with disabilities. *Journal of Tourism Futures*, *2*(2), 196–205. DOI: 10.1108/JTF-03-2015-0010

Celdrán, A. H., Pérez, M. G., Clemente, F. J. G., Ippoliti, F., & Pérez, G. M. (2019). Dynamic network slicing management of multimedia scenarios for future remote healthcare. *Multimedia Tools and Applications*, *78*(17), 24707–24737. DOI: 10.1007/s11042-019-7283-3

Centers for Medicare & Medicaid Services. (2020, March 17). *Medicare telemedicine health care provider fact sheet*. https://www.cms.gov/newsroom/fact-sheets/medicare-telemedicine-health-care-provider-fact-sheet

Chang, H. H., Chou, P. B., & Ramakrishnan, S. (2009). An ecosystem approach for healthcare services cloud. In *2009 IEEE International Conference on e-Business Engineering* (pp. 608–612). IEEE. DOI: 10.1109/ICEBE.2009.98

Char, D. S., Shah, N. H., & Magnus, D. (2018). Implementing machine learning in health care—Addressing ethical challenges. *The New England Journal of Medicine*, *378*(11), 981–983. DOI: 10.1056/NEJMp1714229 PMID: 29539284

Cheng, W., Cao, X., Lian, W., & Tian, J. (2024). An introduction to smart home ward–based hospital-at-home care in China. *JMIR mHealth and uHealth*, *12*, e44422. DOI: 10.2196/44422 PMID: 38298026

Chen, P.-J., Smits, L., Miranda, R., Liao, J.-Y., Petersen, I., Van den Block, L., & Sampson, E. L. (2022). Impact of home healthcare on end-of-life outcomes for people with dementia: A systematic review. *BMC Geriatrics*, *22*(1), 80. DOI: 10.1186/s12877-022-02768-3 PMID: 35081914

Chua, C. M. S., Ko, S. Q., Lai, Y. F., Lim, Y. W., & Shorey, S. (2022). Perceptions of hospital-at-home among stakeholders: A metasynthesis. *Journal of General Internal Medicine*, *37*(3), 637–650. DOI: 10.1007/s11606-021-07065-0 PMID: 34363185

Chwistek, M. (2020). "Are you wearing your white coat?": Telemedicine in the time of pandemic. *Journal of the American Medical Association*, *324*(2), 149–150. DOI: 10.1001/jama.2020.10619 PMID: 32584375

Cingolani, M., Scendoni, R., Fedeli, P., & Cembrani, F. (2023). Artificial intelligence and digital medicine for integrated home care services in Italy: Opportunities and limits. *Frontiers in Public Health*, *10*, 1095001. DOI: 10.3389/fpubh.2022.1095001 PMID: 36684935

Ciuffreda, I., Casaccia, S., & Revel, G. M. (2023). A multi-sensor fusion approach based on PIR and ultrasonic sensors installed on a robot to localise people in indoor environments. *Sensors (Basel)*, *23*(15), 6963. DOI: 10.3390/s23156963 PMID: 37571746

Clark, A. (2003). Artificial intelligence and the many faces of reason. In Stich, S., & Warfield, T. (Eds.), *The Blackwell guide to philosophy of mind* (pp. 309–321). Blackwell Publishing. DOI: 10.1002/9780470998762.ch13

Cloutier, A., Bond, A., Taylor, M. I., Ablett, J., Teubner, A., Farrer, K., Leahy, G., Abraham, A., & Lal, S. (2020). Successful implementation of remote video consultations for patients receiving home parenteral nutrition in a national UK Centre. *Frontline Gastroenterology*, *11*(4), 280–284. DOI: 10.1136/flgastro-2019-101257 PMID: 32587671

Collins, P. F., Huggins, C. E., Booth, A., & Banks, M. (2017). Telehealth dietetic consultation is effective for patients undergoing head and neck cancer treatment. *Journal of Nutrition and Dietetics*, *74*(1), 7–13. DOI: 10.1111/1747-0080.12345

Conway, S. (2016). Teleradiology and telemedicine: They are not equal. *Applied Radiology*, *45*(8), 28–29. https://appliedradiology.com/articles/teleradiology-and-telemedicine-they-are-not-equal. DOI: 10.37549/AR2289

Cortés, U., Annicchiarico, R., Campana, F., Vázquez-Salceda, J., Urdiales, C., Cañamero, L., López, M., Sànchez-Marrè, M., Di Vincenzo, S., & Caltagirone, C. (2004). Artificial intelligence in medicine: Project of a mobile platform in an intelligent environment for the care of disabled and elderly people. *Recenti Progressi in Medicina, 95*(4), 190–195. PMID: 15147063

Crevier, D. (1993). *AI: The tumultuous history of the search for artificial intelligence*. Basic Books.

Crivelli, A., Fabeiro, M., Puga, M., Dieguez, N., Giunta, L., Pochettino, F., Balacco, M., Merlo, G., Garrido, V., Fain, H., Buncuga, M., Martinuzzi, A., Cascarón, M. F., Delgado, N., Capurro, G., Bernardis, V., Ghiglieri, C., Hassam, A., Soria, O., & Fernandez, A. (2022). Care of patients on home parenteral nutrition during the first year of the COVID-19 pandemic: Management of central line-associated bloodstream infections. *Clinical Nutrition ESPEN, 52*, 250–253. DOI: 10.1016/j.clnesp.2022.11.003 PMID: 36513461

Cuerda, M. C., Apezetxea, A., Carrillo, L., Casanueva, F., Cuesta, F., Irles, J. A., Virgili, M., Layola, M., & Lizan, L. (2016). Development and validation of a specific questionnaire to assess health-related quality of life in patients with home enteral nutrition: NutriQoL®. *Patient Preference and Adherence, 10*, 2289–2296. DOI: 10.2147/PPA.S110188 PMID: 27853360

Curioni, C., Silva, A. C., Damião, J., Castro, A., Huang, M., Barroso, T., Araujo, D., & Guerra, R. (2023). The cost-effectiveness of homecare services for adults and older adults: A systematic review. *International Journal of Environmental Research and Public Health, 20*(4), 3373. DOI: 10.3390/ijerph20043373 PMID: 36834068

Czaja, S. J., Charness, N., Fisk, A. D., Hertzog, C., Nair, S. N., Rogers, W. A., & Sharit, J. (2006). Factors predicting the use of technology: Findings from the Center for Research and Education on Aging and Technology Enhancement (CREATE). *Psychology and Aging, 21*(2), 333–352. DOI: 10.1037/0882-7974.21.2.333 PMID: 16768579

Dailah, H. G., Koriri, M., Sabei, A., Kriry, T., & Zakri, M. (2024). Artificial intelligence in nursing: Technological benefits to nurse's mental health and patient care quality. *Health Care, 12*(24), 2555. DOI: 10.3390/healthcare12242555 PMID: 39765983

Danielsen, A., Olofsen, H., & Bremdal, B. A. (2016). Increasing fall risk awareness using wearables: A fall risk awareness protocol. *Journal of Biomedical Informatics, 63*, 184–194. DOI: 10.1016/j.jbi.2016.08.016 PMID: 27544413

Darrat, M., & Flaherty, G. T. (2019). Retrospective analysis of older travellers attending a specialist travel health clinic. *Tropical Diseases, Travel Medicine and Vaccines*, *5*(1), 17. DOI: 10.1186/s40794-019-0094-8 PMID: 31548898

Dartmouth College. (n.d.). *The Dartmouth Summer Research Project on Artificial Intelligence*. https://home.dartmouth.edu

Dash, S., Shakyawar, S. K., Sharma, M., & Kaushik, S. (2019). Big data in healthcare: Management, analysis and future prospects. *Journal of Big Data*, *6*(1), 54. DOI: 10.1186/s40537-019-0217-0

Davenport, T., & Kalakota, R. (2019). The potential for artificial intelligence in healthcare. *Future Healthcare Journal*, *6*(2), 94–98. DOI: 10.7861/futurehosp.6-2-94 PMID: 31363513

Davis, F. D. (1989). Perceived usefulness, perceived ease of use, and user acceptance of information technology. *Management Information Systems Quarterly*, *13*(3), 319–340. DOI: 10.2307/249008

Davis, K., Biddulph, R., & Balashek, S. (1952). Automatic recognition of spoken digits. *The Journal of the Acoustical Society of America*, *24*(6), 637–642. DOI: 10.1121/1.1906946

Debnath, D., Siddique, A. H., Hasan, M., Faisal, F., Karim, A., Azam, S., & De Boer, F. (2021). Smart electrification of rural Bangladesh through smart grids. In *Lecture notes on data engineering and communications technologies* (Vol. 62, pp. 41–55). Springer., DOI: 10.1007/978-981-15-8677-4_4

Dehury, C. K., & Sahoo, P. K. (2016). Design and implementation of a novel service management framework for IoT devices in cloud. *Journal of Systems and Software*, *119*, 149–161. DOI: 10.1016/j.jss.2016.06.059

Demiris, G., & Olson, S. (2010). Information technology and systems in home health care. In *The role of human factors in home health care: Workshop summary* (pp. 173–200). National Academies Press., DOI: 10.17226/12927

Deusdad, B. (2024). Ethical implications in using robots among older adults living with dementia. *Frontiers in Psychiatry*, *15*, 1436273. DOI: 10.3389/fpsyt.2024.1436273 PMID: 39391087

Dias, A., Santinha, G., Rodrigues, M., Queirós, A., Rodrigues, C., & Rocha, N. P. (2021). Smart cities and accessible tourism. In Augusto, J. C. (Ed.), *Handbook of smart cities* (pp. 96–114). Springer., DOI: 10.1007/978-3-030-69698-6_45

Dilbaz, B., Kaplanoğlu, M., & Kaya, D. (2020). Teletıp ve telesağlık: Geçmiş, bugün ve gelecek. *Eurasian Journal of Health Technology Assessment*, *4*(1), 40–56. DOI: 10.5281/zenodo.4321472

Ding, Y., Lin, Y., & Liu, Q. (2010). Developing an accessible transport network for accessible tourism in Beijing. In *TRANSED 2010: 12th International Conference on Mobility and Transport for Elderly and Disabled People*. Hong Kong Society for Rehabilitation; S. K. Yee Medical Foundation; Transportation Research Board.

Diwakar, R., Sharma, R., Nayak, D., & Mohapatra, H. (2025). Optimizing load distribution in big data ecosystems. In *AI and the revival of big data* (pp. 177–200). IGI Global., DOI: 10.4018/979-8-3693-8472-5.ch008

Doğramacı, Y. G. (2020). Telemedicine, health tourism and remote health services: Distance contracts. *İstanbul Hukuk Mecmuası, 78*(2), 657–710. DOI: 10.26650/ihm.2020.78.2.0008

Doi, K. (2007). Computer-aided diagnosis in medical imaging: Historical review, current status and future potential. *Computerized Medical Imaging and Graphics*, *31*(4–5), 198–211. DOI: 10.1016/j.compmedimag.2007.02.002 PMID: 17349778

Domínguez, J. A., Fraiz, J. A., & Alén, E. (2013). Economic profitability of accessible tourism for the tourism industry. *Journal of Tourism and Hospitality Management*, *1*(3), 84–100.

Dong, Y., Scisco, J., Wilson, M., Muth, E., & Hoover, A. (2014). Detecting periods of eating during free-living by tracking wrist motion. *IEEE Journal of Biomedical and Health Informatics*, *18*(4), 1253–1260. DOI: 10.1109/JBHI.2013.2282471 PMID: 24058042

Dorsey, E. R., & Topol, E. J. (2020). State of telehealth. *The New England Journal of Medicine*, *382*(18), 1670–1671. DOI: 10.1056/NEJMp2003107

Drews, W. (2008). A Web 2.0 tourism information system for accessible tourism. In P. O'Connor, W. Höpken, & U. Gretzel (Eds.), *Information and communication technologies in tourism 2008* (pp. 164–174). Springer. DOI: 10.1007/978-3-211-77280-5_15

Dreyfus, H. L. (1965). *Alchemy and artificial intelligence* (Report No. P-3244). RAND Corporation. https://www.rand.org/pubs/papers/P3244.html

Dreyfus, H. L. (1972). *What computers can't do: The limits of artificial intelligence*. Harper & Row.

Dubey, P., & Kumar, M. (2025). Integrating explainable AI with federated learning for next-generation IoT: A comprehensive review and prospective insights. *Computer Science Review*, *56*, 100697. DOI: 10.1016/j.cosrev.2024.100697

Dunn, R. (2019, January 15). 4 promising IoT use cases in agriculture. *IoT For All*. https://www.iotforall.com/4-iot-use-cases-agriculture/

Edirippulige, S., & Armfield, N. R. (2017). Education and training to support the use of clinical telehealth: A review of the literature. *Journal of Telemedicine and Telecare*, *23*(2), 273–282. DOI: 10.1177/1357633X16632968 PMID: 26892005

Eichhorn, V., Miller, G., Michopoulou, E., & Buhalis, D. (2008). Enabling disabled tourists? Accessibility tourism information schemes. *Annals of Tourism Research*, *35*(1), 189–210. DOI: 10.1016/j.annals.2007.07.005

Ekinci, B. (2022). Remote health service delivery (telemedicine) project. *Turkey Health Literacy Journal*, *3*(2), 122–124.

Ercan, F. (2022). Accessible tourism experiences in smart destinations: The case of Breda (Netherlands). In Öztürk, I. E. (Ed.), *Planning and managing the experience economy in tourism* (pp. 274–300). IGI Global., DOI: 10.4018/978-1-7998-8775-1.ch014

Erdelj, M., Król, M., & Natalizio, E. (2017). Wireless sensor networks and multi-UAV systems for natural disaster management. *Computer Networks*, *124*, 72–86. DOI: 10.1016/j.comnet.2017.05.021

Erdinc, O., Paterakis, N. G., Pappi, I. N., Bakirtzis, A. G., & Catalão, J. P. S. (2015). Optimal household appliances scheduling under day-ahead pricing and load-shaping demand response strategies. In *2015 48th Hawaii International Conference on System Sciences* (pp. 1462–1471). IEEE. DOI: 10.1109/HICSS.2015.178

Esteva, A., Kuprel, B., Novoa, R. A., Ko, J., Swetter, S. M., Blau, H. M., & Thrun, S. (2017). Dermatologist-level classification of skin cancer with deep neural networks. *Nature*, *542*(7639), 115–118. DOI: 10.1038/nature21056 PMID: 28117445

Euchi, J. (2021). Do drones have a realistic place in a pandemic fight for delivering medical supplies in healthcare systems problems? *Chinese Journal of Aeronautics*, *34*(2), 182–190. DOI: 10.1016/j.cja.2020.06.006

European Commission. (2021). *Proposal for a regulation of the European Parliament and of the Council laying down harmonised rules on artificial intelligence (Artificial Intelligence Act)*. https://eur-lex.europa.eu/legal-content/EN/TXT/?uri=CELEX%3A52021PC0206

European Parliamentary Technology Assessment. (2019). *Technologies in care for older people*. https://www.europarl.europa.eu/stoa/en/document/EPTA_Report_2019

Ewais, A. M., El-Azab, R., & Adma, M. A. R. (2018). Stand-alone microgrid energy storage schemes: Comparative study. In *2018 Twentieth International Middle East Power Systems Conference (MEPCON)* (pp. 564–569). IEEE. DOI: 10.1109/MEPCON.2018.8635266

Fang, K. Y., Ginige, J. A., Basilakis, J., Bjering, H., & Javadi, B. (2022). Smart homecare research translation into broader practice: Enablers, barriers and directions. *IEEE Access : Practical Innovations, Open Solutions*, *10*, 134726–134743. DOI: 10.1109/ACCESS.2022.3229871

Fathollahi-Fard, A. M., Ahmadi, A., & Karimi, B. (2022). Sustainable and robust home healthcare logistics: A response to the COVID-19 pandemic. *Symmetry*, *14*(2), 193. DOI: 10.3390/sym14020193

Federman, A. D., Soones, T., DeCherrie, L. V., Leff, B., & Siu, A. L. (2018). Association of a bundled hospital-at-home and 30-day postacute transitional care program with clinical outcomes and patient experiences. *JAMA Internal Medicine*, *178*(8), 1033–1040. DOI: 10.1001/jamainternmed.2018.2562 PMID: 29946693

Feigenbaum, E. A., & Feldman, J. (Eds.). (1963). *Computers and thought*. McGraw-Hill.

Ferlito, B., Segers, S., De Proost, M., & Mertes, H. (2024). Responsibility gap(s) due to the introduction of AI in healthcare: An Ubuntu-inspired approach. *Science and Engineering Ethics*, *30*(4), 34. DOI: 10.1007/s11948-024-00501-4 PMID: 39090479

Ferràs, X., Hitchen, E. L., Tarrats-Pons, E., & Serrat, N. (2020). Smart tourism empowered by artificial intelligence: The case of Lanzarote. *Journal of Cases on Information Technology*, *22*(1), 1–13. DOI: 10.4018/JCIT.2020010101

Ferst, M. D. C., & Coutinho, H. R. M. (2021). Impacts of training on perceptions of accessibility in tourism. *Revista Turismo em Análise*, *32*(1), 27–35. DOI: 10.14210/at.v6n1.p27-35

Ferst, M. D. C., dos Anjos, S. J. G., & Kuhn, V. (2023). Valuing accessibility in hospitality and the loyalty of tourists with disabilities. *Turismo: Visão e Ação*, *25*(2), 243–262. DOI: 10.14210/rtva.v25n2.p243-262

Fikes, R. E., & Nilsson, N. J. (1971). STRIPS: A new approach to the application of theorem proving to problem solving. *Artificial Intelligence*, *2*(3–4), 189–208. DOI: 10.1016/0004-3702(71)90010-5

Filipová, I., Dulina, Ľ., Bigošová, E., & Plinta, D. (2021). Modern possibilities of patient transport aids. *Transportation Research Procedia, 55*, 510–517. DOI: 10.1016/j.trpro.2021.07.015

Fortuna, J., Cantwell-Jurkovic, L., Dean, J., Fry, H., & Ross, S. (2024). Staff training on disability awareness in museum settings: A scoping review. *The American Journal of Occupational Therapy*, *78*(5, Supplement_2), 7805205060. DOI: 10.5014/ajot.2024.78S2-PO119 PMID: 39133619

Foster, K. R., & Torous, J. (2019). The opportunity and obstacles for smartwatches and wearable sensors. *IEEE Pulse*, *10*(1), 22–25. DOI: 10.1109/MPULS.2018.2885832 PMID: 30872210

Fradkin, A. (2017). *Search, matching, and the role of digital marketplace design in enabling trade: Evidence from Airbnb* (SSRN Scholarly Paper ID 2939084). Social Science Research Network. DOI: 10.2139/ssrn.2939084

Fraser, D. A. (2017). *Perceptions of risks and barriers to participation in tourism for the disabled* [Unpublished master's thesis]. University of Plymouth.

Free, C., Phillips, G., Watson, L., Galli, L., Felix, L., Edwards, P., Patel, V., & Haines, A. (2013). The effectiveness of mobile-health technologies to improve health care service delivery processes: A systematic review and meta-analysis. *PLoS Medicine*, *10*(1), e1001363. DOI: 10.1371/journal.pmed.1001363 PMID: 23458994

Freer, T. W., & Ulissey, M. J. (2001). Screening mammography with computer-aided detection: Prospective study of 12,860 patients in a community breast center. *Radiology*, *220*(3), 781–786. DOI: 10.1148/radiol.2203001282 PMID: 11526282

French, R. M. (2000). The Turing Test: The first fifty years. *Trends in Cognitive Sciences*, *4*(3), 115–122. DOI: 10.1016/S1364-6613(00)01453-4 PMID: 10689346

Fthenakis, V., & Kim, H. C. (2009). Land use and electricity generation: A life-cycle analysis. *Renewable & Sustainable Energy Reviews*, *13*(6–7), 1465–1474. DOI: 10.1016/j.rser.2008.09.017

Funao, H., Momosaki, R., Tsujikawa, M., Kawamoto, E., Esumi, R., & Shimaoka, M. (2024). Virtual reality–applied home-visit rehabilitation for patients with chronic pain: Protocol for single-arm pre-post comparison study. *JMIR Research Protocols*, *13*, e58734. DOI: 10.2196/58734 PMID: 39753216

Gajarawala, S. N., & Pelkowski, J. N. (2021). Telehealth benefits and barriers. *The Journal for Nurse Practitioners*, *17*(2), 218–221. DOI: 10.1016/j.nurpra.2020.09.013 PMID: 33106751

Galavi, Z., Montazeri, M., & Ahmadian, L. (2022). Barriers and challenges of using health information technology in home care: A systematic review. *The International Journal of Health Planning and Management*, *37*(5), 2542–2568. DOI: 10.1002/hpm.3492 PMID: 35643906

Galvão, D. A., Taaffe, D. R., Hayne, D., Lopez, P., Lyons-Wall, P., Tang, C. I., Chambers, S. K., Devine, A., Spry, N., Jeffery, E., Kudiarasu, C., Joseph, D., & Newton, R. U. (2022). Weight loss for overweight and obese patients with prostate cancer: A study protocol of a randomised trial comparing clinic-based versus Telehealth delivered exercise and nutrition intervention (the telex trial). *BMJ Open*, *12*(6), e058899. DOI: 10.1136/bmjopen-2021-058899 PMID: 35667725

Ganapathy, K. (2020). Space medicine: The ultimate in remote health care. *Telehealth and Medicine Today*, *5*(2), 1–4. DOI: 10.30953/tmt.v5.178

Gao, H., Xu, Y., Yin, Y., Zhang, W., Li, R., & Wang, X. (2020). Context-aware QoS prediction with neural collaborative filtering for Internet-of-Things services. *IEEE Internet of Things Journal*, *7*(5), 4532–4542. DOI: 10.1109/JIOT.2019.2956827

Gao, Z., & Patras, I. (2024). Self-supervised facial representation learning with facial region awareness. In *2024 IEEE/CVF Conference on Computer Vision and Pattern Recognition (CVPR)* (pp. 2081–2092). IEEE. DOI: 10.1109/CVPR52733.2024.00203

Garzotto, F., Comoretto, R. I., Ostermann, M., Nalesso, F., Gregori, D., Bonavina, M. G., Zanardo, G., & Meneghesso, G. (2021). Preventing infectious diseases in intensive care unit by medical devices remote control: Lessons from COVID-19. *Journal of Critical Care*, *61*, 119–124. DOI: 10.1016/j.jcrc.2020.10.014 PMID: 33157307

Gaydos, J. (2019). *Audio visual connection: Brief history of telemedicine*. HMP Global Learning Network. https://www.hmpgloballearningnetwork.com/site/twc/articles/audio-visual-connection-brief-history-telemedicine

Genet, N., Boerma, W. G. W., Kringos, D. S., Bouman, A., Francke, A. L., Fagerström, C., Melchiorre, M. G., Greco, C., & Devillé, W. (2011). Home care in Europe: A systematic literature review. *BMC Health Services Research*, *11*(1), 207. DOI: 10.1186/1472-6963-11-207 PMID: 21878111

Gibson, G. R., & Roberfroid, M. B. (1995). Dietary modulation of the human colonic microbiota: Introducing the concept of prebiotics. *The Journal of Nutrition*, *125*(6), 1401–1412. DOI: 10.1093/jn/125.6.1401 PMID: 7782892

Gillespie, L. D., Robertson, M. C., Gillespie, W. J., Sherrington, C., Gates, S., Clemson, L., & Lamb, S. E. (2012). Interventions for preventing falls in older people living in the community. *Cochrane Database of Systematic Reviews*, *9*(6), CD007146. DOI: 10.1002/14651858.CD007146.pub3 PMID: 22972103

Gillies, R. J., Kinahan, P. E., & Hricak, H. (2016). Radiomics: Images are more than pictures, they are data. *Radiology*, *278*(2), 563–577. DOI: 10.1148/radiol.2015151169 PMID: 26579733

Gilmour, H. (2018). Unmet home care needs in Canada. *Health Reports*, *29*(11), 3–11. PMID: 30485384

Göde, A. (2023). Uzaktan sağlık hizmetlerinin yeri ve geleceği. [The place and future of remote health services] In Söyler, S., & Çavmak, D. (Eds.), *Modern sağlık yönetiminde temel konular* (pp. 183–201). Eğitim Publishing House.

Gökalp, E., Gökalp, M. O., Çoban, S., & Eren, P. E. (2018). Analysing opportunities and challenges of integrated blockchain technologies in healthcare. In S. Wrycza & J. Maślankowski (Eds.), *Information systems: Research, development, applications, education: 11th SIGSAND/PLAIS EuroSymposium 2018* (Lecture Notes in Business Information Processing, Vol. 333, pp. 174–183). Springer. DOI: 10.1007/978-3-030-00060-8_13

Goldrick, M. R., & Gethin, G. T. (2021). Patients' perceptions of, and acceptance toward, using wearable sensor technology in wound care. *Journal of Wound Management*, *22*(1), 13–26. DOI: 10.35279/jowm2021.22.01.04

Götz, F., Reelitz, C., Buck, C., Eymann, T., & Meckl, R. (2022). Potentials of digital business ecosystems in the healthcare market. In Mehdi Khosrow-Pour, D. B. A. (Ed.), *Handbook on digital business ecosystems* (pp. 662–679). Edward Elgar Publishing., DOI: 10.4337/9781839107191.00051

Graboyes, R. F., Bryan, D. S., & Coglianese, J. (2020). Overcoming technological and policy challenges to medical uses of unmanned aerial vehicles. *Mercatus Research Paper*. DOI: 10.2139/ssrn.3561743

Grand View Research. (2025). *Remote healthcare market size, share & trends analysis report*. https://www.grandviewresearch.com/industry-analysis/remote-healthcare-market

Greenblatt, R. D., Eastlake, D. E.III, & Crocker, S. D. (1967). The Greenblatt chess program. *Proceedings of the* November 14–16, 1967, *Fall Joint Computer Conference*, 801–810. DOI: 10.1145/1465611.1465715

Grudin, J. (2018). From tool to partner: The evolution of human-computer interaction. In *Extended Abstracts of the 2018 CHI Conference on Human Factors in Computing Systems* (pp. 1–3). ACM. DOI: 10.1145/3170427.3174358

Gu, D., Humbatova, G., Xie, Y., Yang, X., Zolotarev, O., & Zhang, G. (2021). Different roles of telehealth and telemedicine on medical tourism: An empirical study from Azerbaijan. *Health Care*, *9*(8), 1073. DOI: 10.3390/healthcare9081073 PMID: 34442210

Güdük, Ö. (2025). Telehealth applications in home health services: A bibliometric analysis. *Türkiye Aile Hekimligi Dergisi*, *29*(1), 20–35. DOI: 10.54308/turkjfampract.2025.811

Gulshan, V., Peng, L., Coram, M., Stumpe, M. C., Wu, D., Narayanaswamy, A., Venugopalan, S., Widner, K., Madams, T., Cuadros, J., Kim, R., Raman, R., Nelson, P. C., Mega, J. L., & Webster, D. R. (2016). Development and validation of a deep learning algorithm for detection of diabetic retinopathy in retinal fundus photographs. *Journal of the American Medical Association*, *316*(22), 2402–2410. DOI: 10.1001/jama.2016.17216 PMID: 27898976

Guo, B., Dong, B., Zhang, X., Yang, J., & Wang, Z. (2015). Research on home healthcare management system based on the improved Internet of Things architecture. *International Journal of Smart Home*, *9*(9), 51–62. DOI: 10.14257/ijsh.2015.9.9.06

Haanes, G. G. (2023). Multidisciplinary approaches and community-based interventions: Adaptable strategies for managing sensory impairments in older adults. *Journal of Multidisciplinary Healthcare*, *16*, 2701–2705. DOI: 10.2147/JMDH.S416762 PMID: 37724317

Hadiprawoto, T. R., & Ridley, A. L. (2023). Transparent dashboards: Open data practices for promoting competition-as-motivation in business dashboards. In *2023 IEEE 16th Pacific Visualization Symposium (PacificVis)* (pp. 142–146). IEEE. DOI: 10.1109/PacificVis56936.2023.00023

Haghi, M., Spicher, N., Wang, J., & Deserno, T. M. (2022). Integrated sensing devices for disease prevention and health alerts in smart homes. *Studies in Health Technology and Informatics*, *291*, 39–61. DOI: 10.3233/SHTI220007 PMID: 35593757

Haidari, L. A., Brown, S. T., Ferguson, M., Bancroft, E., Spiker, M., Wilcox, A., Ambikapathi, R., Sampath, V., Connor, D. L., & Lee, B. Y. (2016). The economic and operational value of using drones to transport vaccines. *Vaccine*, *34*(34), 4062–4067. DOI: 10.1016/j.vaccine.2016.06.022 PMID: 27340098

Hall, B. T., Englehart, M. S., Blaseg, K., Wessel, K., Stawicki, S. P. A., & Evans, D. C. (2014). Implementation of a dietitian-led enteral nutrition support clinic results in quality improvement, reduced readmissions, and cost savings. *Nutrition in Clinical Practice*, *29*(5), 649–655. DOI: 10.1177/0884533614538285 PMID: 25606646

Hall, J. L., & McGraw, D. (2014). For telehealth to succeed, privacy and security risks must be identified and addressed. *Health Affairs*, *33*(2), 216–221. DOI: 10.1377/hlthaff.2013.0997 PMID: 24493763

Hamari, J., Koivisto, J., & Sarsa, H. (2014). Does gamification work? A literature review of empirical studies on gamification. In *2014 47th Hawaii International Conference on System Sciences* (pp. 3025–3034). IEEE. DOI: 10.1109/HICSS.2014.377

Hamblin, K., Burns, D., & Goodlad, C. (2025). Technology and homecare in the UK: Policy, storylines and practice. *Journal of Social Policy*, *54*(2), 412–428. DOI: 10.1017/S0047279423000156

Hapsari, A. A., Vresdian, D. J., Dionova, B. W., Zuhriyah, H., Pratama, L. P., & Islami, A. Y. (2024). A systematic review of drone development and innovation helps handling during a pandemic and its challenges for health technology. *Jurnal Teknologi dan Manajemen, 22*(2), 1–10. DOI: 10.52330/jtm.v22i2.246

Hasan, M., Anik, M. H., & Islam, S. (2018). Microgrid energy management system for residential microgrid. In *2018 Fifth HCT Information Technology Trends (ITT)* (pp. 364–367). IEEE. DOI: 10.1109/CTIT.2018.8649518

Hasan, N., & Ahmed, M. F. (2024). Wearable technology for elderly care: Integrating health monitoring and emergency alerts. *Journal of Computer Networks and Communications*, *2024*(1), 5593708. DOI: 10.1155/jcnc/5593708

Haselkorn, A., Coye, M. J., & Doarn, C. R. (2007). The future of remote health services: Summary of an expert panel discussion. *Telemedicine Journal and e-Health*, *13*(3), 341–347. DOI: 10.1089/tmj.2006.0078 PMID: 17603837

Hashimoto, D. A., Rosman, G., Rus, D., & Meireles, O. R. (2018). Artificial intelligence in surgery: Promises and perils. *Annals of Surgery*, *268*(1), 70–76. DOI: 10.1097/SLA.0000000000002693 PMID: 29389679

Hays, R. D., & Skootsky, S. A. (2022). Patient experience with in-person and telehealth visits before and during the COVID-19 pandemic at a large integrated health system in the United States. *Journal of General Internal Medicine*, *37*(4), 847–852. DOI: 10.1007/s11606-021-07196-4 PMID: 34982370

Health Resources & Services Administration. (2022). *What is telehealth?* https://www.hrsa.gov/telehealth/what-is-telehealth

HealthSnap. (2024). *The evolution of remote care management.* https://healthsnap.io/the-evolution-of-remote-care-management/

Helal, S., Mokhtari, M., & Abdulrazak, B. (Eds.). (2008). *The engineering handbook of smart technology for aging, disability, and independence.* John Wiley & Sons., DOI: 10.1002/9780470379424

Hennig, S., Sattler, T., Wasserburger, W., & Wasserburger, M. (2015). How to improve accessibility of natural areas: About the relevance of providing information on accessible services and facilities in natural areas. In M. Schrenk, V. V. Popovich, P. Zeile, P. Elisei, & C. Beyer (Eds.), *PLANNING TIMES – You better keep planning or you get in trouble: Proceedings of 19th International Conference on Urban Planning, Regional Development and Information Society* (pp. 803–812). CORP.

Heratanti, N., Rambi, A. P., & Syarifurrahman, I. (2021). The telehealth effectiveness in home care services: A systematic review. *STRADA Jurnal Ilmiah Kesehatan, 10*(1), 1057–1065. DOI: 10.30994/sjik.v10i1.761

Herbert, J., Schumacher, T., Brown, L. J., Clarke, E. D., & Collins, C. E. (2023). Delivery of telehealth nutrition and physical activity interventions to adults living in rural areas: A scoping review. *The International Journal of Behavioral Nutrition and Physical Activity, 20*(1), 110. DOI: 10.1186/s12966-023-01505-2 PMID: 37715234

Herzfeld, N. (2016). Human and artificial intelligence: A theological response. In *Human identity at the intersection of science, technology and religion* (pp. 117–130). Routledge., DOI: 10.4324/9781315587431-7

Hincapié, M. A., Gallego, J. C., Gempeler, A., Piñeros, J. A., Nasner, D., & Escobar, M. F. (2020). Implementation and usefulness of telemedicine during the COVID-19 pandemic: A scoping review. *Journal of Primary Care & Community Health, 11*, 2150132720980612. DOI: 10.1177/2150132720980612 PMID: 33300414

Hinchliffe, N., Capehorn, M. S., Bewick, M., & Feenie, J. (2022). The potential role of digital health in obesity care. *Advances in Therapy, 39*(10), 4397–4412. DOI: 10.1007/s12325-022-02265-4 PMID: 35925469

Hosny, A., Parmar, C., Quackenbush, J., Schwartz, L. H., & Aerts, H. J. W. L. (2018). Artificial intelligence in radiology. *Nature Reviews. Cancer, 18*(8), 500–510. DOI: 10.1038/s41568-018-0016-5 PMID: 29777175

Hossain, M. N. A., Pal, A., & Hossain, S. K. A. (2015). A wearable sensor based elderly home care system in a smart environment. In *2015 18th International Conference on Computer and Information Technology (ICCIT)* (pp. 329–334). IEEE. DOI: 10.1109/ICCITechn.2015.7488091

Hu, Y., Hu, W., & Quigley, A. (2024). Towards enhanced context awareness with vision-based multimodal interfaces. In *MobileHCI '24: Proceedings of the 26th International Conference on Mobile Human-Computer Interaction* (Article 24, pp. 1–3). ACM. DOI: 10.1145/3640471.3686646

Huang, Y., Hsieh, M.-Y., Chao, H.-C., Hung, S.-H., & Park, J. H. (2009). Pervasive, secure access to a hierarchical sensor-based healthcare monitoring architecture in wireless heterogeneous networks. *IEEE Journal on Selected Areas in Communications, 27*(4), 400–411. DOI: 10.1109/JSAC.2009.090505

Hussain, A., Wenbi, R., da Silva, A. L., Nadher, M., & Mudhish, M. (2015). Health and emergency-care platform for the elderly and disabled people in the Smart City. *Journal of Systems and Software, 110*, 253–263. DOI: 10.1016/j.jss.2015.08.041

Hwei, L. R. Y., & Octavius, G. S. (2021). Potential advantages and disadvantages of telemedicine: A literature review from the perspectives of patients, medical personnel, and hospitals. *Journal of Community Empowerment for Health, 4*(3), 180–186. DOI: 10.22146/jcoemph.64247

Iansiti, M., & Levien, R. (2004). Strategy as ecology. *Harvard Business Review, 82*(3), 68–78. PMID: 15029791

IBM. (n.d.). *The history of artificial intelligence*. https://www.ibm.com/artificial-intelligence/ai-history

İnaç, R. Ç., & Ekmekçi, İ. (2023). Analysis of home healthcare practice to improve service quality: Case study of megacity Istanbul. *Health Care, 11*(3), 319. DOI: 10.3390/healthcare11030319 PMID: 36766894

Institute of Medicine. (1996). *Telemedicine: A guide to assessing telecommunications in health care*. National Academies Press., DOI: 10.17226/5296

Iqbal, O., Iftakhar, T., & Ahmad, S. Z. (2022). Internet of Things for in-home health based monitoring system: Modern advances, challenges and future directions. *Journal on Internet of Things, 4*(1), 35–55. DOI: 10.32604/jiot.2022.022256

Islam, S. M. R., Kwak, D., Kabir, M. H., Hossain, M., & Kwak, K.-S. (2015). The Internet of Things for health care: A comprehensive survey. *IEEE Access : Practical Innovations, Open Solutions, 3*, 678–708. DOI: 10.1109/ACCESS.2015.2437951

Ivanova, M., & Senkiv, G. (2019). Accessible tourism for all in the European Union. *International Journal of Scientific Research and Management, 7*(2), 87–93. DOI: 10.17721/1728-2721.2019.74.12

Iyawa, G. E., Herselman, M., & Botha, A. (2016). Digital health innovation ecosystems: From systematic literature review to conceptual framework. *Procedia Computer Science*, *100*, 244–252. DOI: 10.1016/j.procs.2016.09.149

Jaakkola, H., Henno, J., Mäkelä, J., & Thalheim, B. (2019). Artificial intelligence yesterday, today and tomorrow. In *2019 42nd International Convention on Information and Communication Technology, Electronics and Microelectronics (MIPRO)* (pp. 860–867). IEEE. DOI: 10.23919/MIPRO.2019.8756913

Jacobides, M. G., Cennamo, C., & Gawer, A. (2018). Towards a theory of ecosystems. *Strategic Management Journal*, *39*(8), 2255–2276. DOI: 10.1002/smj.2904

Jalil, S., Bache, S., & Lin, X. (2019). Complementing a clinical trial with human–computer interaction: Patients' user experience with telehealth. *JMIR Human Factors*, *6*(2), e11458. DOI: 10.2196/humanfactors.9481 PMID: 31172958

Javed, I. T., Alharbi, F., Bellaj, B., Margaria, T., Crespi, N., & Qureshi, K. N. (2021). Health-ID: A blockchain-based decentralized identity management for remote healthcare. *Health Care*, *9*(6), 712. DOI: 10.3390/healthcare9060712 PMID: 34200778

Jeri, A., Lambert, K., Mak, M., & Diamantes, M. (2023). Lessons learnt from rapid implementation of telehealth in a paediatric dietetics' outpatient service: Is there a silver lining beyond the coronavirus pandemic to support patient-centred care? *Dietetics*, *2*(3), 267–277. DOI: 10.3390/dietetics2030019

Jha, D., Durak, G., Sharma, V., Keles, E., Cicek, V., Zhang, Z., & Bagci, U. (2025). A conceptual framework for applying ethical principles of AI to medical practice. *Bioengineering (Basel, Switzerland)*, *12*(2), 180. DOI: 10.3390/bioengineering12020180 PMID: 40001699

Jiang, F., Jiang, Y., Zhi, H., Dong, Y., Li, H., Ma, S., Wang, Y., Dong, Q., Shen, H., & Wang, Y. (2017). Artificial intelligence in healthcare: Past, present and future. *Stroke and Vascular Neurology*, *2*(4), 230–243. DOI: 10.1136/svn-2017-000101 PMID: 29507784

Jo, H., Kim, S., & Joo, S. (2013). Smart heating and air conditioning scheduling method incorporating customer convenience for home energy management system. *IEEE Transactions on Consumer Electronics*, *59*(2), 316–322. DOI: 10.1109/TCE.2013.6531112

Johnson, R., & Kent, S. (2007). Designing universal access: Web-applications for the elderly and disabled. *Cognition Technology and Work*, *9*(4), 209–218. DOI: 10.1007/s10111-007-0063-2

Jordanova, M., & Lievens, F. (2011). Global telemedicine and eHealth: A synopsis. In *2011 E-Health and Bioengineering Conference (EHB)* (pp. 1–6). IEEE. DOI: 10.1109/EHB.2011.6107668

Jumper, J., Evans, R., Pritzel, A., Green, T., Figurnov, M., Ronneberger, O., Tunyasuvunakool, K., Bates, R., Žídek, A., Potapenko, A., Bridgland, A., Meyer, C., Kohl, S. A. A., Ballard, A. J., Cowie, A., Romera-Paredes, B., Nikolov, S., Jain, R., Adler, J., & Hassabis, D. (2021). Highly accurate protein structure prediction with AlphaFold. *Nature, 596*(7873), 583–589. DOI: 10.1038/s41586-021-03819-2 PMID: 34265844

Kaganek, K., Ambroży, T., Mucha, D., Jurczak, A., Bornikowska, A., Ostrowski, A., Janiszewska, R., & Mucha, T. (2017). Barriers to participation in tourism in the disabled. *Polish Journal of Sport and Tourism, 24*(3), 121–129. DOI: 10.1515/pjst-2017-0013

Kamanzi, G. N. (2024). Improved access to healthcare, remote monitoring of joint function, and increased patient engagement in managing arthritis symptoms: The role of telehealth in arthritis care. *IDOSR Journal of Scientific Research, 9*(1), 12–24. DOI: 10.59298/IDOSRJSR/2024/9.3.434700

Kamyabi, M., & Alipour, H. (2022). An investigation of the challenges faced by the disabled population and the implications for accessible tourism. *Sustainability (Basel), 14*(8), 4702. DOI: 10.3390/su14084702

Kane, A. (2025). Navigating the transition: Challenges and benefits of shifting from IPv4 to IPv6 in a rapidly evolving internet landscape. *International Journal of Internet and Distributed Systems, 7*(2), 15–26. DOI: 10.4236/ijids.2025.72002

Kang, H. J., Kim, S., & Lee, H. (2019). An ecological approach to smart homes for healthcare services: Conceptual framework of a smart servicescape wheel. *JMIR mHealth and uHealth, 7*(2), e12425. DOI: 10.2196/12425 PMID: 30735145

Kastenholz, E., Eusébio, C., & Figueiredo, E. (2015). Contributions of tourism to social inclusion of people with disability. *Disability & Society, 30*(8), 1259–1281. DOI: 10.1080/09687599.2015.1075868

Keesara, S., Jonas, A., & Schulman, K. (2020). Covid-19 and health care's digital revolution. *The New England Journal of Medicine, 382*(23), e82. DOI: 10.1056/NEJMp2005835 PMID: 32240581

Kelly, J. T., Allman-Farinelli, M., Chen, J., Partridge, S. R., Collins, C., Rollo, M., Haslam, R., Diversi, T., & Campbell, K. L. (2020). Dietitians Australia position statement on telehealth. *Nutrition & Dietetics: the Journal of the Dietitians Association of Australia*, *77*(4), 406–415. DOI: 10.1111/1747-0080.12619 PMID: 32596950

Kelly, J. T., Collins, P. F., McCamley, J., Ball, L., Roberts, S., & Campbell, K. L. (2021). Digital disruption of dietetics: Are we ready? *Journal of Human Nutrition and Dietetics*, *34*(1), 134–146. DOI: 10.1111/jhn.12827 PMID: 33108029

Kelly, J. T., Law, L., Guzman, K. D., Hickman, I. J., Mayr, H., Campbell, K. L., & Erku, D. A. (2022). Are telehealth-delivered nutrition care interventions cost-effective for managing chronic diseases? a systematic review of all payer perspectives. *Current Developments in Nutrition*, *6*, 842. DOI: 10.1093/cdn/nzac065.026

Kelly, J. T., Law, L., Guzman, K. R. D., Hickman, I. J., Mayr, H. L., Campbell, K. L., & Erku, D. A. (2023). Cost-effectiveness of telehealth-delivered nutrition interventions: A systematic review of randomized controlled trials. *Nutrition Reviews*, *81*(12), 1599–1611. DOI: 10.1093/nutrit/nuad032 PMID: 37016937

Khan, M., Manduchi, B., Rodríguez, V., Fitch, M., Barbon, C., McMillan, H., Hutcheson, K. A., & Martino, R. (2022). Exploring patient experiences with a telehealth approach for the pro-active trial intervention in head and neck cancer patients. *BMC Health Services Research*, *22*(1), 1218. DOI: 10.1186/s12913-022-08554-6 PMID: 36180905

Kim, S. J., Lim, G. J., Cho, J., & Côté, M. J. (2017). Drone-aided healthcare services for patients with chronic diseases in rural areas. *Journal of Intelligent & Robotic Systems*, *88*(1), 163–180. DOI: 10.1007/s10846-017-0548-z

Kim, S., Zhang, Y., Mauldin, K., & Limketkai, B. N. (2024). Advances in Digital Health for Gastrointestinal Nutrition. *Current Treatment Options in Cardiovascular Medicine*, *22*(4), 267–278. DOI: 10.1007/s11938-024-00458-0

Klimova, B. (2019). Exploring eLearning for dementia care. In J. J. Park, L. T. Yang, Y. S. Jeong, & F. Hao (Eds.), *Advanced multimedia and ubiquitous engineering* (Lecture Notes in Electrical Engineering, Vol. 518, pp. 341–346). Springer. DOI: 10.1007/978-981-13-1328-8_44

Koçaş, M. (2022). Sağlık hizmetleri ve yönetiminde Nesnelerin İnterneti. In Yeşilyurt, Ö. (Ed.), *Sağlık yönetiminde yenilikçi yaklaşımlar* (pp. 19–37). Efeakademi Yayınları.

Ko, M., Azzopardi, M., Loizou, C., Logeswaran, A., Ng, B., Pacho, A., & Chong, Y. J. (2025). Telehealth and people with disabilities in the United Kingdom: A scoping review. *Frontiers in Public Health, 13*, 1433755. DOI: 10.3389/fpubh.2025.1504318 PMID: 40013026

Kosinski, K., Bucher, G., Szczerba, P., Weiss, E., Burch, C., & Chan, P. (2025). Exploring robotic solutions for home health care: A research study on robot assistants in home health-care delivery. *Mental Health and Digital Technologies*. DOI: 10.1108/MHDT-12-2024-0083

Kraśnik, W., Jankowska, O., Kurzeja, J., Piotrowicz, K., Piotrowicz, H., Bajkacz, A., Rogala, A., & Osmólska, J. (2024). The benefits and challenges of virtual reality application in rehabilitation for chronic conditions. *Journal of Education, Health and Sport, 75*, 56379–56379. DOI: 10.12775/JEHS.2024.75.56379

Krupinski, E. A., & Bernard, J. (2014). Standards and guidelines in telemedicine and telehealth. *Health Care, 2*(1), 74–93. DOI: 10.3390/healthcare2010074 PMID: 27429261

Kruse, C. S., Krowski, N., Rodriguez, B., Tran, L., Vela, J., & Brooks, M. (2017). Telehealth and patient satisfaction: A systematic review and narrative analysis. *BMJ Open, 7*(8), e016242. DOI: 10.1136/bmjopen-2017-016242 PMID: 28775188

Kruse, C. S., Soma, M., Pulluri, D., Nemali, N. T., & Brooks, M. (2017). The effectiveness of telemedicine in the management of chronic heart disease—A systematic review. *JRSM Open, 8*(3), 2054270416681747. DOI: 10.1177/2054270416681747 PMID: 28321319

Kulikowski, C. A. (2019). Beginnings of artificial intelligence in medicine (AIM): Computational artifice assisting scientific inquiry and clinical art—With reflections on present AIM challenges. *Yearbook of Medical Informatics, 28*(1), 249–256. DOI: 10.1055/s-0039-1677895 PMID: 31022744

Kumar, S., Mohapatra, H., & Dalai, A. K. (2024). Enhancing energy efficiency in wireless sensor networks via clustering approach. In *2024 4th International Conference on Artificial Intelligence and Signal Processing (AISP)* (pp. 1–6). IEEE. DOI: 10.1109/AISP61711.2024.10870799

Kumar, N. M., & Mallick, P. K. (2018). Blockchain technology for security issues and challenges in IoT. *Procedia Computer Science, 132*, 1815–1823. DOI: 10.1016/j.procs.2018.05.140

Kutlusoy, Z. (2019). Felsefe açısından yapay zeka. [Artificial intelligence from a philosophical perspective] In Telli, G. (Ed.), *Yapay zeka ve gelecek* (pp. 25–43). Doğu Kitapevi.

Ku, W., Lim, S. S., Look, K. S., & Tan, W. H. (2019). Investigating tourists' behavioral intentions using stimulus-organism-response theory. *Asia Pacific Journal of Tourism Research*, *24*(7), 689–702. DOI: 10.1080/10941665.2019.1622638

Kvedar, J. C., Fogel, A. L., Elenko, E., & Zohar, D. (2016). Digital medicine's march on chronic disease. *Nature Biotechnology*, *34*(3), 239–246. DOI: 10.1038/nbt.3495 PMID: 26963544

Kyung, R., & Park, C. S. (2020). How artificial intelligence and virtual reality benefit the elderly and individuals with disabilities. *Journal of Gerontology and Medicine*, *1*(2), 1–7. DOI: 10.30564/jgm.v1i2.1824

Lakhwani, T. S., Sinjana, Y., & Kapoor, A. P. (2025). Beyond numbers: A novel IoT and drone framework for enhancing healthcare logistics. *Discover Health Systems*, *4*(1), 19. DOI: 10.1007/s44250-025-00187-w

Lal, S., Van Gossum, A., Joly, F., Bozzetti, F., Cuerda, C., Lamprecht, G., Mundi, M. S., Staun, M., Szczepanek, K., Wanten, G., Wheatley, C., & Pironi, L. (2020). Considerations for the management of home parenteral nutrition during the SARS-CoV-2 pandemic: A position paper from the Home Artificial Nutrition and Chronic Intestinal Failure Special Interest Group of ESPEN. *Clinical Nutrition (Edinburgh, Lothian)*, *39*(7), 1988–1991. DOI: 10.1016/j.clnu.2020.05.023 PMID: 32487434

Lawrence, J., Truong, D., Dao, A., & Bryant, P. A. (2023). Virtual hospital-level care—Feasibility, acceptability, safety and impact of a pilot hospital-in-the-home model for COVID-19 infection. *Frontiers in Digital Health*, *5*, 1068444. DOI: 10.3389/fdgth.2023.1068444 PMID: 37090066

LeCun, Y., Bengio, Y., & Hinton, G. (2015). Deep learning. *Nature*, *521*(7553), 436–444. DOI: 10.1038/nature14539 PMID: 26017442

Ledley, R. S., & Lusted, L. B. (1959). Reasoning foundations of medical diagnosis. *Science*, *130*(3366), 9–21. DOI: 10.1126/science.130.3366.9 PMID: 13668531

Lee, W., Cho, S., Chu, P., Vu, H., Helal, S., Song, W., Jeong, Y., & Cho, K. (2016). Automatic agent generation for IoT-based smart house simulator. *Neurocomputing*, *209*, 14–24. DOI: 10.1016/j.neucom.2015.04.130

Lei, M., Shiyan, L., Chuanwen, J., Hongling, L., & Yan, Z. (2009). A review on the forecasting of wind speed and generated power. *Renewable & Sustainable Energy Reviews*, *13*(4), 915–920. DOI: 10.1016/j.rser.2008.02.002

Levesque, H. J. (2017). *Common sense, the Turing Test, and the quest for real AI.* MIT Press. DOI: 10.7551/mitpress/10909.001.0001

Li, X., & Xu, Y. (2022). Role of human-computer interaction healthcare system in the teaching of physiology and medicine. *Computational Intelligence and Neuroscience, 2022*, Article 5849736. (Retraction published *Computational Intelligence and Neuroscience, 2023*, Article 9812579. https://doi.org/)DOI: 10.1155/2022/5849736

Li, Y., Zhang, Y., & Lv, B. (2017). A health monitoring system based on wearable equipment. *MATEC Web of Conferences, 139*, Article 00164. DOI: 10.1051/matecconf/201713900164

Liasidou, S., Umbelino, J., & Panão, M. J. (2019). Revisiting tourism studies curriculum to highlight accessible tourism issues. *European Journal of Tourism Research, 21*, 103–106. DOI: 10.54055/ejtr.v21i.357

Li, C. Z., & Borycki, E. M.Li Cindy ZhiruiBorycki Elizabeth M. (2019). Smart homes for healthcare. *Studies in Health Technology and Informatics*, *257*, 283–287. DOI: 10.3233/978-1-61499-951-5-283 PMID: 30741210

Lighthill, J. (1973). Artificial intelligence: A general survey. In *Artificial intelligence: A paper symposium* (pp. 1–20). Science Research Council.

Li, K. F. (2013). Smart home technology for telemedicine and emergency management. *Journal of Ambient Intelligence and Humanized Computing*, *4*(5), 535–546. DOI: 10.1007/s12652-012-0129-8 PMID: 32218875

Limketkai, B. N., Mauldin, K., Manitius, N., Jalilian, L., & Salonen, B. R. (2021). The age of artificial intelligence: Use of digital technology in clinical nutrition. *Current Surgery Reports*, *9*(7), 20. DOI: 10.1007/s40137-021-00297-3 PMID: 34123579

Lim, L. J., Tison, G. H., & Delling, F. N. (2020). Artificial intelligence in cardiovascular imaging. *Methodist DeBakey Cardiovascular Journal, 16*(2), 138–145. DOI: 10.14797/mdcj-16-2-138 PMID: 32670474

Lin, G., Li, J. Y., Fazly, A., Pavlovic, V., & Truong, K. (2023). Identifying multimodal context awareness requirements for supporting user interaction with procedural videos. In *CHI '23: Proceedings of the 2023 CHI Conference on Human Factors in Computing Systems* (Article 186, pp. 1–17). ACM. DOI: 10.1145/3544548.3581006

Lin, K. Y., Chang, K. H., Lin, Y. W., & Wu, M. J. (2025). Exploring key considerations for artificial intelligence robots in home healthcare using the unified theory of acceptance and use of technology and the fuzzy analytical hierarchy process method. *Systems*, *13*(1), 25. DOI: 10.3390/systems13010025

Lister, C., West, J. H., Cannon, B., Sax, T., & Brodegard, D. (2014). Just a fad? Gamification in health and fitness: A systematic review. *JMIR Serious Games*, *2*(2), e9. DOI: 10.2196/games.3413 PMID: 25654660

Liu, L., Stroulia, E., Nikolaidis, I., Miguel-Cruz, A., & Rios Rincon, A. (2016). Smart homes and home health monitoring technologies for older adults: A systematic review. *International Journal of Medical Informatics*, *91*, 44–59. DOI: 10.1016/j.ijmedinf.2016.04.007 PMID: 27185508

Lodwick, G. S., Haun, C. L., Smith, W. E., Keller, R. F., & Robertson, E. D. (1963). Computer diagnosis of primary bone tumors: A preliminary report. *Radiology*, *80*(2), 273–275. DOI: 10.1148/80.2.273

Luccio, F. L., & Beltrame, L. (2018). Accessible tourism for users with hearing loss. In *Proceedings of the 4th EAI International Conference on Smart Objects and Technologies for Social Good* (pp. 243–248). ACM. DOI: 10.1145/3284869.3284909

Lyapina, M., & Kisselova-Yaneva, A. (2017). Why new regulations of the European Parliament on medical devices are needed. *Medical Informatics*, *4*(1), 591–596. DOI: 10.18044/Medinform.201741.591

Madsen, C., Poropatich, R., & Koehlmoos, T. P. (2023). Telehealth in the Military Health System: Impact, obstacles, and opportunities. *Military Medicine*, *188*(Supplement_1), 15–23. DOI: 10.1093/milmed/usac207 PMID: 36882030

Maelen, C. V., Lievens, E., Vermeulen, J., & Milkaite, I. (2021). AI and data protection: The case of smart home assistants. In *Artificial intelligence and the law* (pp. 173–206). Intersentia., DOI: 10.1017/9781839701047.009

Magade, K., & Sharma, A. (2024). Significant role of IoT in cyber-physical systems, context awareness, and ambient intelligence. In *The next generation innovation in IoT and cloud computing with applications* (pp. 16–34). CRC Press., DOI: 10.1201/9781003406723-2

Mahmoudzadeh, M., & Sarjaz, M. B. (2018). Environmental barriers to tourism development for people with disabilities. *Tourism Planning & Development*, *15*(3), 288–305. DOI: 10.1080/21568316.2017.1331252

Mandel, J. C., Kreda, D. A., Mandl, K. D., Kohane, I. S., & Ramoni, R. B. (2016). SMART on FHIR: A standards-based, interoperable apps platform for electronic health records. *Journal of the American Medical Informatics Association : JAMIA*, *23*(5), 899–908. DOI: 10.1093/jamia/ocv189 PMID: 26911829

Mangone, E. R., Agarwal, S., L'Engle, K., Lasway, C., Zan, T., van Beijma, H., Orkis, J., & Karam, R. (2016). Sustainable cost models for mHealth at scale: Modeling program data from m4RH Tanzania. *PLoS One*, *11*(1), e0148011. DOI: 10.1371/journal.pone.0148011 PMID: 26824747

Mansour, M. B., Ayman, A., & Yehia, M. (2024). E-healthcare system using IoT-based wearable device. *International Journal of Fuzzy Logic and Intelligent Systems*, *24*(3), 295–305. DOI: 10.5391/IJFIS.2024.24.3.295

Marcus, G., Rossi, F., & Veloso, M. (2016). Beyond the Turing Test. *AI Magazine*, *37*(1), 3–4. DOI: 10.1609/aimag.v37i1.2650

Marescaux, J., Leroy, J., Gagner, M., Rubino, F., Mutter, D., Vix, M., Butner, S. E., & Smith, M. K. (2001). Transatlantic robot-assisted telesurgery. *Nature*, *413*(6854), 379–380. DOI: 10.1038/35096636 PMID: 11574874

Marston, S., Li, Z., Bandyopadhyay, S., Zhang, J., & Ghalsasi, A. (2011). Cloud computing—The business perspective. *Decision Support Systems*, *51*(1), 176–189. DOI: 10.1016/j.dss.2010.12.006

Martin, K., & Gardner, G. (2017). Home enteral nutrition: Updates, trends, and challenges. *Nutrition in Clinical Practice*, *32*(6), 712–721. DOI: 10.1177/0884533617701401 PMID: 28437132

Martin, K., & McGinnis, C. (2016). Home nutrition support: Ethics and reimbursement. *Nutrition in Clinical Practice*, *31*(3), 325–333. DOI: 10.1177/0884533616639128 PMID: 27072855

Marwah, R., Thakur, J. S., & Tanwar, P. (2024). Augmented reality assistive technologies for disabled individuals. *arXiv*. /arXiv.2402.17256DOI: 10.48550

Marwah, K., & Hajati, F. (2021). A survey on Internet of Things in telehealth. In *Lecture notes in networks and systems* (Vol. 204, pp. 235–248). Springer., DOI: 10.1007/978-3-030-75025-1_22

Mathews, D., Abernethy, A., Butte, A. J., Glicksberg, B. S., & Kulikowski, C. (2023). *Telehealth and mobile health case study for understanding and anticipating emerging science and technology* (NAM Perspectives). National Academy of Medicine. DOI: 10.31478/202311e

Mauldin, K., Gieng, J., Saarony, D., & Hu, C. (2021). Performing nutrition assessment remotely via telehealth. *Nutrition in Clinical Practice*, *36*(4), 751–768. DOI: 10.1002/ncp.10682 PMID: 34101249

Ma, Y., Zhang, L., Liu, W., & Chen, X. (2025). Telemedicine-supported home enteral nutrition service (HENST): A five-year regional experience in China. *Asia Pacific Journal of Clinical Nutrition*, *34*(1), 87–95. DOI: 10.1016/j.apjcn.2025.01.010

Mazen, R., Radwan, M., & Abdel-Samiea, M. (2013). Utilization of biomass energy in high-rise buildings. In *2013 4th International Youth Conference on Energy (IYCE)* (pp. 1–3). IEEE. DOI: 10.1109/IYCE.2013.6604200

McAllister, R. (2024, November 22). *State-by-state breakdown—Average cost of hospital stays in the U.S.* North American Community Hub. https://nchstats.com/average-cost-of-hospital-stays-in-us/

McBain, R. K., Cantor, J., Pera, M. F., Breslau, J., Bravata, D. M., & Whaley, C. M. (2023, January). Mental health service utilization rates among commercially insured adults in the US during the first year of the COVID-19 pandemic. [). American Medical Association.]. *JAMA Health Forum*, *4*(1), e224936–e224936. DOI: 10.1001/jamahealthforum.2022.4936 PMID: 36607697

McCarthy, J. (1959). Programs with common sense. In *Mechanisation of thought processes* (Vol. 2, pp. 77–84). Her Majesty's Stationery Office.

McCarthy, J., Minsky, M. L., Rochester, N., & Shannon, C. E. (1955). *A proposal for the Dartmouth Summer Research Project on Artificial Intelligence* Dartmouth College.

McCulloch, W. S., & Pitts, W. (1943). A logical calculus of the ideas immanent in nervous activity. *The Bulletin of Mathematical Biophysics*, *5*(4), 115–133. DOI: 10.1007/BF02478259

McFarlane, D. C., & Latorella, K. A. (2002). The scope and importance of human interruption in human-computer interaction design. *Human-Computer Interaction*, *17*(1), 1–61. DOI: 10.1207/S15327051HCI1701_1

McKinney, S. M., Sieniek, M., Godbole, V., Godwin, J., Antropova, N., Ashrafian, H., Back, T., Chesus, M., Corrado, G. S., Darzi, A., Etemadi, M., Garcia-Vicente, F., Gilbert, F. J., Halling-Brown, M., Hassabis, D., Jansen, S., Karthikesalingam, A., Kelly, C. J., King, D., & Shetty, S. (2020). International evaluation of an AI system for breast cancer screening. *Nature*, *577*(7788), 89–94. DOI: 10.1038/s41586-019-1799-6 PMID: 31894144

Megido, I., Sela, Y., & Grinberg, K. (2023). Cost effectiveness of home care versus hospital care: A retrospective analysis. *Cost Effectiveness and Resource Allocation : C/E*, *21*(1), 13. DOI: 10.1186/s12962-023-00424-0 PMID: 36732792

Mehta, P., Stahl, M. G., Germone, M. M., Nagle, S., Guigli, R., Thomas, J., Shull, M., & Liu, E. (2020). Telehealth and nutrition support during the COVID-19 pandemic. *Journal of the Academy of Nutrition and Dietetics, 120*(12), 1953–1957. DOI: 10.1016/j.jand.2020.07.013 PMID: 32792328

Mei, C., Zhang, Y., Liu, H., & Wang, Z. (2024). Understanding versus imitation: Evaluating AI chatbots against human-like dialogue. *Journal of Artificial Intelligence Research.* Advance online publication.

Menachemi, N., & Collum, T. H. (2011). Benefits and drawbacks of electronic health record systems. *Risk Management and Healthcare Policy, 4*, 47–55. DOI: 10.2147/RMHP.S12985 PMID: 22312227

Mennella, C., Maniscalco, U., De Pietro, G., & Esposito, M. (2024). Ethical and regulatory challenges of AI technologies in healthcare: A narrative review. *Heliyon, 10*(4), e26297. DOI: 10.1016/j.heliyon.2024.e26297 PMID: 38384518

Merih, Y. D., Ertürk, N., Yemenici, M., & Satman, İ. (2021). Evde sağlık hizmetlerinde teknoloji kullanımı. *Journal of Health Institutes of Türkiye, 4*(3), 76–89. DOI: 10.54537/tusebdergisi.1037224

Mihaela, D. (2019). Accessibility in tourism – Need and opportunity. *Journal of Tourism Research, 21*, 12–18.

Miller, R. A., Pople, H. E.Jr, & Myers, J. D. (1982). INTERNIST-1, an experimental computer-based diagnostic consultant for general internal medicine. *The New England Journal of Medicine, 307*(8), 468–476. DOI: 10.1056/NEJM198208193070803 PMID: 7048091

Minsky, M. (1961). Steps toward artificial intelligence. *Proceedings of the IRE, 49*(1), 8–30. DOI: 10.1109/JRPROC.1961.287775

Minsky, M., & Papert, S. (1969). *Perceptrons: An introduction to computational geometry.* MIT Press.

Mishra, A. R., & Garg, P. (2024). Recent advancements in text summarization with natural language processing. In *A handbook of computational linguistics: Artificial intelligence in natural language processing* (pp. 15–37). Bentham Science Publishers., DOI: 10.2174/9789815238488124020004

Mohapatra, H. (2021). Socio-technical challenges in the implementation of smart city. In *2021 International Conference on Innovation and Intelligence for Informatics, Computing, and Technologies (3ICT)* (pp. 57–62). IEEE. DOI: 10.1109/3ICT53449.2021.9581905

Moore, J. F. (2006). Business ecosystems and the view from the firm. *Antitrust Bulletin*, *51*(1), 31–75. DOI: 10.1177/0003603X0605100103

Moor, J. H. (2001). The status and future of the Turing Test. *Minds and Machines*, *11*(1), 77–93. DOI: 10.1023/A:1011218925467

Moris, M. I., Alakhras, H., Eid, N. G., & Higazy, M. (2019). Human resources capacity building in accessible tourism in Egypt. *Journal of Association of Arab Universities for Tourism and Hospitality*, *17*(3), 82–89. DOI: 10.21608/jaauth.2019.92004

Morita, P. P., West, R., Da Costa, D., Michalski, A., Kalesnikava, V., Kuziemsky, C., & St-Amant, O. (2023). Health monitoring using smart home technologies: Scoping review. *JMIR mHealth and uHealth*, *11*, e37347. DOI: 10.2196/37347 PMID: 37052984

Morley, J., Machado, C. C. V., Burr, C., Cowls, J., Joshi, I., Taddeo, M., & Floridi, L. (2020). The ethics of AI in health care: A mapping review. *Social Science & Medicine*, *260*, 113172. DOI: 10.1016/j.socscimed.2020.113172 PMID: 32702587

Mosa, A. S. M., Yoo, I., & Sheets, L. (2012). A systematic review of healthcare applications for smartphones. *BMC Medical Informatics and Decision Making*, *12*(1), 67. DOI: 10.1186/1472-6947-12-67 PMID: 22781312

Mourtzis, D., Angelopoulos, J., & Panopoulos, N. (2023). The future of the human–machine interface (HMI) in society 5.0. *Future Internet*, *15*(5), 162. DOI: 10.3390/fi15050162

Muck, T. R., & Frohlich, A. A. (2013). Seamless integration of HW/SW components in a HLS-based SoC design environment. In *2013 International Symposium on Rapid System Prototyping (RSP)* (pp. 109–115). IEEE. DOI: 10.1109/RSP.2013.6683966

Mulherin, D. W., Walker, R., Holcombe, B., & Guenter, P. (2020). Aspen report on nutrition support practice processes with covid-19: The first response. *Nutrition in Clinical Practice*, *35*(5), 783–791. DOI: 10.1002/ncp.10553 PMID: 32671870

Munawar, H. S., Akram, J., Khan, S. I., Ullah, F., & Choi, B. J. (2023). Drone-as-a-service (DaaS) for COVID-19 self-testing kits delivery in smart healthcare setups: A technological perspective. *ICT Express*, *9*(4), 748–753. DOI: 10.1016/j.icte.2022.09.008

Mundi, M. S., Elfadil, O. M., Bonnes, S. L., Salonen, B. R., & Hurt, R. T. (2021). Use of telehealth in home nutrition support: Challenges and advantages. *Nutrition in Clinical Practice*, *36*(4), 775–784. DOI: 10.1002/ncp.10736 PMID: 34245465

Munnecke, T. H., & Kuhn, I. M. (1989). Large-scale portability of hospital information system software within the Veterans Administration. In *Proceedings of the Annual Symposium on Computer Application in Medical Care* (pp. 133–137). American Medical Informatics Association., https://www.ncbi.nlm.nih.gov/pmc/articles/PMC2244995/ DOI: 10.1007/978-1-4612-3488-3_8

Muñoz-Bonet, J. I., López-Prats, J. L., Flor-Macián, E. M., Cantavella, T., Domínguez, A., Vidal, Y., & Brines, J. (2020). Medical complications in a telemedicine home care programme for paediatric ventilated patients. *Journal ofTelemedicine and Telecare*, *26*(7–8), 462–473. DOI: 10.1177/1357633X19843761 PMID: 31023136

Munyewende, P. O., Rispel, L. C., & Chirwa, T. (2014). Positive practice environments influence job satisfaction of primary health care clinic nursing managers in two South African provinces. *Human Resources for Health*, *12*(1), 27. DOI: 10.1186/1478-4491-12-27 PMID: 24885785

Mustafa, M., Alshare, M., Bhargava, D., Neware, R., Singh, B., & Ngulube, P. (2022). Perceived security risk based on moderating factors for blockchain technology applications in cloud storage to achieve secure healthcare systems. *Computational and Mathematical Methods in Medicine*, *2022*, 6112815. DOI: 10.1155/2022/6112815 PMID: 35096132

Naik, D. B., Sri, S. N., Priya, G. M., & Priya, P. S. (2023). Machine learning boosting algorithms to detect the fake user profiles on Instagram. In *2023 International Conference on Quantum Technologies, Communications, Computing, Hardware and Embedded Systems Security (iQ-CCHESS)* (pp. 1–7). IEEE. DOI: 10.1109/iQ-CCHESS56596.2023.10391800

Nair, K., Kulkarni, J., Warde, M., Dave, Z., Rawalgaonkar, V., Gore, G., & Joshi, J. (2015). Optimizing power consumption in IoT based wireless sensor networks using Bluetooth Low Energy. In *2015 International Conference on Green Computing and Internet of Things (ICGCIoT)* (pp. 589–593). IEEE. DOI: 10.1109/ICGCIoT.2015.7380533

Nasr, M. M., Islam, M. M., Shehata, S., Karray, F., & Quintana, Y. (2021). Smart healthcare in the age of AI: Recent advances, challenges, and future prospects. *IEEE Access : Practical Innovations, Open Solutions*, *9*, 145248–145270. DOI: 10.1109/ACCESS.2021.3118960

National Consortium of Telehealth Resource Centers. (2021). *History of telehealth.* https://telehealthresourcecenter.org/wp-content/uploads/2021/11/History_of_Telehealth.pdf

Naureen, A., Vamshi, K., Krishna, K. C., & Hussain, M. M. (2024). Healthcare 5.0 fundamentals. In Hassan, A., Prasad, V. K., Bhattacharya, P., Dutta, P., & Damaševičius, R. (Eds.), *Federated learning and AI for Healthcare 5.0* (pp. 1–33). IGI Global., DOI: 10.4018/978-1-6684-9510-0.ch001

NEJM Catalyst. (2018). What is telehealth? *NEJM Catalyst Innovations in Care Delivery*, *4*(2). DOI: 10.1056/CAT.18.0268

Nelson, E., Yadrich, D. M., Thompson, N., Wright, S., Stone, K. J., Adams, N., Werkowitch, M., & Smith, C. E. (2017). Telemedicine support groups for home parenteral nutrition users. *Nutrition in Clinical Practice*, *32*(6), 789–798. DOI: 10.1177/0884533617735527 PMID: 29016235

Nesbitt, T. S. (2012). The evolution of telehealth: Where have we been and where are we going? In Lustig, T. A. (Ed.), *The role of telehealth in an evolving health care environment* (pp. 11–16). National Academies Press.

Newell, A., Shaw, J. C., & Simon, H. A. (1959). Report on a general problem-solving program. In *Proceedings of the International Conference on Information Processing* (pp. 256–264). UNESCO.

Newell, A., & Simon, H. A. (1956). The logic theory machine: A complex information processing system. *IEEE Transactions on Information Theory*, *2*(3), 61–79. DOI: 10.1109/TIT.1956.1056797

Newell, A., & Simon, H. A. (1976). Computer science as empirical inquiry: Symbols and search. *Communications of the ACM*, *19*(3), 113–126. DOI: 10.1145/360018.360022

Nguyen, G., Furness, K., Croagh, D., Haines, T., & Hanna, L. (2024). Supplemental tube feeding: Qualitative study of patient perspectives in advanced pancreatic cancer. BMJ Supportive &Amp. *Palliative Care*, *14*(e3), e3002–e3010. DOI: 10.1136/spcare-2024-004836 PMID: 38580394

Nibbelink, C. W., & Brewer, B. B. (2018). Decision-making in nursing practice: An integrative literature review. *Journal of Clinical Nursing*, *27*(5–6), 917–928. DOI: 10.1111/jocn.14151 PMID: 29098746

Nichols, T., Calder, R., Morgan, M., Lawn, S., Beauchamp, A., Trezona, A., & Klepac Pogrmilovic, B. (2020). *Self-care for health: A national policy blueprint* (Policy Paper 2020-01). Mitchell Institute, Victoria University. https://www.vu.edu.au/sites/default/files/self-care-for-health-national-policy-blueprint-mitchell-institute.pdf

Nielsen, J. (1994). *Usability engineering*. Morgan Kaufmann.

Nilsson, N. J. (1984). *Shakey the Robot* (Technical Note 323). SRI International.

Nimmy, K., Sankaran, S., Achuthan, K., & Calyam, P. (2022). Lightweight and privacy-preserving remote user authentication for smart homes. *IEEE Access : Practical Innovations, Open Solutions*, *10*, 176–190. DOI: 10.1109/ACCESS.2021.3137175

Norman, C. D., & Skinner, H. A. (2006). eHealth literacy: Essential skills for consumer health in a networked world. *Journal of Medical Internet Research*, *8*(2), e9. DOI: 10.2196/jmir.8.2.e9 PMID: 16867972

Norouzi, S., Majd, F. A., Rostami, S., Mirzaee, M., Sistani, S., & Ahmadian, L. (2024). Tele-medical nutrition therapy to promote healthy eating and nutrition adherence of chronic patients in the covid-19 pandemic: A pragmatically before-after trial. *Health Science Reports*, *7*(11), e70193. DOI: 10.1002/hsr2.70193 PMID: 39540025

Nouri, S., Khoong, E. C., Lyles, C. R., & Karliner, L. (2020). Addressing equity in telemedicine for chronic disease management during the Covid-19 pandemic. *NEJM Catalyst Innovations in Care Delivery*, *1*(3). DOI: 10.1056/CAT.20.0123

Obermeyer, Z., Powers, B., Vogeli, C., & Mullainathan, S. (2019). Dissecting racial bias in an algorithm used to manage the health of populations. *Science*, *366*(6464), 447–453. DOI: 10.1126/science.aax2342 PMID: 31649194

Odeh, B., Philip, N., & Kayyali, R. (2014). Acceptability of telehealth by elderly patients. *Age and Ageing*, *43*(Suppl_2), ii13. DOI: 10.1093/ageing/afu036.4

Oelschlägel, L., Christensen, V. L., Moen, A., Heggdal, K., Österlind, J., Dihle, A., & Steindal, S. A. (2023). Patients' experiences with a welfare technology application for remote home care: A longitudinal study. *Journal of Clinical Nursing*, *32*(17–18), 6545–6558. DOI: 10.1111/jocn.16592 PMID: 36437490

Oelschlägel, L., Moen, A., Dihle, A., Christensen, V. L., Heggdal, K., Österlind, J., & Steindal, S. A. (2024). Implementation of remote home care: Assessment guided by the RE-AIM framework. *BMC Health Services Research*, *24*(1), 145. DOI: 10.1186/s12913-024-10625-9 PMID: 38287394

Önder, E. (2021). Geçmişten günümüze evde sağlık hizmetleri. In Özaydın, Ö., & Güdük, Ö. (Eds.), *Evde sağlık hizmetlerinde teknoloji kullanımı* (pp. 203–224). Nobel Akademik Yayıncılık.

Ong, T., Barrera, J. F., Sunkara, C., Soni, H., Ivanova, J., Cummins, M. R., Schuler, K. R., Wilczewski, H., Welch, B. M., & Bunnell, B. E. (2024). Mental health providers are inexperienced but interested in telehealth-based virtual reality therapy: Survey study. *Frontiers in Virtual Reality*, *5*, 1332874. DOI: 10.3389/frvir.2024.1332874 PMID: 39228388

Onofri, A., Ullmann, N., Verrillo, E., Paglietti, M. G., Pavone, M., & Cutrera, R. (2025). Televisit with TytoHome™ device in medically complex child in long-term mechanical ventilation: A pilot study. *Italian Journal of Pediatrics, 51*(1), 45. DOI: 10.1186/s13052-025-01885-0 PMID: 39939975

Padhan, S., Mohapatra, A., Ramasamy, S. K., & Agrawal, S. (2023). Artificial intelligence (AI) and robotics in elderly healthcare: Enabling independence and quality of life. *Cureus, 15*(8), e42905. DOI: 10.7759/cureus.42905 PMID: 37664381

Pallotta, G. (2021). *Analysis and development of a tele-health system to support remote areas* [Doctoral dissertation, University of Camerino]. UniCam Eprints. https://pubblicazioni.unicam.it/retrieve/0bdcc121-fde0-4c54-bfbf-4a3927e33f7d/PALLOTTA%20GRAZIANO%20PHD%20THESIS%2023.06.pdf

Pandey, R., Rajput, I. S., Tyagi, S., Koranga, M., & Sharma, P. K. (2024). Enhancing smart city resilience. In *Advances in computational intelligence and robotics* (pp. 77–90). IGI Global. DOI: 10.4018/979-8-3693-2373-1.ch005

Panyadee, C., Krajangchom, S., Sangkakorn, K., & Intawong, K. (2023). Smart wellness technology for tourism destination. *TEM Journal, 12*(2), 456–467. DOI: 10.18421/TEM122-03

Paputungan, I. V., Al Fitri, M. R., & Oktiawati, U. Y. (2019). Motion and movement detection for DIY home security system. In *2019 IEEE Conference on Sustainable Utilization and Development in Engineering and Technologies (CSUDET)* (pp. 122–125). IEEE. DOI: 10.1109/CSUDET47057.2019.9214684

Paré, G., Jaana, M., & Sicotte, C. (2007). Systematic review of home telemonitoring for chronic diseases: The evidence base. *Journal of the American Medical Informatics Association : JAMIA, 14*(3), 269–277. DOI: 10.1197/jamia.M2270 PMID: 17329725

Patel, A., & Champaneria, T. A. (2016). Fuzzy logic-based algorithm for context awareness in IoT for smart home environment. In *2016 IEEE Region 10 Conference (TENCON)* (pp. 1057–1060). IEEE. DOI: 10.1109/TENCON.2016.7848168

Patel, S. Y., Mehrotra, A., Huskamp, H. A., Uscher-Pines, L., Ganguli, I., & Barnett, M. L. (2021). Variation in telemedicine use and outpatient care during the COVID-19 pandemic in the United States. *Health Affairs, 40*(2), 349–358. DOI: 10.1377/hlthaff.2020.01786 PMID: 33523745

Paterakis, N. G., Erdinç, O., Bakirtzis, A. G., & Catalão, J. P. S. (2015). Optimal household appliances scheduling under day-ahead pricing and load-shaping demand response strategies. *IEEE Transactions on Industrial Informatics, 11*(6), 1509–1519. DOI: 10.1109/TII.2015.2438534

Pearl, J. (1988). *Probabilistic reasoning in intelligent systems: Networks of plausible inference*. Morgan Kaufmann.

Peng, I. (2022). *A history of telemedicine in America*. RexMD. https://rexmd.com/learn/a-history-of-telemedicine-in-america

Pentiuk, S. S., O'Flaherty, T., Santoro, K., Willging, P., & Kaul, A. (2011). Pureed by gastrostomy tube diet improves gagging and retching in children with fundoplication. *JPEN. Journal of Parenteral and Enteral Nutrition*, *35*(3), 375–379. DOI: 10.1177/0148607110377797 PMID: 21527599

Persoon, A., Huisman-de Waal, G., Naber, T. A., Schoonhoven, L., Tas, T., Sauerwein, H., & van Achterberg, T. (2005). Impact of long-term HPN on daily life in adults. *Clinical Nutrition (Edinburgh, Lothian)*, *24*(2), 304–313. DOI: 10.1016/j.clnu.2004.12.009 PMID: 15784493

Picard, R. W. (2000). *Affective computing*. MIT Press. DOI: 10.7551/mitpress/1140.003.0008

Picozzi, P., Nocco, U., Puleo, G., Labate, C., & Cimolin, V. (2023). Telemedicine and robotic surgery: A narrative review to analyze advantages, limitations and future developments. *Electronics (Basel)*, *13*(1), 124. DOI: 10.3390/electronics13010124

Pironi, L., Arends, J., Bozzetti, F., Cuerda, C., Gillanders, L., Jeppesen, P. B., Joly, F., Kelly, D., Lal, S., Staun, M., Szczepanek, K., Van Gossum, A., Wanten, G., & Schneider, S. M. (2016). ESPEN guidelines on chronic intestinal failure in adults. *Clinical Nutrition (Edinburgh, Lothian)*, *35*(2), 247–307. DOI: 10.1016/j.clnu.2016.01.020 PMID: 26944585

Poli, M. (2019). Tourism, design and disability? In D. Gursoy & R. Nunkoo (Eds.), *Strategic innovative marketing and tourism: 7th ICSIMAT, Athenian Riviera, Greece, 2018* (pp. 603–611). Springer. DOI: 10.1007/978-3-030-12453-3_69

Popiel, M. (2016). Barriers in undertaking tourist activity by disabled people. *Journal of Kinesiology and Exercise Sciences*, *15*(74), 103–110.

Porteny, T., Brophy, S. A., & Burroughs, E. (2025). Experiences of telehealth reimbursement policies in federally qualified health centers. *JAMA Network Open*, *8*(2), e2459554–e2459554. DOI: 10.1001/jamanetworkopen.2024.59554 PMID: 39937474

Pramanik, P. K. D., Pareek, G., & Nayyar, A. (2019). Security and privacy in remote healthcare: Issues, solutions, and standards. In Tripathy, B. K., & Acharjya, D. P. (Eds.), *Telemedicine technologies* (pp. 201–225). Academic Press., DOI: 10.1016/B978-0-12-816948-3.00014-3

Prat, V. D., Pedrazzoli, P., & Caccialanza, R. (2024). Nutritional care for cancer patients: Are we doing enough? *Frontiers in Nutrition*, *11*, 1361800. DOI: 10.3389/fnut.2024.1361800 PMID: 38721029

Procter, R., Tolmie, P., & Rouncefield, M. (2023). Holding AI to account: Challenges for the delivery of trustworthy AI in healthcare. *ACM Transactions on Computer-Human Interaction*, *30*(2), 26. DOI: 10.1145/3577009

Pruszyński, J., Jasik, A., Marcinowska-Suchowierska, E., Puzianowska-Kuźnicka, M., & Zgliczyński, W. S. (2022). New technologies in elderly care. *Wiedza Medyczna*, *4*(1), 43–52. DOI: 10.36553/wm.131

Puja, D., Upadhyay, S., Agrawal, S., Goswami, J. K., & Singh, S. K. (2023). A healthcare system for patients based on IoT. *Scandinavian Journal of Information Systems*, *35*(1), 446–456. DOI: 10.5281/SJIS.7752846

Puri, V. (2021). Telemedicine history and its advantages. *General Medicine: Open Access*, *9*(10), 1–2. DOI: 10.35248/2327-5146.21.9.351

Putri, D., & Taufik, D. N. (2024). Development of disabled-friendly tourism infrastructure. *SocioVoyage: International Journal of Social Dynamics in Tourism*, *1*(3), 26–35. DOI: 10.56910/sociovoyage.v1i3.4

Rabearison, H. M., Razafison, F., Razafimanjato, N., Zafintsalama, M., & Andriatsihoarana, H. (2025). Architecture and organizational protocol of a connected medical monitoring device. *International Journal of Scientific Research and Technology*, *2*(4), 204–216. DOI: 10.5281/zenodo.15191781

Rai, H. K., Cavalcanti Barroso, A., Yates, L., Schneider, J., & Orrell, M. (2020). Involvement of people with dementia in the development of technology-based interventions: Narrative synthesis review and best practice guidelines. *Journal of Medical Internet Research*, *22*(12), e17531. DOI: 10.2196/17531 PMID: 33270034

Raja, A., Lakshmi, K. U., Chaitanya, K., Kavya, M., Mahammed, N., & Palankaiah, C. C. (2025). IoT based wearable ECG monitoring system for patient emergency condition. *International Journal for Modern Trends in Science and Technology*, *11*(3), 136–142. DOI: 10.5281/zenodo.15084903

Rajasekharan, J., & Koivunen, V. (2014). Optimal energy consumption model for smart grid households with energy storage. *IEEE Journal of Selected Topics in Signal Processing*, *8*(6), 1154–1166. DOI: 10.1109/JSTSP.2014.2361315

Raj, S., Sheel, S., Singh, R., Ashar, S., & Mohapatra, H. (2025). Securing smart cities. In *New horizons in leadership* (pp. 487–512). IGI Global., DOI: 10.4018/979-8-3693-6437-6.ch021

Ramirez-Vega, D., Salinas-Cortes, M., Melendez-Coral, M., Cordell, G. A., & Rodriguez-Garcia, A. (2022). The evolution of nutrition intervention during the COVID-19 pandemic. *Ciencia & Saude Coletiva*, *27*(8), 3053–3061. DOI: 10.1590/1413-81232022278.04082021 PMID: 35894318

Ramlee, R., Tang, D. H., & Ismail, M. M. (2012). Smart home system for disabled people via wireless Bluetooth. In *2012 International Conference on System Engineering and Technology (ICSET)* (pp. 1–4). IEEE. DOI: 10.1109/ICSEngT.2012.6339347

Reddy, P., & Malone, M. (1998). Cost and outcome analysis of home parenteral and enteral nutrition. *JPEN. Journal of Parenteral and Enteral Nutrition*, *22*(5), 302–310. DOI: 10.1177/0148607198022005302 PMID: 9739034

Remillard, E. T., Rogers, W. A., & Ruiz, S. (2019). Utilizing technology networks to support social networks for people aging with disability. *Innovation in Aging*, *3*(Suppl_1), S758–S759. DOI: 10.1093/geroni/igz038.2787

Ribeiro, F., Metrôlho, J., Leal, J., Martins, H., & Bastos, P. (2018). A mobile application to provide personalized information for mobility impaired tourists. In *ICT tools and applications for accessible tourism* (pp. 171–191). IGI Global., DOI: 10.4018/978-1-7998-6428-8.ch008

Rinde, E., & Balteskard, L. (2002). Is there a future for telemedicine? *Lancet*, *359*(9322), 1957–1958. DOI: 10.1016/S0140-6736(02)08845-1 PMID: 12076546

Roberts, N., Carrigan, A., Hibbert, P., Williams, R. C., Austin, E., Pulido, D. F., Meulenbroeks, I., Nguyen, H. M., Hatem, S., Maka, K., Loy, G., & Braithwaite, J. (2023). Consumer and provider perspectives on hospital in the home: A qualitative study. *Health & Social Care in the Community*, *2023*, 7105751. DOI: 10.1155/2023/7105751

Robinson, H., MacDonald, B., & Broadbent, E. (2014). The role of healthcare robots for older people at home: A review. *International Journal of Social Robotics*, *6*(4), 575–591. DOI: 10.1007/s12369-014-0242-2

Robles, T., Bordel, B., Alcarria, R., & Sánchez-de-Rivera, D. (2020). Enabling trustworthy personal data protection in eHealth and well-being services through privacy-by-design. *International Journal of Distributed Sensor Networks*, *16*(5), 1550147720912110. DOI: 10.1177/1550147720912110

Rochester, N., Holland, J. H., Haibt, L. H., & Duda, W. L. (1956). Tests on a cell assembly theory of the action of the brain, using a large digital computer. *IEEE Transactions on Information Theory*, *2*(3), 80–93. DOI: 10.1109/TIT.1956.1056810

Rosa, M. P., & Lopes, J. D. C. (2019). Senior tourists' perceptions of bus stop environments used in collaborative design. *WIT Transactions on the Built Environment, 186*, 121–132. DOI: 10.2495/UT190111

Rosa, M., Gameiro, C., Sousa, C., & Pinto, P. (2020). An analysis of elderly tourists' constraints in the use of public transport. *Transport Development and Integration, 4*(2), 163–178. DOI: 10.2495/TDI-V4-N2-163-178

Rosa, M., Pinto, A., & Assunção, P. (2020). An evaluation of the universal accessibility of bus stop infrastructure. *International Journal of Sustainable Development and Planning, 15*(6), 835–840. DOI: 10.18280/ijsdp.150606

Rosenblatt, F. (1958). The perceptron: A probabilistic model for information storage and organization in the brain. *Psychological Review, 65*(6), 386–408. DOI: 10.1037/h0042519 PMID: 13602029

Rouidi, M., Hamdoune, A., Choujtani, K., & Chati, A. (2022). TAM-UTAUT and the acceptance of remote healthcare technologies by healthcare professionals: A systematic review. *Informatics in Medicine Unlocked, 32*, 101008. DOI: 10.1016/j.imu.2022.101008

Roy, J., Levy, D. R., & Senathirajah, Y. (2022). Defining telehealth for research, implementation, and equity. *Journal of Medical Internet Research, 24*(4), e35037. DOI: 10.2196/35037 PMID: 35416778

Rumetshofer, H., & Wöß, W. (2004). Tourism information systems promoting barrier-free tourism. In *ICCSA 2004: International Conference on Computer Science and its Applications* (pp. 280–286). Springer. DOI: 10.1007/978-3-540-24707-4_35

Rural Telehealth Evaluation Center. (2022). *Telehealth: Current definitions and future trends*. University of Arkansas for Medical Sciences. https://idhi.uams.edu/rtec/wp-content/uploads/sites/4/2022/05/Telehealth-Definitions-Paper-06MAY2022-1.pdf

Ryu, S. (2010). History of telemedicine: Evolution, context, and transformation. *Healthcare Informatics Research, 16*(1), 65–66. DOI: 10.4258/hir.2010.16.1.65 PMID: 22509475

Sabetsarvestani, P., Mohammadi, F., Tehranineshat, B., Bijani, M., & Fereidouni, Z. (2022). Barriers to efficient management of in-home care: A qualitative content analysis. *Nursing Open, 9*(2), 1200–1209. DOI: 10.1002/nop2.1161 PMID: 34908248

Saeed, S. A., & Masters, R. M. (2021). Disparities in health care and the digital divide. *Current Psychiatry Reports, 23*(9), 61. DOI: 10.1007/s11920-021-01274-4 PMID: 34297202

Saif, S., Biswas, S., & Chattopadhyay, S. (2020). Intelligent, secure big health data management using deep learning and blockchain technology: An overview. In Dash, S., Acharya, B. R., Mittal, M., Abraham, A., & Kelemen, A. (Eds.), *Deep learning techniques for biomedical and health informatics* (pp. 187–209). Springer., DOI: 10.1007/978-3-030-33966-1_10

Salha, R. A., Jawabrah, M. Q., Badawy, U., Jarada, A., & Alastal, A. I. (2020). Towards smart, sustainable, accessible and inclusive city for people with disability by taking into account checklists tools. *Journal of Geographic Information System*, *12*(4), 348–371. DOI: 10.4236/jgis.2020.124022

Samuel, A. L. (1959). Some studies in machine learning using the game of checkers. *IBM Journal of Research and Development*, *3*(3), 210–229. DOI: 10.1147/rd.33.0210

Sancho-Esper, F., Ostrovskaya, L., Rodriguez-Sanchez, C., & Campayo-Sanchez, F. (2022). Virtual reality in retirement communities: Technology acceptance and tourist destination recommendation. *Journal of Vacation Marketing*, *28*(4), 370–385. DOI: 10.1177/13567667211066387

Sanz, M. F., Ferrandis, E. D., & Ferrer, J. G. (2013). Involving elderly and disabled tourists as active participants in energy savings. *Journal of Sustainable Tourism*, *21*(2), 256–272. DOI: 10.1080/09669582.2012.709211

Saqui, O., Sinha, R., & Ethans, K. (2007). Telehealth in the management of home parenteral nutrition patients in rural Ontario: A five-year experience. *JPEN. Journal of Parenteral and Enteral Nutrition*, *31*(4), 300–305. DOI: 10.1177/0148607107031004300

Sari, S., & Ünüvar, Ş. (2019). Hotel managers and staff's attitudes towards accessible tourism. *Journal of Tourism and Gastronomy Studies*, *7*(4), 3060–3087. DOI: 10.21325/jotags.2019.516

Sarmento, E., Brás, C., & Vargas de Oliveira, C. (2016). Issues and challenges of accessibility for senior tourism. *European Journal of Tourism Research*, *14*, 7–26. DOI: 10.54055/ejtr.v14i.251

Sasegbon, A., Dupont, C., Nguyen, T., & Martin, A. (2025). Telemedicine in Home Parenteral Nutrition: A Multinational Survey of Physician Perspectives During the COVID-19 Pandemic. *Clinical Nutrition ESPEN*, *57*, 112–119. DOI: 10.1016/j.clnesp.2025.03.006

Saygılı, T., Oymak Yalçın, S., & Özsarı, H. (2021). Advanced age and disabled health tourism: Concept, problems and solution suggestions. *International Journal of Health Management and Tourism*, *6*(2), 492–514. DOI: 10.31201/ijhmt.918595

Schneider, S. M., Raina, C., Pugliese, P., Pouget, I., Rampal, P., & Hebuterne, X. (2001). Outcome of patients treated with home enteral nutrition. *JPEN. Journal of Parenteral and Enteral Nutrition*, *25*(4), 203–209. DOI: 10.1177/0148607101025004203 PMID: 11434651

Schönenberger, K. A., Herren, L., Lutz, T., & Ballmer, P. E. (2022). Attitudes and expectations of patients receiving home parenteral nutrition towards eHealth: A Swiss multicenter survey study. *Clinical Nutrition ESPEN*, *47*, 314–320. DOI: 10.1016/j.clnesp.2022.01.025

Scott, A. F., Ayers, S., Pluye, P., Grad, R., Sztramko, R., Marr, S., Papaioannou, A., Clark, S., Gerantonis, P., & Levinson, A. J. (2022). Impact and perceived value of iGeriCare e-learning among dementia care partners and others: Pilot evaluation using the IAM4all questionnaire. *JMIR Aging*, *5*(4), e40357. DOI: 10.2196/40357 PMID: 36150051

Seivert, S., & Badowski, M. E. (2021). The rise of telemedicine: Lessons from a global pandemic. *European Medical Journal. Innovations*, *5*(1), 64–69. DOI: 10.33590/emjinnov/20-00239

Selfridge, O. G. (1959). Pandemonium: A paradigm for learning. In *Mechanisation of thought processes* (pp. 511–529). Her Majesty's Stationery Office.

Senillosa, M. B., Saimovici, J., Mandirola Brieux, H. F., Rabinovich, D., Galván, C., Jauregui, O. I., Rizzato Lede, D. A., Otero, C. M., & Luna, D. R. (2022). Mobile application for home healthcare: Physician's expectations and perceptions. *Studies in Health Technology and Informatics*, *290*, 197–199. DOI: 10.3233/SHTI220060 PMID: 35672999

Senyo, P. K., Liu, K., & Effah, J. (2019). Digital business ecosystem: Literature review and a framework for future research. *International Journal of Information Management*, *47*, 52–64. DOI: 10.1016/j.ijinfomgt.2019.01.002

Sesha Bhargavi, V.Sesha Bhargavi Velagaleti. (2024). Empathetic algorithms: The role of AI in understanding and enhancing human emotional intelligence. *Journal of Electrical Systems*, *20*(3s), 2051–2060. DOI: 10.52783/jes.1806

Shachar, C., Engel, J., & Elwyn, G. (2020). Implications for telehealth in a post-pandemic future: Regulatory and privacy issues. *Journal of the American Medical Association*, *323*(23), 2375–2376. DOI: 10.1001/jama.2020.7943 PMID: 32421170

Shah, N., Krupinski, E., Bernard, J., & Moyer, M. (2021). The evolution and utilization of telehealth in ambulatory nutrition practice. *Nutrition in Clinical Practice*, *36*(4), 739–749. DOI: 10.1002/ncp.10641 PMID: 33734469

Shahriyar, F., Islam, M., Chakraborty, A., Hasan, M., Zaman, H. U., & Siddique, A. H. (2021). Fault and system analysis model of voltage source control based HVDC transmission system. In *2021 12th International Conference on Computing Communication and Networking Technologies (ICCCNT)* (pp. 1–6). IEEE. DOI: 10.1109/ICCCNT51525.2021.9579990

Shamsabadi, A., Mehraeen, E., & Pashaei, Z. (2023). *Perspective chapter: telehealth technologies for the elderly people*. Geriatric Medicine and Healthy Aging., DOI: 10.5772/intechopen.105568

Shanimon, S., & Hameedu, M. S. (2013). Foreign direct investment and accessible tourism in India. *International Journal of Scientific and Research Publications*, *3*(12), 1–5.

Shannon, C. E. (1950). Programming a computer for playing chess. *The London, Edinburgh and Dublin Philosophical Magazine and Journal of Science*, *41*(314), 256–275. DOI: 10.1080/14786445008521796

Shapiro, S. C. (1992). Artificial intelligence. In Shapiro, S. C. (Ed.), *Encyclopedia of artificial intelligence* (Vol. 1, pp. 54–57). Wiley.

Sharkey, A., & Sharkey, N. (2012). Granny and the robots: Ethical issues in robot care for the elderly. *Ethics and Information Technology*, *14*(1), 27–40. DOI: 10.1007/s10676-010-9234-6

Sharma, A., Pesarlanka, D. B., & Sharma, S. (2025). Integrating machine learning, artificial intelligence, deep learning, and IoT in remote patient monitoring. In Tyagi, A. K., & Rajest, S. S. (Eds.), *Future innovations in the convergence of AI and Internet of Things in medicine* (pp. 285–318). IGI Global., DOI: 10.4018/979-8-3693-7703-1.ch011

Sharma, K., Singh, H., Sharma, D. K., Kumar, A., Nayyar, A., & Krishnamurthi, R. (2021). Dynamic models and control techniques for drone delivery of medications and other healthcare items in COVID-19 hotspots. In Gupta, B. B., Agrawal, P., Hassanien, A. E., & Abraham, A. (Eds.), *Emerging technologies for battling COVID-19: Applications and innovations* (pp. 1–34). Springer., DOI: 10.1007/978-3-030-60039-6_1

Sheth, A., Jaimini, U., & Yip, H. Y. (2018). How will the Internet of Things enable augmented personalized health? *IEEE Intelligent Systems*, *33*(1), 89–97. DOI: 10.1109/MIS.2018.012001556 PMID: 29887765

Shetty, E. A., & McIntosh, A. (2020). Online communications of accessibility in hotel restaurants. *Hospitality Insights*, *4*(2), 7–8. DOI: 10.24135/hi.v4i2.87

Shidende, D., Kessel, T., Treydte, A., & Moebs, S. (2023). A systematic literature review of accessibility evaluation methods for augmented reality applications. *Studies in Health Technology and Informatics*, *306*, 575–582. DOI: 10.3233/SHTI230681 PMID: 37638964

Shiferaw, F., & Zolfo, M. (2012). The role of information communication technology (ICT) towards universal health coverage: The first steps of a telemedicine project in Ethiopia. *Global Health Action*, *5*(1), 15638. DOI: 10.3402/gha.v5i0.15638 PMID: 22479235

Shigekawa, E., Fix, M., Corbett, G., Roby, D. H., & Coffman, J. (2018). The current state of telehealth evidence: A rapid review. *Health Affairs*, *37*(12), 1975–1982. DOI: 10.1377/hlthaff.2018.05132 PMID: 30633674

Shirvanian, N., Shams, M., Rahmani, A. M., Lansky, J., Mildeova, S., & Hosseinzadeh, M. (2025). The Internet of Things in elderly healthcare applications: A systematic review and future directions. *IEEE Access : Practical Innovations, Open Solutions*, *13*, 71335–71373. DOI: 10.1109/ACCESS.2025.3562147

Shirzadfar, H., & Lotfi, F. (2017). The evolution and transformation of telemedicine. *International Journal of Biosensors & Bioelectronics*, *3*(4), 303–306. DOI: 10.15406/ijbsbe.2017.03.00070

Shortliffe, E. H. (1976). *Computer-based medical consultations: MYCIN*. Elsevier.

Shurson, L., Pilon, B., Ketel, C., & Anthamatten, A. (2019). Development of an interprofessional home healthcare management service within an urban housing development. *Home Healthcare Now*, *37*(5), 285–291. DOI: 10.1097/NHH.0000000000000817 PMID: 31483361

Simon, H. A. (1965). *The shape of automation for men and management*. Harper & Row.

Şimşir, İ., & Mete, B. (2021). Sağlık hizmetlerinin geleceği: Dijital sağlık teknolojileri. *Journal of Innovative Healthcare Practices*, *2*(1), 33–39.

Singh, R., Seniaray, S., & Das, P. (2022). Role of IoT in universal design. In Kumar, A., Maurer, J. L., & Kadry, S. (Eds.), *Handbook of smart materials, technologies, and devices* (pp. 709–728). Springer., DOI: 10.1007/978-3-030-84205-5_128

SINPE – Italian Society of Parenteral and Enteral Nutrition. (2014). Home artificial nutrition in Italy: Annual report and national registry data analysis (2005–2012). *Clinical Nutrition (Edinburgh, Lothian)*, *33*(5), 755–761. DOI: 10.1016/j.clnu.2014.01.012

Sitges-Maciá, E., Bonete-López, B., Sánchez-Cabaco, A., & Oltra-Cucarella, J. (2021). Effects of e-health training and social support interventions for informal caregivers of people with dementia—A narrative review. *International Journal of Environmental Research and Public Health, 18*(15), 7728. DOI: 10.3390/ijerph18157728 PMID: 34360020

Sivakumar, V. G., Baskar, V. V., Vadivel, M., Vimal, S. P., & Murugan, S. (2023). IoT and GIS integration for real-time monitoring of soil health and nutrient status. In *2023 International Conference on Self Sustainable Artificial Intelligence Systems (ICSSAS)* (pp. 1265–1270). IEEE. DOI: 10.1109/ICSSAS57918.2023.10331694

Smirek, L., Zimmermann, G., & Beigl, M. (2016). Just a smart home or your smart home – A framework for personalized user interfaces based on Eclipse Smart Home and Universal Remote Console. *Procedia Computer Science, 98*, 107–116. DOI: 10.1016/j.procs.2016.09.018

Smith, J. D., Margolis, S. A., Ayton, J., Ross, V., Chalmers, E., Giddings, P., Baker, L., Kelly, M., & Love, C. (2008). Defining remote medical practice. *The Medical Journal of Australia, 188*(3), 159–161. DOI: 10.5694/j.1326-5377.2008.tb01561.x PMID: 18241174

Smolić, Š., Blaževski, N., & Fabijančić, M. (2022). Remote healthcare during the COVID-19 pandemic: Findings for older adults in 27 European countries and Israel. *Frontiers in Public Health, 10*, 927367. DOI: 10.3389/fpubh.2022.921379 PMID: 35910874

Snoswell, C. L., Taylor, M. L., Comans, T. A., Smith, A. C., Gray, L. C., & Caffery, L. J. (2020). Determining if telehealth can reduce health system costs: Scoping review. *Journal of Medical Internet Research, 22*(10), e17298. DOI: 10.2196/17298 PMID: 33074157

Sockolow, P. S., Bowles, K. H., Topaz, M., Koru, G., Hellesø, R., O'Connor, M., & Bass, E. J. (2021). The time is now: Informatics research opportunities in home health care. *Applied Clinical Informatics, 12*(1), 100–106. DOI: 10.1055/s-0040-1722222 PMID: 33598906

Solomonoff, R. J. (1964). A formal theory of inductive inference. *Information and Control, 7*(1), 1–22. DOI: 10.1016/S0019-9958(64)90223-2

Soriano, G. P., Yasuhara, Y., Ito, H., Matsumoto, K., Osaka, K., Kai, Y., Locsin, R., Shoenhofer, S., & Tanioka, T. (2022). Robots and robotics in nursing. *Health Care, 10*(8), 1571. DOI: 10.3390/healthcare10081571 PMID: 36011228

Soussi, O., Lemiere, P., Millot, S., & others. (2024). Beyond telehealth in heart failure: How a nurse-led mobile team unit improves management. *European Heart Journal, 45*(Suppl_1), Article ehae758.2623. DOI: 10.1093/eurheartj/ehae758.2623

Stavropoulos, T. G., Papastergiou, A., Mpaltadoros, L., Nikolopoulos, S., & Kompatsiaris, I. (2020). IoT wearable sensors and devices in elderly care: A literature review. *Sensors (Basel), 20*(10), 2826. DOI: 10.3390/s20102826 PMID: 32429331

Steindal, S. A., Nes, A. A. G., Godskesen, T. E., Dihle, A., Lind, S., Winger, A., & Klarare, A. (2020). Patients' experiences of telehealth in palliative home care: Scoping review. *Journal of Medical Internet Research, 22*(5), e16218. DOI: 10.2196/16218 PMID: 32369037

Steindal, S. A., Nes, A. A. G., Godskesen, T. E., Holmen, H., Winger, A., Österlind, J., Dihle, A., & Klarare, A. (2023). Advantages and challenges of using telehealth for home-based palliative care: Systematic mixed studies review. *Journal of Medical Internet Research, 25*, e43684. DOI: 10.2196/43684 PMID: 36912876

Steinhubl, S. R., Waalen, J., Edwards, A. M., Ariniello, L. M., Mehta, R. R., Ebner, G. S., Carter, C., Baca-Motes, K., Felicione, E., Sarich, T., & Topol, E. J. (2018). Effect of a home-based wearable continuous ECG monitoring patch on detection of undiagnosed atrial fibrillation: The mSToPS randomized clinical trial. *Journal of the American Medical Association, 320*(2), 146–155. DOI: 10.1001/jama.2018.8102 PMID: 29998336

Stock, S. E., Davies, D. K., Herold, R. G., & Wehmeyer, M. L. (2019). Technology to support transportation needs assessment, training, and pre-trip planning by people with intellectual disability. *Advances in Neurodevelopmental Disorders, 3*(3), 319–324. DOI: 10.1007/s41252-019-00117-x

Su, Z., Liang, F., Sheng, W., & Bishop, A. (2024). Robot-assisted homecare for older adults: A user study on needs and challenges. *Cobot, 2*, 100013. DOI: 10.12688/cobot.17644.2

Swanepoel, L., Spencer, J., & Draper, D. (2020). Education and training for disability awareness of hospitality staff. *African Journal of Hospitality, Tourism and Leisure, 9*(4), 402–417. DOI: 10.46222/ajhtl.19770720-36

Szanton, S. L., Leff, B., Wolff, J. L., Roberts, L., & Gitlin, L. N. (2016). Home-based care program reduces disability and promotes aging in place. *Health Affairs, 35*(9), 1558–1563. DOI: 10.1377/hlthaff.2016.0140 PMID: 27605633

Szewczyka, I., & Zontek, E. L. (2018). Adjustment for elderly and disabled tourists in Polish hotels. *New Trends and Issues Proceedings on Humanities and Social Sciences*, *5*(2), 160–170. DOI: 10.18844/prosoc.v5i2.3667

Szewczyk, I. (2020). Problems of collective transport management – Obstacles to access for disabled people. *Transportation Research Procedia*, *45*, 78–86. DOI: 10.1016/j.trpro.2020.02.064

Tachibana, T., Furuichi, T., & Mineno, H. (2016). Implementing and evaluating priority control mechanism for heterogeneous remote monitoring IoT system. In *MobiQuitous '16: Adjunct proceedings of the 13th International Conference on Mobile and Ubiquitous Systems: Computing, Networking and Services* (pp. 239–244). ACM. DOI: 10.1145/3004010.3004040

Talal, M., Zaidan, A. A., Zaidan, B. B., Albahri, A. S., Alamoodi, A. H., Albahri, O. S., Alsalem, M. A., Lim, C. K., Tan, K. L., Shir, W. L., & Mohammed, K. I. (2019). Smart home-based IoT for real-time and secure remote health monitoring of triage and priority system using body sensors: Multi-driven systematic review. *Journal of Medical Systems*, *43*(3), 42. DOI: 10.1007/s10916-019-1158-z PMID: 30648217

Tanaka, M., Ishii, S., Matsuoka, A., Tanabe, S., Matsunaga, S., Rahmani, A., Dutt, N., Rasouli, M., & Nyamathi, A. (2024). Perspectives of Japanese elders and their healthcare providers on use of wearable technology to monitor their health at home: A qualitative exploration. *International Journal of Nursing Studies*, *152*, 104691. DOI: 10.1016/j.ijnurstu.2024.104691 PMID: 38262231

Tao, M., Ota, K., & Dong, M. (2017). Ontology-based data semantic management and application in IoT- and cloud-enabled smart homes. *Future Generation Computer Systems*, *76*, 528–539. DOI: 10.1016/j.future.2016.11.012

Tenner, E. (2015). The design of everyday things by Donald Norman [Review of the book The design of everyday things, by D. A. Norman]. *Technology and Culture*, *56*(3), 785–787. DOI: 10.1353/tech.2015.0104

Tewksbury, C., Deleener, M. E., Dumon, K. R., & Williams, N. N. (2021). Practical considerations of developing and conducting a successful telehealth practice in response to covid-19. *Nutrition in Clinical Practice*, *36*(4), 769–774. DOI: 10.1002/ncp.10742 PMID: 34156725

Thacharodi, A., Singh, P., Meenatchi, R., Tawfeeq Ahmed, Z. H., Kumar, R. R. S., v, N., Kavish, S., Maqbool, M., & Hassan, S. (2024). Revolutionizing healthcare and medicine: The impact of modern technologies for a healthier future—A comprehensive review. *Health Care Science*, *3*(5), 329–349. DOI: 10.1002/hcs2.115 PMID: 39479277

Thayer, J., & Dreisbach-Williams, S. (2023). Early innovations in maritime telemedical services: The KDKF Radio Medico Station. *Journal of the Medical Library Association: JMLA*, *111*(1–2), 625–630. DOI: 10.5195/jmla.2023.1567 PMID: 37312806

Thiels, C. A., Aho, J. M., Zietlow, S. P., & Jenkins, D. H. (2015). Use of unmanned aerial vehicles for medical product transport. *Air Medical Journal*, *34*(2), 104–108. DOI: 10.1016/j.amj.2014.10.011 PMID: 25733117

Thomas, A., & Wee, H. (2022). Educational tourist motivations, destination image, and destination selection behavior in an extended S-O-R model. *International Journal of Academic Research in Business & Social Sciences*, *12*(10), 2198–2210. DOI: 10.6007/IJARBSS/v12-i10/14849

Tian, Y. J., Wong, T., Chen, Q., & Denver, L. (2024). Benefits and barriers associated with the use of smart home health technologies in the care of older persons: A systematic review. *BMC Geriatrics*, *24*(1), 152. DOI: 10.1186/s12877-024-04702-1 PMID: 38355464

tom Dieck, M. C., Jung, T., & Michopoulou, E. (2019). Experiencing virtual reality in heritage attractions: Perceptions of elderly users. In tom Dieck, M. C., & Jung, T. (Eds.), *Augmented reality and virtual reality* (pp. 89–98). Springer., DOI: 10.1007/978-3-030-06246-0_7

Topol, E. J. (2019). *Deep medicine: How artificial intelligence can make healthcare human again*. Basic Books.

Topol, E. J. (2019). High-performance medicine: The convergence of human and artificial intelligence. *Nature Medicine*, *25*(1), 44–56. DOI: 10.1038/s41591-018-0300-7 PMID: 30617339

Torab-Miandoab, A., Samad-Soltani, T., Jodati, A., & Rezaei-Hachesu, P. (2023). Interoperability of heterogeneous health information systems: A systematic literature review. *BMC Medical Informatics and Decision Making*, *23*(1), 18. DOI: 10.1186/s12911-023-02115-5 PMID: 36694161

Tornvall, I., Kenny, D., Wubishet, B. L., Russell, A., Menon, A., & Comans, T. (2025). Economic evaluations of mHealth interventions for the management of type 2 diabetes: A scoping review. *Journal of Diabetes Science and Technology*, *19*(1), 179–190. DOI: 10.1177/19322968231183956 PMID: 37395212

Totten, A. M., Womack, D. M., Eden, K. B., McDonagh, M. S., Griffin, J. C., Grusing, S., & Hersh, W. R. (2016). *Telehealth: Mapping the evidence for patient outcomes from systematic reviews* (Technical Brief No. 26). Agency for Healthcare Research and Quality. https://www.ncbi.nlm.nih.gov/books/NBK379320/

Trout, K. E., Rampa, S., Wilson, F. A., & Stimpson, J. P. (2017). Legal mapping analysis of state telehealth reimbursement policies. *Telemedicine Journal and e-Health, 23*(10), 805–814. DOI: 10.1089/tmj.2017.0016 PMID: 28430029

Tsai, C.-H., Zdravkovic, J., & Stirna, J. (2020). Capability management of digital business ecosystems—A case of resilience modeling in the healthcare domain. In Herbaut, N., & La Rosa, M. (Eds.), *Advanced information systems engineering* (pp. 126–137). Springer., DOI: 10.1007/978-3-030-58135-0_11

Tsvetanov, F. (2024). Integrating AI technologies into remote monitoring patient systems. *Engineering Proceedings, 70*(1), 54. DOI: 10.3390/engproc2024070054

Tuna, A., Das, R., & Tuna, G. (2015). Integrated smart home services and smart wearable technology for the disabled and elderly. In *Proceedings of the 7th International Conference on Computer Supported Education* (pp. 173–177). SCITEPRESS. DOI: 10.5220/0005552001730177

Turing, A. M. (1936). On computable numbers, with an application to the Entscheidungsproblem. *Proceedings of the London Mathematical Society, 2*(42), 230–265. DOI: 10.1112/plms/s2-42.1.230

Turing, A. M. (1950). Computing machinery and intelligence. *Mind, 59*(236), 433–460. DOI: 10.1093/mind/LIX.236.433

Turner, K., Bobonis Babilonia, M., Naso, C., Nguyen, O., Gonzalez, B. D., Oswald, L. B., Robinson, E., Elston Lafata, J., Ferguson, R. J., Alishahi Tabriz, A., Patel, K. B., Hallanger-Johnson, J., Aldawoodi, N., Hong, Y.-R., Jim, H. S. L., & Spiess, P. E. (2022). Health care providers' and professionals' experiences with telehealth oncology implementation during the COVID-19 pandemic: A qualitative study. *Journal of Medical Internet Research, 24*(1), e29635. DOI: 10.2196/29635 PMID: 34907900

Ultimate Care. (2025). *The impact of home care on reducing healthcare costs.* https://www.ultimatecareny.com/resources/the-impact-of-home-care-on-reducing-healthcare-costs

Ulutas, I., & Omeroglu, E. (2012). Maternal attitudes, emotional intelligence and home environment and their relations with emotional intelligence of sixth years old children. In *Emotional intelligence: New perspectives and applications* (pp. 117–132). IntechOpen., DOI: 10.5772/32926

Vaartio-Rajalin, H., & Fagerström, L. (2019). Professional care at home: Patient-centeredness, interprofessionality and effectivity? A scoping review. *Health & Social Care in the Community, 27*(4), e270–e288. DOI: 10.1111/hsc.12731 PMID: 30843316

Vaartio-Rajalin, H., Näsman, Y., Santamäki-Fischer, R., & Hemberg, J. (2019). Working in home healthcare and suggestions for development. *Home Health Care Services Quarterly*, *38*(4), 257–269. DOI: 10.1080/01621424.2019.1641450 PMID: 31295058

Van de Voorde, P., Gautama, S., Momont, A., Ionescu, C. M., De Paepe, P., & Fraeyman, N. (2017). The drone ambulance [A-UAS]: Golden bullet or just a blank? *Resuscitation*, *116*, 46–48. DOI: 10.1016/j.resuscitation.2017.04.037 PMID: 28487253

Vargemidis, D., Gerling, K., Spiel, K., Vanden Abeele, V., & Geurts, L. (2020). Wearable physical activity tracking systems for older adults—A systematic review. *ACM Transactions on Computing for Healthcare*, *1*(4), 25. DOI: 10.1145/3402523

Vegesna, A., Tran, M., Angelaccio, M., & Arcona, S. (2017). Remote patient monitoring via non-invasive digital technologies: A systematic review. *Telemedicine Journal and e-Health*, *23*(1), 3–17. DOI: 10.1089/tmj.2016.0051 PMID: 27116181

Venkatesh, V., Morris, M. G., Davis, G. B., & Davis, F. D. (2003). User acceptance of information technology: Toward a unified view. *Management Information Systems Quarterly*, *27*(3), 425–478. DOI: 10.2307/30036540

Verma, G. K. (2023). Multimodal fusion framework: Emotion recognition from physiological signals. In *Multimodal affective computing: Affective information representation, modelling, and analysis* (pp. 115–127). Bentham Science Publishers., DOI: 10.2174/9789815124453123010012

Viswanadham, N. (2021). Ecosystem model for healthcare platform. *Sadhana*, *46*(4), 188. DOI: 10.1007/s12046-021-01708-y

Vo, D. K., & Trinh, K. T. L. (2024). Advances in wearable biosensors for healthcare: Current trends, applications, and future perspectives. *Biosensors (Basel)*, *14*(11), 560. DOI: 10.3390/bios14110560 PMID: 39590019

Voigt, P., & von dem Bussche, A. (2017). *The EU General Data Protection Regulation (GDPR): A practical guide*. Springer., DOI: 10.1007/978-3-319-57959-7

Wai-leung, B. C. (2004). Accessible tourism in Hong Kong: An untapped market. In *10th International Conference on Mobility and Transport for Elderly and Disabled People*. Japan Society of Civil Engineers; Transportation Research Board.

Wakerman, J. (2004). Defining remote health. *The Australian Journal of Rural Health*, *12*(5), 210–214. DOI: 10.1111/j.1440-1854.2004.00607.x PMID: 15588265

Wan, C., Zhao, J., Song, Y., Xu, Z., Lin, J., & Hu, Z. (2015). Photovoltaic and solar power forecasting for smart grid energy management. *CSEE Journal of Power and Energy Systems*, *1*(4), 38–46. DOI: 10.17775/CSEEJPES.2015.00046

Wang, J., Sun, Z., Zhou, Y., & Dai, J. (2012). Optimal dispatching model of smart home energy management system. In *2012 IEEE Innovative Smart Grid Technologies - Asia (ISGT Asia)* (pp. 1–5). IEEE. DOI: 10.1109/ISGT-Asia.2012.6303266

Wang, P. (2024). The integration and innovation of smart tourism management and big data technology. In *2023 3rd International Conference on Artificial Intelligence, Automation, and High-Performance Computing (AIAHPC)* (pp. 45–51). IEEE. DOI: 10.1109/AIARS63200.2024.00118

Wang, J., Chen, W., Wang, L., Ren, Y., & Sherratt, R. S. (2020). Blockchain-based data storage mechanism for industrial Internet of Things. *Intelligent Automation & Soft Computing*, *26*(5), 1157–1172. DOI: 10.32604/iasc.2020.012174

Wang, N., Cao, Z., Zhang, J., & Fuh, Y.-C. (2024). Perceptions and satisfaction with the use of digital medical services in urban older adults of China: Mixed methods study. *Journal of Medical Internet Research*, *26*, e48654. DOI: 10.2196/48654 PMID: 39303282

Warshaw, E. M., Lederle, F. A., Grill, J. P., Gravely, A. A., Bangerter, A. K., Fortier, L. A., Bohjanen, K. A., Chen, K., Lee, P. K., Rabinovitz, H. S., Johr, R. H., Kaye, V. N., Bowers, S., Wenner, R., Askari, S. K., Kedrowski, D. A., & Nelson, D. B. (2009). Accuracy of teledermatology for nonpigmented neoplasms. *Journal of the American Academy of Dermatology*, *60*(4), 579–588. DOI: 10.1016/j.jaad.2008.11.892 PMID: 19217689

Weizenbaum, J. (1966). ELIZA—A computer program for the study of natural language communication between man and machine. *Communications of the ACM*, *9*(1), 36–45. DOI: 10.1145/365153.365168

Weng, S. F., Reps, J., Kai, J., Garibaldi, J. M., & Qureshi, N. (2017). Can machine-learning improve cardiovascular risk prediction using routine clinical data? *PLoS One*, *12*(4), e0174944. DOI: 10.1371/journal.pone.0174944 PMID: 28376093

Whende, M. C. (2019). Artificial intelligence, critical thinking and the nursing process. *On-Line Journal of Nursing Informatics*, *23*(1).

Wiener, N. (1948). *Cybernetics: Or control and communication in the animal and the machine*. MIT Press.

Wiener, N. (1960). Some moral and technical consequences of automation. *Science*, *131*(3410), 1355–1358. DOI: 10.1126/science.131.3410.1355 PMID: 17841602

Williams, K. S., Singh, M. J., Elumn, J. E., Threats, M., Sha, Y., McCall, T., Wang, K., Massey, B., Peng, M. L., & Wiley, K. (2024). Enhancing healthcare accessibility through telehealth for justice impacted individuals. *Frontiers in Public Health*, *12*, 1401950. DOI: 10.3389/fpubh.2024.1401950 PMID: 39175903

Wilson, F. A., Rampa, S., Trout, K. E., & Stimpson, J. P. (2017). Reimbursements for telehealth services are likely to be lower than non-telehealth services in the United States. *Journal of Telemedicine and Telecare*, *23*(4), 497–500. DOI: 10.1177/1357633X16652288 PMID: 27260264

Winograd, T. (1972). *Understanding natural language*. Academic Press. DOI: 10.1016/0010-0285(72)90002-3

Wood, S., Khong, C., Dirlikov, B., & Shem, K. (2021). Nutrition counseling and monitoring via tele-nutrition for healthy diet for people with spinal cord injury: A case series analyses. *The Journal of Spinal Cord Medicine*, *45*(4), 547–555. DOI: 10.1080/10790268.2021.1871824 PMID: 33606588

Woo, K., Song, J., Adams, V., Block, L. J., Currie, L. M., Shang, J., & Topaz, M. (2022). Exploring prevalence of wound infections and related patient characteristics in homecare using natural language processing. *International Wound Journal*, *19*(1), 211–221. DOI: 10.1111/iwj.13623 PMID: 34105873

Wootton, R., Geissbuhler, A., Jethwani, K., Kovarik, C., Person, D. A., Vladzymyrskyy, A., Zanaboni, P., & Zolfo, M. (2012). Long-running telemedicine networks delivering humanitarian services: Experience, performance and scientific output. *Bulletin of the World Health Organization*, *90*(5), 341–347. DOI: 10.2471/BLT.11.099143 PMID: 22589567

World Health Organization. (2010). *Telemedicine: Opportunities and developments in Member States*. https://www.who.int/goe/publications/goe_telemedicine_2010.pdf

World Health Organization. (2020). *Global strategy on digital health 2020–2025*. https://www.who.int/docs/default-source/documents/gs4dhdaa2a9f352b0445bafbc79ca799dce4d.pdf

World Health Organization. (2024, October 1). *Ageing and health*. https://www.who.int/news-room/fact-sheets/detail/ageing-and-health

Wu, S., & Wang, S. (2025). Exploring the impact of AI-enhanced virtual tourism on tourists' pro-environmental behavior: A stimulus-organism-response model perspective. *Acta Psychologica*, *253*, 104773. DOI: 10.1016/j.actpsy.2025.104773 PMID: 39904230

Wu, X., & Lai, I. K. W. (2022). The use of 360-degree virtual tours to promote mountain walking tourism: Stimulus–organism–response model. *Information Technology & Tourism, 24*(1), 85–107. DOI: 10.1007/s40558-021-00218-1

Wylde, V., Rawindaran, N., Lawrence, J., Balasubramanian, R., Prakash, E., Jayal, A., Khan, I., Hewage, C., & Platts, J. (2022). Cybersecurity, data privacy and blockchain: A review. *SN Computer Science, 3*(2), 127. DOI: 10.1007/s42979-022-01020-4 PMID: 35036930

Xu, M. (2023). Research on smart tourism system based on artificial intelligence. In *2023 IEEE 3rd International Conference on Information Technology, Big Data and Artificial Intelligence (ICIBA)* (pp. 201–205). IEEE. DOI: 10.1109/ICIBA56860.2023.10165293

Xu, X., Lu, Y., Vogel-Heuser, B., & Wang, L. (2021). Industry 4.0 and Industry 5.0—Inception, conception and perception. *Journal of Manufacturing Systems, 61*, 530–535. DOI: 10.1016/j.jmsy.2021.10.006

Yampolskiy, R. V. (2013). Turing Test as a defining feature of AI-completeness. In Duch, W., & Mańdziuk, J. (Eds.), *Artificial intelligence, evolutionary computing and metaheuristics* (pp. 3–17). Springer., DOI: 10.1007/978-3-642-29694-9_1

Yang, G., Pang, Z., Jamal Deen, M., Dong, M., Zhang, Y.-T., Lovell, N., & Rahmani, A. M. (2020). Homecare robotic systems for Healthcare 4.0: Visions and enabling technologies. *IEEE Journal of Biomedical and Health Informatics, 24*(9), 2535–2549. DOI: 10.1109/JBHI.2020.2990529 PMID: 32340971

Yu, J., Kim, S., Hailu, T. B., Park, J., & Han, H. (2024). The effects of virtual reality (VR) and augmented reality (AR) on senior tourists' experiential quality. *Current Issues in Tourism, 27*(3), 464–478. DOI: 10.1080/13683500.2023.2165483

Yuksel, O. (2024). An overview of health services in the Industry 5.0 era. *International Journal of Engineering and Innovative Research, 6*(3), 222–237. DOI: 10.47933/ijeir.1537942

Zagmutt, F. J., Pouzou, J. G., & Costard, S. (2020). The EAT-Lancet Commission's dietary composition may not prevent noncommunicable disease mortality. *The Journal of Nutrition, 150*(5), 985–988. DOI: 10.1093/jn/nxaa020 PMID: 32061173

Zahari, N. F., Kamarudin, H., Zawawi, Z. A., Rashid, R. B. A., & Bahari, M. M. (2023). Heritage tourism: A disabled person's rights to engage in social activity. *Planning Malaysia, 21*(5), 484–494. DOI: 10.21837/pm.v21i25.1252

Zajadacz, A. (2015). The contribution of the geography of disability to the development of accessible tourism. *Turyzm (Lódz), 25*(1), 19–27. DOI: 10.2478/tour-2014-0016

Zeevi, D., Korem, T., Zmora, N., Israeli, D., Rothschild, D., Weinberger, A., Ben-Yacov, O., Lador, D., Avnit-Sagi, T., Lotan-Pompan, M., Suez, J., Mahdi, J. A., Matot, E., Malka, G., Kosower, N., Rein, M., Zilberman-Schapira, G., Dohnalová, L., Pevsner-Fischer, M., & Segal, E. (2015). Personalized nutrition by prediction of glycemic responses. *Cell*, *163*(5), 1079–1094. DOI: 10.1016/j.cell.2015.11.001 PMID: 26590418

Zenginis, I., Vardakas, J. S., Koltsaklis, N. E., & Verikoukis, C. (2022). Smart home's energy management through a clustering-based reinforcement learning approach. *IEEE Internet of Things Journal*, *9*(17), 16363–16371. DOI: 10.1109/JIOT.2022.3152586

Zhai, S., Chu, F., Tan, M., Chi, N. C., Ward, T., & Yuwen, W. (2023). Digital health interventions to support family caregivers: An updated systematic review. *Digital Health*, *9*, 20552076231171967. DOI: 10.1177/20552076231171967 PMID: 37223775

Zhang, W., & Li, W. (2019). A deep reinforcement learning based human behavior prediction approach in smart home environments. In *2019 International Conference on Robots & Intelligent System (ICRIS)* (pp. 59–62). IEEE. DOI: 10.1109/ICRIS.2019.00024

Zheng, Y., Head, B. A., & Schapmire, T. J. (2016). A systematic review of telehealth in palliative care: Caregiver outcomes. *Telemedicine Journal and e-Health*, *22*(4), 288–294. DOI: 10.1089/tmj.2015.0090 PMID: 26360181

Zundel, K. M. (1996). Telemedicine: History, applications, and impact on librarianship. *Bulletin of the Medical Library Association*, *84*(1), 71–79. https://www.ncbi.nlm.nih.gov/pmc/articles/PMC226126/ PMID: 8938332

About the Contributors

Haşim Çapar holds a Ph.D. in Health Management. He is currently an Asst. Prof. Dr. at the Health Management, Dicle University in Diyarbakır, Türkiye. His research interests and expertise in health management and health economics are particularly interested in medical tourism. He is the Editor-in-Chief of the Journal of Health and Social Welfare Research. He also has professional experience in health management.

Mehmet Aziz Çakmak holds a master's degree in Health Management. He currently works as a lecturer at the Artuklu University Technology Transfer Office in Mardin, Türkiye. He is interested in artificial intelligence in health and home health. ÇAKMAK, who is also the ranger manager of a company related to artificial intelligence, has a nationally accepted patent registration. ÇAKMAK, who has written many books, articles and papers, is also the secretary of the Journal of Health and Social Welfare Research.

***

Çağlar Akçalı completed her bachelor's and master's degrees in Nutrition and Dietetics, with a particular focus on sustainable nutrition, health communication, and public health. She has engaged in research and academic activities that integrate these fields, contributing to both theoretical and applied aspects. Akçalı currently serves as a faculty member in the Department of Nutrition and Dietetics at the Faculty of Health Sciences, Mardin Artuklu University, where she delivers courses at undergraduate and graduate levels. Her academic interests include the development of sustainable food systems, the role of nutrition in public health, and the use of effective communication strategies to promote healthy lifestyles. She has participated in various projects, conferences, and publications in these domains, aiming to bridge scientific knowledge with practical health interventions.

Mohammad Nabil Almunawar is currently a professor at the School of Business and Economics, Universiti of Brunei Darussalam (UBDSBE), Brunei Darussalam. He was the former dean of UBDSBE. He received his bachelor's degree in 1983 from Bogor Agricultural University, Indonesia, master's degree (MSc) from the Department of Computer Science, University of Western Ontario, London, Canada in 1991, and Ph.D in Computer Science/Information Systems from the University of New South Wales in 1998. Dr. Almunawar has published more than 250 papers in refereed journals, books, book chapters, encyclopedias, and international conference proceedings. He has more than 30 years of teaching experience in the area of information systems. His overall research interests include applications of IT in management, e-business/commerce, digital marketplace/platform, digital business ecosystem, health informatics, information security, and cloud computing. Currently, he focuses his research on digital transformation, digital marketplace, digital platform, and digital business ecosystem.

Yasin Aras works as Asst. Prof. in the Department of Health Management at Aksaray University. Having completed his bachelor's, master's, and doctoral studies in health management, Aras conducts research primarily in the areas of health policies, healthcare management, performance evaluation, and quality in health services. With publications in national and international peer-reviewed journals, Aras participates in various projects as a researcher in addition to his academic activities, working to improve the effectiveness and efficiency of health services.

İlknur Arslan Aras is an academic specializing in health management. She completed her undergraduate education in health institutions management and obtained her master's and Ph.D. degrees in health management. Her academic work focuses on health economics, digital health, health policies, and particularly on the use of Data Envelopment Analysis (DEA). She actively participates in national and international conferences and has published various articles and book chapters. She currently works as an Assistant Professor in the Department of Health Management at the Faculty of Health Sciences, Yüksek İhtisas University.

Çağla Çetinkaya holds a Ph.D. in Tourism and currently serves as an Assistant Professor at Istanbul Nişantaşı University, Faculty of Applied Sciences, Department of Tourism and Hotel Management. Her areas of expertise include health tourism, agricultural tourism, tourism marketing, and artificial intelligence applications in tourism. Dr. Çetinkaya has previously worked in the hospitality industry, including positions at Hilton Hotels, and integrates practical experience with academic research.She has contributed extensively to the field through academic publications, book chapters, and national/international conference presentations. Her recent studies focus on visitor experiences, smart tourism technologies, and inclusive tourism practices, particularly in museum settings.

Murat Konca completed his undergraduate, graduate, and doctoral studies in the field of health management. His academic work focuses on health economics, performance evaluation in healthcare systems, health technologies, and remote healthcare.

Hitesh Mohapatra received the B.E. degree in Information Technology from Biju Patnaik University of Technology (BPUT), Odisha in 2006, and the MTech. Degree in CSE from Odisha University of Technology and Research (OUTR) University, Odisha in 2009. He received his Ph.D. in Computer Science & Engineering in 2021 from Veer Surendra Sai University of Technology (VSSUT), Burla, India. He has contributed 50+ SCI and Scopus indexed research articles. He has authored two books on Software Engineering and C Programming respectively. He has 15 years of teaching experience both in industry and academia. He has served the research community with various capacities like session chair, technical chair, keynote speaker etc. His research interests include wireless sensor network, smart city, smart grid and smart water. Currently he is working as Associate professor at School of Computer Engineering, KIIT Deemed to be University, Bhubaneswar, and Odisha.

Mehmet Özyurt is a Research Assistant at the Department of Health Management at Mardin Artuklu University and is pursuing his doctoral studies in Health Management at the Institute of Health Sciences at Marmara University. He completed his master's degree in Health Economics at Istanbul University-Cerrahpaşa and his bachelor's degree in Health Institution Management at Eskişehir Osmangazi University with honors. His research focuses on health management, health economics, digital health applications, and sustainable development goals.

Yiğit Kerem YILDIZ holds a Ph.D. in Health Management. He currently works as a lecturer at the Istanbul Nisantasi University in Istanbul, Türkiye. His research interests and expertise are in health management, digital health and innovation. He has publications scanned in different indexes.

Mustafa Z. Younis is an internationally recognized scholar and tenured professor at Jackson State University, Mississippi, USA. In addition, Prof. Younis has held visiting professor positions at universities such as Tsinghua University, China, and Jena University, Germany. Prof. Younis has authored and published over 100 articles, 150 abstracts and presentations in refereed journals and meetings and universities in Europe, China and the Middle East. He has also presented at various national and international conferences. Prof. Younis' co-authored articles appeared in leading journals such as "Nature", "The Lancet" and "JAMA" and the European Journal of Health Economics.

Index

T

U

V

www.ingramcontent.com/pod-product-compliance
Lightning Source LLC
LaVergne TN
LVHW081524300926
849161LV00006B/1285
* 9 7 9 8 3 3 7 3 3 0 9 9 0 *